D1256119

Diagnosis and Treatment of Aortic and Peripheral Arterial Aneurysms

Diagnosis and Treatment of Aortic and Peripheral Arterial Aneurysms

Keith D. Calligaro, M.D.

Associate Clinical Professor of Surgery
University of Pennsylvania School of Medicine

Chief, Section of Vascular Surgery
Pennsylvania Hospital
Philadelphia, Pennsylvania

Matthew J. Dougherty, M.D.

Clinical Assistant Professor of Surgery
University of Pennsylvania School of Medicine

Section of Vascular Surgery
Pennsylvania Hospital
Philadelphia, Pennsylvania

Larry H. Hollier, M.D.

Julius H. Jacobson II, M.D., Professor
Chairman, Mount Sinai School of Medicine of the
City University of New York
Surgeon-in-Chief, Chairman, Department of Surgery
The Mount Sinai Hospital
New York, New York

W.B. SAUNDERS COMPANY

A Division of Harcourt Brace & Company
Philadelphia   London   Toronto   Montreal   Sydney   Tokyo

W.B. SAUNDERS COMPANY
A Division of Harcourt Brace & Company

The Curtis Center
Independence Square West
Philadelphia, Pennsylvania 19106

Library of Congress Cataloging-in-Publication Data

Diagnosis and treatment of aortic and peripheral arterial aneurysms /
[edited by] Keith D. Calligaro, Matthew J. Dougherty, Larry H. Hollier.

p.   cm.

ISBN 0–7216–7675–8

1. Aortic aneurysms—Surgery.   2. Aneurysms—Surgery.   I. Calligaro,
    Keith D.   II. Dougherty, Matthew J.   III. Hollier, Larry H.   [DNLM:
    1. Aortic Aneurysm, Abdominal—surgery.   2. Aortic Aneurysm,
    Abdominal—diagnosis.   3. Aortic Aneurysm, Thoracic—
    surgery.   4. Aneurysm—surgery.   WG 410 D5355 1999]

RD598.6.D53   1999

617.4'13—dc21

DNLM/DLC   98–5823

DIAGNOSIS AND TREATMENT OF AORTIC AND PERIPHERAL
ARTERIAL ANEURYSMS   ISBN 0–7216–7675–8

Printed in the United States of America.

Last digit is the print number: 9   8   7   6   5   4   3   2   1

Contributors

Enrico Ascher, M.D.

Professor, Department of Surgery, State University of New York Health Science Center at Brooklyn College of Medicine; Division of Vascular Surgery, Maimonides Medical Center, Brooklyn, New York

Treatment of Carotid Artery Aneurysms and Aortic Arch Vessel Aneurysms

David C. Brewster, M.D.

Clinical Professor of Surgery, Harvard Medical School; Senior Attending Surgeon and Director, Endovascular Surgery, Massachusetts General Hospital, Boston, Massachusetts

Treatment of Type B Aortic Dissections

Keith D. Calligaro, M.D.

Associate Clinical Professor of Surgery, University of Pennsylvania School of Medicine; Chief, Section of Vascular Surgery, Pennsylvania Hospital, Philadelphia, Pennsylvania

Preoperative Pulmonary Evaluation for Aortic Aneurysm Surgery; Venous Anomalies Encountered During Abdominal Aortic Surgery

Matthew P. Campbell, M.D.

Assistant Professor of Surgery, Baylor College of Medicine; Houston, Texas

Thoracoabdominal Aortic Aneurysm Repair

Gabriel Carabello, M.D.

Assistant Professor of Surgery, University of California, Los Angeles, UCLA School of Medicine, Los Angeles, California

Treatment of Chylous Ascites After Abdominal Aortic Aneurysm Repair

Jeffrey P. Carpenter, M.D.

Associate Professor of Surgery, Department of Surgery, University of Pennsylvania School of Medicine, Philadelphia, Pennsylvania

Popliteal Artery Aneurysms

Benjamin B. Chang, M.D.

Associate Professor of Surgery, Albany Medical College; Attending, Albany Medical Center Hospital, Albany, New York

Alternative Approach for Management of Infected Aortic Grafts

John D. Corson, M.B., Ch.B.

Professor of Surgery, University of Iowa College of Medicine; Director, Vascular Surgery Section, University of Iowa Hospitals and Clinics, Iowa City, Iowa

Aortic Ligation and Aneurysm Exclusion as Treatment Options for Abdominal Aortic Aneurysms

Jacob Cynamon, M.D.

Associate Professor of Radiology, Albert Einstein College of Medicine of Yeshiva University; Director, Vascular and Interventional Radiology, Montefiore Medical Center, Bronx, New York

Transluminally Placed Endovascular Grafts for the Treatment of Aortoiliac Aneurysms

Rahul Dandora, B.A.

Section of Vascular Medicine, Pennsylvania Hospital, Philadelphia, Pennsylvania

Preoperative Pulmonary Evaluation for Aortic Aneurysm Surgery

R. Clement Darling III, M.D.

Assistant Professor of Surgery, Albany Medical College; Chief, Vascular Surgery, Attending, Albany Medical Center Hospital, Albany, New York

Alternative Approach for Management of Infected Aortic Grafts

Dominic A. DeLaurentis, M.D.

Professor of Surgery, University of
Pennsylvania School of Medicine;
Attending Surgeon, Pennsylvania
Hospital, Philadelphia, Pennsylvania

*Preoperative Pulmonary Evaluation for
Aortic Aneurysm Surgery; Venous
Anomalies Encountered During
Abdominal Aortic Surgery*

Matthew J. Dougherty, M.D.

Clinical Assistant Professor of Surgery,
University of Pennsylvania School of
Medicine; Attending Surgeon, Section of
Vascular Surgery, Pennsylvania
Hospital, Philadelphia, Pennsylvania

*Preoperative Pulmonary Evaluation for
Aortic Aneurysm Surgery; Venous
Anomalies Encountered During
Abdominal Aortic Surgery*

James I. Fann, M.D.

Clinical Assistant Professor, Department
of Cardiothoracic Surgery, Stanford
University School of Medicine, Stanford,
California; Cardiovascular Surgeon, VA
Medical Center, Palo Alto, California

*Endovascular Treatment of Thoracic
Aortic Aneurysms and Dissection*

Paul Finn, M.D.

Professor of Radiology, Department of
Radiology, Northwestern University
Medical School, Chicago, Illinois

*Preoperative Imaging Studies of
Abdominal Aortic Aneurysms: When
Are Computed Tomography,
Arteriography, or New Modalities
Indicated?*

Jonathan P. Gertler, M.D.

Associate Professor of Surgery, Harvard
Medical School; Associate
Director—Vascular Laboratory, Vascular
Surgeon, Massachusetts General
Hospital, Boston, Massachusetts

*Concomitant Aortic Aneurysm Repair
and Coronary Artery Bypass*

Jerry Goldstone, M.D.

Professor of Surgery, University of
California, San Francisco, School of
Medicine; Chief, Vascular Surgery, San
Francisco General Hospital, San
Francisco, California

*Prevention and Treatment of Aortic
Graft–Enteric Fistula*

Richard Green, M.D.

Professor of Surgery, University of
Rochester School of Medicine and
Dentistry; Attending, Chief of Vascular
Surgery, Strong Memorial Hospital,
Rochester, New York

*Complicated Abdominal Aortic
Aneurysm Repair*

Roy Greenberg, M.D.

Fellow of Vascular Surgery, University
of Rochester School of Medicine and
Dentistry, Rochester, New York

*Complicated Abdominal Aortic
Aneurysm Repair; Prevention and
Treatment of Spinal Cord Ischemia
Associated With Aortic Aneurysm
Repair*

John W. Hallett, Jr., M.D.

Professor of Surgery, Dean of Faculty
Affairs, Mayo Medical School; Chair,
Executive Committee, Mayo Gonda
Vascular Center, Mayo Clinic, Rochester,
Minnesota

*Concomitant Aortic Aneurysm Repair
and Other Abdominal Surgery*

Ian N. Hamilton, Jr., M.D.

Assistant Professor, Department of
Surgery, University of Tennessee School
of Medicine, Chattanooga Unit; Staff
Surgeon, Erlanger Medical Center,
Chattanooga, Tennessee

*Optimal Repair Methods for
Thoracoabdominal Aortic Aneurysms:
Spinal Damage, Bypass, and
Intraoperative Drugs*

Anil Hingorani, M.D.

Attending, Staff, Maimonides Medical
Center, Brooklyn, New York

*Treatment of Carotid Artery Aneurysms
and Aortic Arch Vessel Aneurysms*

Jamal J. Hoballah, M.D.

Associate Professor of Surgery,
University of Iowa College of Medicine;
Chief, Vascular Surgery Section, VAMC;
Attending Surgeon, University of Iowa
Hospitals and Clinics, Iowa City, Iowa

*Aortic Ligation and Aneurysm
Exclusion as Treatment Options for
Abdominal Aortic Aneurysms*

Larry H. Hollier, M.D.

Julius H. Jacobson II, M.D., Professor, Chairman, Mount Sinai School of Medicine of the City University of New York; Surgeon-in-Chief, Chairman, Department of Surgery, The Mount Sinai Hospital, New York, New York

Optimal Repair Methods for Thoracoabdominal Aortic Aneurysms: Spinal Drainage, Bypass, and Intraoperative Drugs

Gordon L. Hyde, M.D., F.A.C.S.

Professor Emeritus, Vascular Surgery, University of Kentucky College of Medicine, Lexington, Kentucky

Treatment of Sciatic Artery Aneurysms

Dimitrios C. Iliopoulos, M.D.

Assistant Professor of Surgery, Baylor College of Medicine, Houston, Texas

Thoracoabdominal Aortic Aneurysm Repair

Kaj Johansen, M.D., Ph.D.

Professor of Surgery, University of Washington School of Medicine; Director of Surgical Education, Providence Seattle Medical Center, Seattle, Washington

Management of Ruptured Abdominal Aortic Aneurysms

Peter G. Kalman, M.D., F.R.C.S.

Associate Professor, Department of Surgery, University of Toronto Faculty of Medicine; Director, The Toronto Hospital Vascular Center, The Toronto Hospital—General Division, Toronto, Ontario, Canada

Natural History of Abdominal Aortic Aneurysms: Do Size, Sex, Age, and Family Matter?

Edouard Kieffer, M.D.

Professor of Vascular Surgery, Chief, Department of Vascular Surgery, Pitié-Salpêtrière University Hospital, Paris, France

Surgical Management of Aneurysms of Aberrant Subclavian Arteries

Paul B. Kreienberg, M.D.

Associate Professor of Surgery, Albany Medical College; Attending, Albany Medical College, Albany, New York

Alternative Approach for Management of Infected Aortic Grafts

Gregory J. Landry, M.D.

Fellow, Division of Vascular Surgery, Oregon Health Sciences University School of Medicine, Portland, Oregon

Preoperative Cardiac Evaluation for Aortic Aneurysm Surgery

Eugene S. Lee, M.D.

Resident, Department of Surgery, University of Minnesota Medical School—Minneapolis, Minneapolis, Minnesota

Prevention and Treatment of Aortic Graft–Enteric Fistula

Alan B. Lumsden, M.B., Ch.B.

Associate Professor of Surgery, Emory University School of Medicine; Associate Head General Vascular Surgery, Emory University Hospital, Atlanta, Georgia

Paraanastomotic Aortic Aneurysms: A Continuing Surgical Challenge; Treatment of Visceral Artery Aneurysms

Michael L. Marin, M.D.

Associate Professor of Surgery, The Mount Sinai School of Medicine of the City University of New York; Director, Endovascular Surgical Development, Associate Professor of Surgery, The Mount Sinai Hospital, Bronx, New York

Transluminally Placed Endovascular Grafts for the Treatment of Aortoiliac Aneurysms

Louis M. Messina, M.D.

Professor of Surgery, University of California, San Francisco, School of Medicine; Chief, Division of Vascular Surgery, The Medical Center at the University of California, San Francisco, California

The Isolated Hypogastric Artery Aneurysm

Charles C. Miller III, Ph.D.

Assistant Professor, Baylor College of Medicine, Houston, Texas

Thoracoabdominal Aortic Aneurysm Repair

D. Craig Miller, M.D.

Professor, Department of Cardiothoracic Surgery, Stanford University School of Medicine; Cardiovascular Surgeon, Stanford University Medical Center, Stanford, California

Endovascular Treatment of Thoracic Aortic Aneurysms and Dissection

Marc E. Mitchell, M.D.

Assistant Professor of Surgery, Georgetown University School of Medicine; Chief, Section of Vascular Surgery, VA Medical Center, Washington, D.C.

Popliteal Artery Aneurysms

Takao Ohki, M.D.

Assistant Professor of Surgery, Albert Einstein College of Medicine of Yeshiva University; Chief, Endovascular Program, Attending Surgeon, Montefiore Medical Center, Bronx, New York

Transluminally Placed Endovascular Grafts for the Treatment of Aortoiliac Aneurysms

Kenneth Ouriel, M.D.

Associate Professor of Surgery and Radiology, University of Rochester School of Medicine and Dentistry, Rochester, New York

Prevention and Treatment of Spinal Cord Ischemia Associated With Aortic Aneurysm Repair

Frank T. Padberg, Jr., M.D., F.A.C.S.

Professor of Surgery, New Jersey Medical School, University of Medicine and Dentistry of New Jersey, Newark, New Jersey; Chief, Section of Vascular Surgery, New Jersey Veterans Healthcare System, Lyons and East Orange, New Jersey

Treatment of Infected False Aneurysm of the Femoral Artery

Philip S. K. Paty, M.D.

Associate Professor of Surgery, Albany Medical College; Attending, Albany Medical Center Hospital, Albany, New York

Alternative Approach for Management of Infected Aortic Grafts

William H. Pearce, M.D.

Professor of Surgery, Northwestern University Medical School; Director, Noninvasive Blood Flow Laboratory, Chief, Division of Vascular Surgery, Northwestern Memorial Hospital, Chicago, Illinois

Preoperative Imaging Studies of Abdominal Aortic Aneurysms: When Are Computed Tomography, Arteriography, or New Modalities Indicated?

John M. Porter, M.D.

Professor of Surgery, Head, Division of Vascular Surgery, Oregon Health Sciences University School of Medicine, Portland, Oregon

Preoperative Cardiac Evaluation for Aortic Aneurysm Surgery

William J. Quiñones-Baldrich, M.D.

Professor of Surgery, Section of Vascular Surgery, University of California, Los Angeles, School of Medicine, Los Angeles, California

Treatment of Chylous Ascites After Abdominal Aortic Aneurysm Repair

Carol A. Raviola, M.D.

Assistant Professor of Surgery, University of Pennsylvania School of Medicine and Jefferson Medical College of Thomas Jefferson University; Section of Vascular Surgery, Pennsylvania Hospital, Philadelphia, Pennsylvania

Preoperative Pulmonary Evaluation for Aortic Aneurysm Surgery

Linda Reilly, M.D.

Associate Program Director for General Surgery Program, Associate Professor in Residence, University of California, San Francisco, School of Medicine, San Francisco, California

The Isolated Hypogastric Artery Aneurysm

Ignacio Rua, M.D.

Attending Vascular and General Surgeon, Baptist Hospital of Miami, Miami, Florida

Preoperative Pulmonary Evaluation for Aortic Aneurysm Surgery

Hazim J. Safi, M.D.

Professor of Surgery, Baylor College of Medicine; Houston, Texas

Thoracoabdominal Aortic Aneurysm Repair

Luis A. Sanchez, M.D.

Division of Vascular Surgery, Albert Einstein College of Medicine of Yeshiva University, Bronx, New York

Transluminally Placed Endovascular Grafts for the Treatment of Aortoiliac Aneurysms

Steven M. Santilli, M.D., Ph.D.

Assistant Professor of Surgery, University of Minnesota Medical School—Minneapolis; Chief, Vascular Surgery, VA Medical Center, Minneapolis, Minnesota

Prevention and Treatment of Aortic Graft–Enteric Fistula

Marcel Scheinman, M.D.

Vascular Research Resident, Maimonides Medical Center, Brooklyn, New York

Treatment of Carotid Artery Aneurysms and Aortic Arch Vessel Aneurysms

Sherry D. Scovell, M.D.

Resident, Department of Surgery, Temple University School of Medicine, Philadelphia, Pennsylvania

Etiology of Abdominal Aortic Aneurysms: The Structural Basis for Aneurysm Formation

James M. Seeger, M.D.

Professor, Department of Surgery, Chief, Section of Vascular Surgery, University of Florida College of Medicine; Chief, Vascular Surgery Section, Veterans Affairs Medical Center, Gainesville, Florida

Prevention of Sigmoid and Pelvic Ischemia During Abdominal Aortic Aneurysm Surgery

Dhiraj M. Shah, M.D.

Professor of Surgery, Albany Medical College; Head, Department of General Surgery, Attending, Albany Medical Center Hospital, Albany, New York

Alternative Approach for Management of Infected Aortic Grafts

Gregorio A. Sicard, M.D.

Chief, Division of General and Vascular Surgery, Professor of Surgery, Washington University School of Medicine; Director, Vascular Surgery Service, Barnes Hospital, St. Louis, Missouri

Midline Versus Retroperitoneal Approach for Abdominal Aortic Aneurysm Surgery

Suzanne M. Slonim, M.D.

Assistant Professor, Department of Radiology, Stanford University School of Medicine, Stanford, California; Chief, Section of Interventional Radiology, VA Medical Center, Palo Alto, California

Endovascular Treatment of Thoracic Aortic Aneurysms and Dissection

Robert B. Smith III, M.D.

John E. Skandalakis Professor of Surgery, Emory University School of Medicine; Head, General Vascular Surgery, Emory University Hospital, Atlanta, Georgia

Paraanastomotic Aortic Aneurysms: A Continuing Surgical Challenge; Treatment of Visceral Artery Aneurysms

Ronald J. Stoney, M.D.

Professor Emeritus, University of California, San Francisco, School of Medicine, San Francisco, California

The Isolated Hypogastric Artery Aneurysm

William D. Suggs, M.D.

Associate Professor of Surgery, Albert Einstein College of Medicine of Yeshiva University; Vascular Surgery Services, Montefiore Medical Center, Bronx, New York

Transluminally Placed Endovascular Grafts for the Treatment of Aortoiliac Aneurysms

Brian V. Taylor, M.Sc.

University of Toronto, Toronto, Ontario, Canada

Natural History of Abdominal Aortic Aneurysms: Do Size, Sex, Age, and Family Matter?

Boulos Toursarkissian, M.D.

Assistant Professor, University of Texas

Medical School at San Antonio; University Hospital, San Antonio, Texas

Midline Versus Retroperitoneal Approach for Abdominal Aortic Aneurysm Surgery

Frank J. Veith, M.D.

Professor of Surgery, Albert Einstein College of Medicine of Yeshiva University; Chief, Vascular Surgical Services, Montefiore Medical Center, Bronx, New York

Transluminally Placed Endovascular Grafts for the Treatment of Aortoiliac Aneurysms

Reese A. Wain, M.D.

Assistant Professor of Surgery, Albert Einstein College of Medicine of Yeshiva University, Bronx, New York

Transluminally Placed Endovascular Grafts for the Treatment of Aortoiliac Aneurysms

John V. White, M.D.

Professor of Surgery, Temple University School of Medicine; Division of Vascular Surgery, Temple University Hospital, Philadelphia, Pennsylvania

Etiology of Abdominal Aortic

Aneurysms: The Structural Basis for Aneurysm Formation

W. Kent Williamson, M.D.

Resident, Department of Surgery, Oregon Health Sciences University School of Medicine, Portland, Oregon

Preoperative Cardiac Evaluation for Aortic Aneurysm Surgery

Douglas J. Wirthlin, M.D.

Fellow of Vascular Surgery, Harvard Medical School, Boston, Massachusetts

Concomitant Aortic Aneurysm Repair and Coronary Artery Bypass

Chester C. Yavorski, M.D.

Vascular Fellow, University of Kentucky College of Medicine, Lexington, Kentucky

Treatment of Sciatic Artery Aneurysms

Richard A. Yeager, M.D.

Associate Professor of Surgery, Division of Vascular Surgery, Oregon Health Sciences University School of Medicine, Portland, Oregon

Preoperative Cardiac Evaluation for Aortic Aneurysm Surgery

Preface

Beginning with Hunter's classic report, arterial aneurysm was among the first of conditions to be addressed in the modern surgical era. The epidemiology, clinical presentation, and treatment of aneurysmal disease continue to evolve 300 years later. In the last half of this century, basic science research has helped define the genetics, histopathology, and etiology of arterial aneurysm. Developments in imaging technology have allowed the delineation of the prevalence and the natural history of aneurysmal disease. Advancements in critical care have allowed the widespread application of classic surgical techniques in the treatment of aneurysms. Indications for surgery have changed as the morbidity of aneurysms has dropped. As with other manifestations of atherosclerotic disease, the prevalence of aneurysm in our aging population is rising. Superimposed on this already dynamic paradigm are the explosive developments occurring with the application of endovascular technology in the treatment of arterial aneurysms.

This book is intended to provide a survey of current concepts in the diagnosis and treatment of arterial aneurysmal disease, excluding intracerebral pathology. Contributors regarded as experts in specific areas related to aneurysms have provided data, illustrations, experience, and insight, which in aggregate provide a compendium that serves as a valuable resource to students and practitioners of vascular medicine and surgery.

KEITH D. CALLIGARO, M.D.
MATTHEW J. DOUGHERTY, M.D.
LARRY H. HOLLIER, M.D.

Contents

Part 3

**Surgical Approaches and Techniques for Treating
Challenging Abdominal Aortic Aneurysms**

Part 4

**Prevention and Treatment of Complications of
Abdominal Aortic Aneurysm Surgery**

Part 5
Management of Nonaortic Arterial Aneurysms

Etiology, Natural History, and Preoperative Evaluation of Patients Undergoing Aortic Aneurysm Surgery

Etiology of Abdominal Aortic Aneurysms: The Structural Basis for Aneurysm Formation

John V. White, M.D., and Sherry D. Scovell, M.D.

The incidence of aortic aneurysmal disease continues to increase, and its associated mortality has risen concomitantly over the past decade. Though studies have identified many promising causative factors, none has completely explained the pathogenesis and progression of aneurysmal disease. The cause of aortic aneurysm probably is multifactorial, with significant genetic, epidemiologic, and behavioral influences.[1] Whatever the combination of causative agents and events, all eventually manifest through the same pathway: the destruction of vital aortic wall structural components and aneurysm formation.

Aneurysm formation represents the loss of structural integrity of the aortic wall. The consequences of this loss are well recognized by surgeons, physicians, and the family members of patients who succumbed to aneurysm rupture. Prevention of rupture is the primary goal of intervention in aneurysmal disease. To accomplish this goal, it is necessary to define the structural defect that results in the loss of aortic wall biomechanical function and leads to the uncontrolled expansion of this vessel. Understanding the process of structural component failure requires knowledge of the composition of the normal aortic wall and the biomechanical function of those components as they are organized.

Aortic Wall Structure

Intima

The intima is defined by the layer of endothelial cells attached to an underlying basement membrane. The endothelial cells mediate interactions between blood and blood vessels. These interactions regulate activation of the clotting and fibrinolytic systems and coordinate systemic and local vascular resistance through intercellular communication with the smooth muscle cells of the media. The endothelial cells sit on a collagen substructure and the internal elastic lamina, which defines the junction of the intima and the media. This substructure contains numerous lymphatic pores or pits that allow transport through the arterial wall (Fig. 1–1) of various substances, including cellular messengers that pass through the layers of the aortic wall within this intramural lymphatic network.[2] Loss of endothelial cells initiates a sequence of events that may result in atherosclerotic plaque formation mediated by platelet-derived growth factors.[3] Endothelial cells may also play a role in

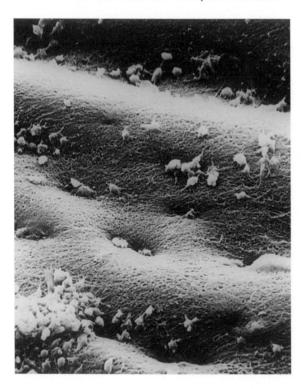

Figure 1–1. Subendothelial collagen lies on top of the internal elastine membrane. Numerous lymphatic pits penetrate this layer and allow passage of substances from the intima into the media.

accelerating the destruction of aortic wall components in aneurysmal disease through activation of the lytic pathway.[4, 5]

Disruption of the intima does not decrease arterial wall biomechanical function, as is demonstrated by the large number of uncomplicated endarterectomies performed each year. The absence of this layer in aortic aneurysms is more likely the manifestation of altered aortic wall metabolism rather than the primary structural defect in this pathologic process.

Media

The media is composed largely of smooth muscle cells within an elastin and collagen substructure. The smooth muscle cells are oriented obliquely to form layers that spiral down the long axis of the vessel.[6] Interspersed with the layers of smooth muscle cells are concentric elastic lamellae (Fig. 1–2). Thin, transversely directed elastic fibers and collagen fibers provide a structural link between these two major media components. These fine fibers travel from the surface of the elastin lamella to the outer surface of the smooth muscle cell membrane in an area of contractile elements.[7] This relationship permits transmission of the contractile force of the smooth muscle cell to the elastin and collagen substructure. This represents the contractile unit of the media.[8]

Elastic lamellae maintain the flow of blood during diastole. The radial vectors of systolic pressure increase the diameter of these lamellae, effectively stretching them.[9] These elastic fibers passively recoil during diastole, providing sufficient excursion toward the lumen in a bellows-like fashion to continue the movement of blood. The role of the smooth muscle cells is far more complex; the contractility of these cells to alter vascular resistance is perhaps the most fundamental activity throughout the arterial tree. A variety of

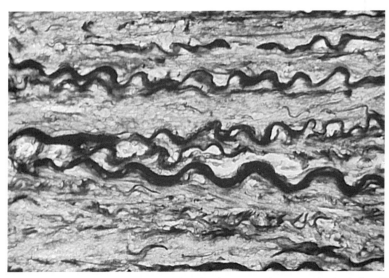

Figure 1-2. Within the media, smooth muscle cells alternate with concentric elastic lamellae that provide passive elastic recoil during systole.

other functions also have been identified. Subsets of these cells can have macrophage-like functions, scavenging bacteria and debris and releasing degradative enzymes within the media.[10, 11] These cells may be integrally involved in destruction of aortic wall components. Other medial smooth muscle cells can provide significant synthetic function, producing collagen in large quantities when stimulated.[12] Though these cells are capable of producing elastic fibers, humans lose this ability early in life.[13] Little elastin synthesis within the aortic wall can be detected beyond infancy.

Despite the presence of contractile elements, smooth muscle cells do not regulate the maximal outer diameter of the aorta. The role of smooth muscle contraction in limiting the maximal aortic outer diameter was evaluated in our laboratories. We used a laser scanner to measure outer diameter and construct pressure-diameter curves for infrarenal aortic segments.[14] After baseline pressure-diameter measurements were taken, the canine infrarenal aortas were randomly divided into two groups. Group I vessels were bathed for 1 hour in a solution of nifedipine and nitroprusside to block smooth muscle cell contractile function without cell injury. The aortas in group II were soaked in elastase (20 μg/mL) for 1 hour. The aortas of both groups were then returned to the laser scanner for repeat pressure-diameter measurements. Although smooth muscle cell contraction was inhibited in group I aortas, the biomechanical behavior of these vessels did not differ from those of controls ($P = 0.4$, group I versus control) (Fig. 1–3). The elastase treatment of group II aortic segments induced a significant change in the pressure-diameter profile ($P = 0.2$, group II versus control).

Results of our studies and those cited earlier suggest that medial smooth muscle cells may play a role in the formation of abdominal aortic aneurysm formation and growth through their degradative and synthetic functions but not through loss of contractile function. The connective tissue elements of the media also do not limit maximal aortic outer diameter. Analysis of the bursting pressures of the individual aortic layers documented that the media ruptures at relatively low pressures.[15, 16] These investigations strongly suggest that loss of the structural integrity of the adventitia, not the media, is required for aneurysm formation.

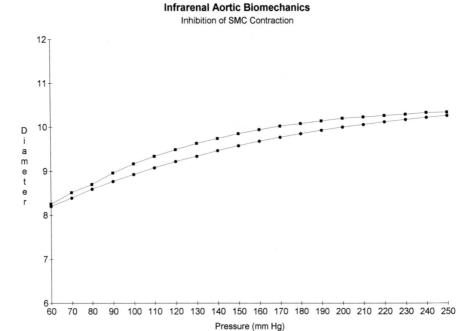

Figure 1–3. Pressure-diameter curves of normal canine infrarenal aortic segments (control) and segments incubated in nifedipine and nitroprusside to block smooth muscle cell contraction (group I). Despite inhibition of smooth muscle cell contraction, the maximal outer aortic diameter did not significantly increase.

Adventitia

The architecture of the adventitia differs significantly from the other layers of the aortic wall. This mostly acellular layer of the aortic wall, composed of large amounts of elastin and collagen, is particularly well suited to limit the maximal aortic outer diameter. Its construction is a model of strength and limited elasticity. Distribution of the elastin and collagen components is not uniform throughout the adventitia. The inner third of the adventitia, adjacent to the media, consists of densely compacted elastin and collagen fibers.[17] The density of elastin fibers decreases from the inner to the outer portion of the adventitia, and the collagen components become more loosely woven toward the outer adventitial surface. These outermost, loosely woven collagen fibers appear to interweave with the perivascular collagen-containing tissue to link the aorta to its anatomic environment.

Elastin fiber density is greatest within the inner third of the adventitia, where thick elastic fibers, oriented longitudinally in the direction of blood flow, are closely applied, forming sheets (Fig. 1–4). The fibers separate only to form fenestrae that permit the passage of the vasa vasorum into the aortic wall. These concentric elastin sheets, or lamellae, entirely surround the aorta. The thick elastic fibers within each sheet appear to be linked by thin elastic fibers that run circumferentially around the aorta. The adventitial elastin lamellae alternate with lamellae of collagen composed of fibers that travel circumferentially around the aortic wall, with a predominant axis of orientation of these fibers perpendicular to that of the thick elastic fibers. These alternating lamellae are tightly juxtaposed and appear to be interconnected by small radial fibrils (Fig. 1–5).

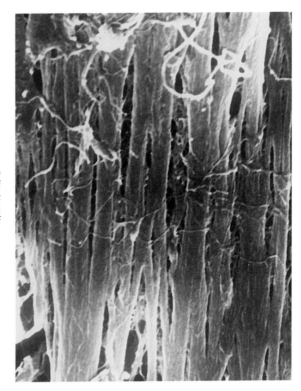

Figure 1–4. The elastic lamellae reside within the inner third of the adventitia. The thick elastic fibers are closely juxtaposed and oriented in the direction of blood flow.

The biomechanical function of the adventitia appears to be maintenance of the maximal aortic outer diameter. Previous studies have demonstrated that the adventitia contains elastin and collagen that provide resistance to the radial stresses of flowing blood.[15, 16] To confirm this finding, our laboratory performed pressure-diameter measurements of whole-vessel infrarenal aortas and endarterectomized aortic segments containing only adventitia.[14] Explanted canine infrarenal aortas were immediately placed into the sampling

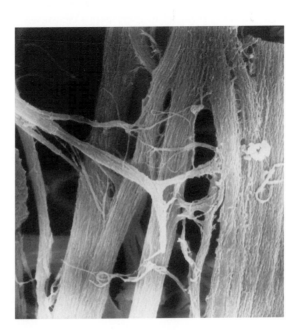

Figure 1–5. The thick elastic fibers within the inner third of the adventitia appear to be interconnected by small radial fibrils and separate to permit passage of the vasa vasorum.

chamber of a laser scanner capable of detecting a 5 μm change in the outer aortic diameter. The vessels were slowly pressurized from 50 to 250 mm Hg with warmed saline introduced through an inflow port while pressure was recorded through a distal cannula. These continuous pressure-diameter measurements confirmed that the adventitia alone is capable of maintaining normal maximal aortic outer diameter, even at extremely high pressures (Fig. 1–6). Treating the adventitial sleeves with elastase produced a significant loss of structural integrity, pathologic dilation, and a pressure-diameter relationship consistent with aneurysm formation.

Dobrin and colleagues[18] studied the contributions of elastin and collagen to the maintenance of arterial wall biomechanical function. Assessing pressure-diameter relationships of arterial segments, they demonstrated that destruction of elastin results in pathologic dilation of the vessel, whereas destruction of the collagen within the vessel wall results in rupture. They concluded from these series of studies that aneurysmal disease was a process of elastin degradation and that rupture was related to collagen disruption. Taken together, these findings strongly implicate adventitial elastin and structural organization of the adventitia as the critical structures in maintenance of aortic wall biomechanical integrity and prevention of aneurysm formation.

Aneurysm Formation

In Vivo Model of Aneurysm Formation

To confirm the role of adventitial elastin degradation in aneurysm formation, a model of selective adventitial elastin degradation was created.[19] The infrarenal aorta of a rabbit was surgically exposed, and pancreatic elastase was dripped over the exposed adventitial surface. Within 1 hour, an aneurysm was grossly evident, with a greater than 100% increase in maximal aortic outer diameter. Histologic analysis and grading of the structural injury (Table 1–1) created in this model revealed a nearly selective adventitial elastin-based injury.[20] The amount of elastin was slightly reduced in the outermost portion of the media, but no specific collagen fiber damage was observed, and the smooth muscle architecture of the media was intact. The aneurysms formed in this model continued to increase in diameter, consistent with the progression observed in human aneurysmal disease.

These data strongly support the concept that adventitial elastin degradation is the critical structural defect required for aneurysm formation. After aneu-

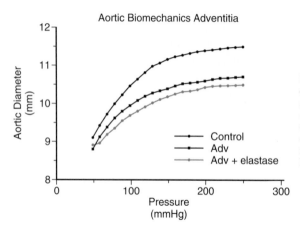

Figure 1–6. Pressure-diameter curves of whole infrarenal aortic segments and adventitial sleeves demonstrate that the adventitia is capable of maintaining maximal outer aortic diameter within a normal range, even at extremely high pressures.

Table 1-1.
In Vivo Model of Aneurysm Formation: Histologic Injury Severity Scores

Aortic Wall Layer	Injury Score* (Mean ± SD)
Intima	
Internal elastic membrane	3.01 ± 0.66
Media	
Thickness	2.97 ± 0.61
Smooth muscle cells	2.97 ± 0.61
Elastin	1.86 ± 0.91
Adventitia	
Collagen	1.81 ± 0.27
Elastin	0.78 ± 0.53

*Injury score scale: 0, complete loss of the structural element; 1, loss of more than half of the structural element; 2, loss of less than half of the structural element; 3, minimal loss of the structural element; 4, no injury.

rysm formation occurs, a series of pathologic events within the aortic wall begins, marked by the continued synthesis and degradation of collagen components that permit aneurysm growth.

Adventitial Elastin Degradation and Aneurysm Formation in Patients

The importance of adventitial elastin degradation in human aneurysmal disease was investigated in a study of normal aortic and aneurysm walls. The study was conducted to determine whether the process of elastin degradation parallels aneurysm growth or is complete before aneurysm formation. The aneurysm walls of 12 patients undergoing elective repair of asymptomatic infrarenal aortic aneurysms were studied with light and scanning microscopy.[21] Aneurysms were classified as small (diameter <5 cm), moderate (diameter between 5 and 7 cm), or large (diameter >7 cm). The structural findings were compared with normal control values obtained from evaluation of infrarenal aortic walls removed at autopsy from six cadavers without evidence of aneurysmal disease. Using quantitative videomicroscopy, the amount of elastin within the inner third of the adventitia was assessed and compared with that in normal aortic walls.

Anatomic assessment of the normal human aortic wall, especially the adventitial ultrastructure, revealed it to be remarkably similar to the canine aorta. The intima and media were remarkable only in that even grossly normal aortic wall demonstrated some subendothelial thickening. The inner third of the adventitia from the normal aortas of control patients were composed of densely compacted, alternating layers of elastin and collagen (Fig. 1–7). The adventitial elastin layers were composed of thick elastic fibers whose long axes were parallel to the direction of blood flow and alternated with collagen lamellae composed of fibers directed circumferentially.

The architectural appearance of all aneurysm specimens, even those with small diameters, was drastically altered. The intima was absent, and virtually all of the media was replaced by thrombus and atheromatous debris (Fig. 1–8). Little elastin remained within the adventitia, and the thick elastic lamellae of the inner third of the adventitia were totally degraded. Only scattered, isolated deposits of elastin remained within this inner adventitia. These deposits contained elastic fibers that were disorganized, tortuous, and without a pre-

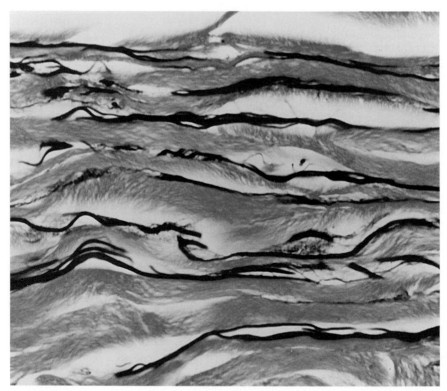

Figure 1-7. The inner third of the adventitia of the normal human infrarenal aorta demonstrates the characteristic densely compacted, alternating layers of elastin and collagen.

dominant axis of orientation (Fig. 1–9). The fibers had no relationship to the surrounding collagen. There were areas of newly synthesized collagen but not elastin, suggesting that the aortic wall response to elastin degradation is collagen synthesis. These findings demonstrate a complete loss of structural integrity and a subsequent structural reorganization within the adventitia resulting from elastin degradation and collagen deposition.

Quantitative assessment of the elastic remnants documented that the elastin content within the inner third of the adventitia of all aneurysms was reduced by $81.6 \pm 2.1\%$ compared with normal controls. The elastin content did not differ among small, moderate, and large aneurysms; all aneurysm wall specimens demonstrated diffuse loss of elastin. This information suggests that elastin degradation does not parallel aneurysm growth, because nearly all of the elastin lamellae within the inner third of the adventitia are degraded before clinically detectable aneurysm formation.

Hypothesis of Aneurysm Formation and Growth

Based on the information in the previous sections, a more comprehensive hypothesis of abdominal aortic aneurysm formation has been constructed. Because the intima and media can be removed from the aorta without the loss of structural integrity, aneurysmal disease must be a disorder of the adventitia. The relationship of the structural components of this layer must be maintained for the preservation of aortic wall biomechanics.

The elastic lamellae of the adventitia maintain adventitial collagen architecture in a manner that permits minimal deformation of the aortic wall despite

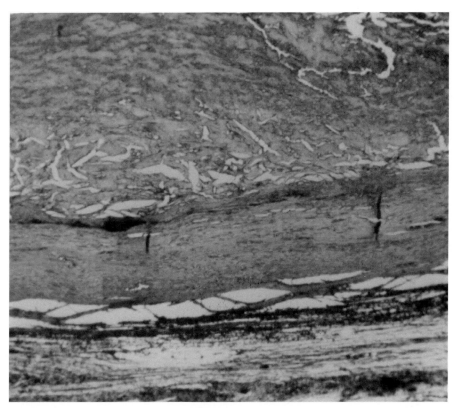

Figure 1–8. The adventitia remaining within the aneurysm wall demonstrates essentially complete absence of the intima and media and layering of the flow surface with thrombus and atheromatous debris.

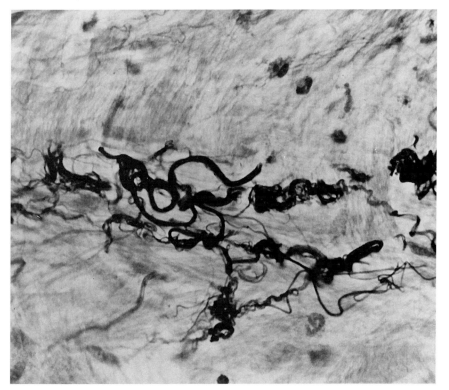

Figure 1–9. The wall of the aneurysm contains small deposits of elastin that is composed of degraded and tortuous elastic fibers with no axis of orientation or relation to the surrounding collagen.

high intraluminal pressures and wall stresses. Elastin degradation may be induced through a variety of initiators, including genetic predisposition, environmental factors, and elastin fatigue. Elastin degradation of the aortic wall manifests first in the intima and media, causing deterioration of these layers. The disruption of medial architecture does not directly result in the loss of biomechanical function of the aortic wall or in clinically detectable aortic dilation. Ultimately, however, the forces that caused medial elastin degradation also cause degradation of the elastic lamellae within the inner third of the adventitia. The loss of the adventitial elastic lamellae permits loosening and stretching of adventitial collagen, resulting in aortic wall weakening and clinically apparent aneurysm formation.

Aneurysm growth results from the continuous opposing forces of collagen deposition and degradation. Aneurysm rupture occurs when the rate of collagen degradation exceeds the rate of collagen deposition within the aneurysm wall or when wall stresses exceed the tolerable limits of the collagen components.

References

1. Powell J, Greenhalgh RM. Cellular, enzymatic, and genetic factors in the pathogenesis of abdominal aortic aneurysms. J Vasc Surg 1989;9:297–304.
2. Jellinek H, Detre Z. Role of the altered transmural permeability in the pathomechanism of atherosclerosis. Pathol Res Pract 1986;181:693–712.
3. Walker LN, Bowen-Pope DF, Ross R, Reidy MA. Production of platelet-derived growth factor–like molecules by cultured arterial smooth muscle cells accompanies proliferation after arterial injury. Proc Natl Acad Sci USA 1986;83:7311–7315.
4. Furchgott RF. Role of endothelium in responses of vascular smooth muscle. Circ Res 1983;53:557–573.
5. Modur V, Feldhaus MJ, Weyrich AS, et al. Oncostatin M is a proinflammatory mediator: in vivo effects correlate with endothelial cell expression of inflammatory cytokines and adhesion molecules. J Clin Invest 1997;100:158–168.
6. Rhodin JAG. Architecture of the vessel wall. *In* Bohr D, Somlyo AP, Sparko HV (eds). Handbook of Physiology. Section 2: The Cardiovascular System. Bethesda: The American Physiological Society, 1980:1–31.
7. Davis EC. Smooth muscle cell to elastic lamina connections in developing mouse aorta: role in aortic medial organization. Lab Invest 1993;68:89–99.
8. Wolinsky H, Glagov S. A lamellar unit of aortic medial structure and function in mammals. Circ Res 1967;20:99–111.
9. Dobrin PB. Mechanical properties of arteries. Physiol Rev 1978;58:397–460.
10. Garfield RE, Chako S, Blose S. Phagocytosis by muscle cells. Lab Invest 1975;33:418–427.
11. Yanagi H, Sasaguri Y, Sugama R, et al. Production of tissue collagenase (matrix metalloproteinase 1) by human aortic smooth muscle cells in response to platelet-derived growth factor. Atherosclerosis 1991;3:207–216.
12. Leung DYM, Glagov S, Matthews MB. Cyclic stretching stimulates synthesis of matrix components by arterial smooth muscle cells in vitro. Science 1976;191:475–477.
14. White JV. Role of adventitial defects in the pathogenesis of aortic aneurysms. *In* Veith F (ed). Current Critical Problems in Vascular Surgery, vol 5. St. Louis: Quality Medical Publishing, 1993:293–301.
15. Butcher HR. The elastic properties of human aortic intima, media and adventitia: the initial effect of thromboendarterectomy. Ann Surg 1960;151:480–489.
16. Sumner DS, Hokanson DE, Strandness DE. Arterial walls before and after endarterectomy: stress-strain characteristics and collagen-elastin content. Arch Surg 1969;99:606–611.
17. Haas KS, Phillips SJ, Comerota AJ, White JV. The architecture of adventitial elastin in the canine infrarenal aorta. Anat Rec 1991;230:86–96.
18. Dobrin PB, Baker WH, Gley WC. Elastolytic and collagenolytic studies of arteries. Arch Surg 1984;119:405–409.
19. White JV. Aneurysm formation in vivo by the topical degradation of adventitial elastin. J Vasc Surg 1994;20:153–155.
20. Campbell C, Oh J, White JV. The critical aortic wall structural defect in abdominal aortic aneurysm formation. Surg Forum 1994;45:372–375.
21. White JV, Haas K, Phillips SJ, Comerota AJ. Adventitial elastolysis is a primary event in aneurysm formation. J Vasc Surg 1993;17:371–381.

Natural History of Abdominal Aortic Aneurysms: Do Size, Sex, Age, and Family Matter?

Peter G. Kalman, M.D., and Brian V. Taylor, M.Sc.

The importance of continuous advancement of our knowledge regarding the natural history of abdominal aortic aneurysms is demonstrated by the threatened risk of rupture. In two institutional experiences, the overall 30-day mortality rate for patients presenting to the hospital with rupture was between 50% and 70%.[1, 2] These mortality rates may be low estimates, because only persons who arrive in the emergency department after rupture in time for a diagnosis to be made are included. The true mortality for all ruptured aneurysms is undoubtedly higher and may be as high as 90% to 95%.

The prevalence of small and large abdominal aneurysms appears to be increasing, a finding that may be the result of improved imaging techniques and increased physician awareness.[3] The first report of a successful abdominal aneurysm repair was made more than four decades ago,[4] but disagreement continues regarding the risk of rupture and indications for elective surgery.[5] Seventy-five percent of abdominal aneurysms are asymptomatic when first detected on routine physical examinations or as incidental findings on ultrasonographic studies or computed tomography (CT) scans. Most of those identified are small, usually less than 5 cm in diameter. This chapter summarizes the influences of size, sex, age, and family history on the natural history of abdominal aneurysms.

Contributing Factors

Size

In a landmark study published in 1966, Szilagyi and colleagues[6] reported their observations of a large cohort of patients with asymptomatic abdominal aneurysms and concluded that the 5-year survival and risk of rupture were related to aneurysm size. For aneurysms less than or equal to 6 cm in diameter, the 5-year survival rate was 48% and the risk of rupture was 20%, compared with the 5-year survival rate of 6% and a rupture incidence of 43% for aneurysms larger than 6 cm.[6] This report greatly influenced decision making by vascular surgeons for several years and was the basis for using a 6-cm cutoff as the indication for elective repair. This became the central dogma despite the extreme variations in aneurysm measurement used in this study (eg, physical examination, plain radiography, at laparotomy or autopsy).[6]

The next study that had an impact on surgical decision making was reported in 1977 by Darling and associates.[7] In this study, 24,000 consecutive autopsies at the Massachusetts General Hospital were reviewed over a 23-year period.[7] The findings supported the contention that aneurysm rupture was related to size, but it was noteworthy that rupture was also found in aneurysms that were less than 4 cm in diameter. Based on these observations, the investigators recommended that even small aneurysms should be repaired because they were all potentially lethal.[7] The critical limitation of this and other autopsy studies for the purpose of defining natural history is the inaccuracy of size determination when the aneurysm is not measured under conditions of physiologic blood pressure. This situation results in underestimating the size of the aneurysm and therefore in overestimating the risk correlated with a given size.

The consensus among vascular surgeons is that the most significant predictor of rupture is size. The 5-year risk for aneurysms between 5.0 and 5.9 cm in diameter is approximately 20% to 25%; for 6 cm, the risk is 35% to 40%; and for those larger than 7 cm, the rupture risk is more than 75%. Most surgeons agree that repair is indicated when, on balance, the risk of operation is less than the risk of rupture for each size range.

Although Scott and coworkers[8] stated that surgery was detrimental for aneurysms smaller than 6 cm in diameter, a report from a subcommittee of the Joint Council of the Society for Vascular Surgery and the International Society for Cardiovascular Surgery recommended that asymptomatic aneurysms between 4 and 5 cm in diameter be considered for elective repair, provided the patient has an acceptably low operative risk and the surgeon has documented low morbidity and mortality rates for elective surgery.[5]

Advocates of small aneurysm (<5 cm) repair cite a lower operative mortality when the patient is younger and healthier, because the operative risk increases with age. It has been suggested that elective repair improves late survival,[9] and using a Markov decision tree analysis of data obtained from reports in the literature, Katz and Cronenwett[10] concluded that small aneurysm repair was cost effective for patients with an acceptable operative risk.

Although many vascular surgeons claim to have witnessed ruptures of small aneurysms, the risk of rupture generally is considered to be small or negligible, falling below the expected operative mortality risk for elective repair.[11–16] Sterpetti and colleagues[11] reviewed 40,000 autopsies from two hospitals in Rome and found that only 5% of ruptured aneurysms were smaller than 5 cm in diameter. Their study[11] and the autopsy study by Darling[7] overestimated the rupture risk of small aneurysms, largely because the proportion of ruptures identified at autopsy represents the prevalence of all ruptured aneurysms rather than the incidence that would be observed in a normal population.[12] Moreover, accurate measurement of aneurysm size at autopsy is difficult because of tissue shrinkage, and underestimating the true measurement overestimates the rupture risk.[12]

Two regional referral centers reported 5-year risks of rupture for small aneurysms of 2% and 0%, respectively.[13, 14] The results from studying referral-based cohorts have been criticized because the rupture risk in this patient population is potentially overestimated; return to the referral center often depends on development of new symptoms or a significant change in size that prompts referral.[12]

Some reports that originate from population-based studies are free from autopsy and referral center bias.[12, 15] At the Mayo Clinic, Nevitt and associates[12] found that the risk of rupture for small aneurysms at 5 years was 0%. Similarly, results from a population-based study in Sweden[15] demonstrated that the risk of rupture was 2.5% at 7 years, and none of the ruptures was identified in aneurysms that were smaller than 5 cm in diameter.

Improved late survival has been used as the justification for early repair of small aneurysms, and it has even been suggested to be cost-effective procedure.[10] Hallett and colleagues[16] summarized findings for a population-based cohort from the Mayo Clinic and observed that the 5-year survival rate for patients undergoing aneurysm repair was 62%, compared with the expected survival of 83% for the general population. The decreased survival primarily resulted from the prevalence of coronary disease in the former group, and this finding questions the rationale for elective surgery in this group, particularly for patients with small aneurysms.[16] An almost identical late survival rate (68% at 5 years) was observed for the patient population described in the Canadian Aneurysm Study.[17]

Because initial aneurysm size alone has been insufficient to reliably predict risk, the growth rate of small aneurysms was analyzed. Bernstein and Chan[18] followed 99 high-risk patients for an average of 2.4 years (range, 1 to 9 years) with serial ultrasonographic studies at 3-month intervals. For aneurysms initially smaller than 6 cm, the mean expansion rate was 0.4 cm/year,[18] and the rupture risk for aneurysms smaller than 6 cm in diameter was less than 5% during the follow-up period, which supported the idea of continuing with a conservative approach. The study protocol dictated that surgery was indicated when the aneurysm reached 6 cm or expanded rapidly (>0.4 cm/year) between consecutive ultrasonographic follow-up assessments. The results of this study had a long-lasting influence on vascular surgeons, for whom an expansion rate of 0.5 cm between consecutive 6-month assessments was considered a strong indication for elective surgery. Later studies, however, failed to demonstrate this relation between expansion at follow-up and risk of rupture.[12, 19]

Whether or not aneurysm expansion is related to rupture risk, significant variability is observed in growth rates.[18, 20, 21] In the Kingston aneurysm study, Brown and associates[14] found that the mean growth rate of aneurysms with an initial diameter of 4.5 to 4.9 cm was 0.7 cm/year, and they recommended that low-risk patients be considered for elective repair because of the inevitable expansion to 5 cm. Sterpetti and coworkers[20] observed a mean expansion of 0.48 cm/year, but individual rates were extremely variable. Using Cox regression, Cronenwett and colleagues[19] conducted a multivariate analysis of the variables predictive of small aneurysm rupture. The combination of diastolic blood pressure, initial anteroposterior diameter, and degree of chronic obstructive pulmonary disease best predicted aneurysm rupture at 5 years.[19] The growth rate of small aneurysms at The Toronto Hospital was determined from a registry of 430 patients, 214 of whom had more than three evaluations at 6-month intervals. Patients were monitored for an average of 3.3 years, and the average initial aneurysm size was 4 cm (Kalman PG: unpublished data). During follow-up, 58.4% of patients had no change or a decrease in aneurysm size, 25.3% had aneurysm expansions between 0.1 to 0.25 cm, 12.6% had increases greater than 0.25 cm, and only 3.7% had a growth rate greater than 0.5 cm.

One pitfall of the studies looking at the natural history of aneurysm expansion and rupture is the data source; data can originate from a variety of study designs (eg, autopsy data, referral-based and population-based studies). The true risk of rupture for small aneurysms remains unknown, and this question is unlikely to be answered until well-designed, prospective, randomized trials are completed.[22–24]

Sex

In reports of patients undergoing elective and emergency aneurysm repair, between 15% and 20% are women. As with cardiac disease, it has been suggested that gender bias may exist in patient selection for aneurysm repair.[25] Physicians are less likely to conduct aggressive investigation of coronary artery disease followed by surgical intervention for women than for men.[26] Data illustrate that women with chronic angina and significant disability are less likely to undergo cardiac catheterization or surgical revascularization than men.[27] Similarly, women who have suffered acute myocardial infarction are less likely to be evaluated for or selected for revascularization than men.[28] These studies and others have raised the possibility of gender bias in the management of patients with coronary artery disease.

Similar trends are observed in the epidemiology of gender-related management of abdominal aneurysms. Caution must be exercised when interpreting reported results regarding the prevalence of aneurysms, and results differ depending on the source of the data. Johnston[25] summarized the sex distribution from surgical series in the literature and found that 18.5% of 7084 elective aneurysm repairs were in women. This percentage of women is generally less than that observed from reported autopsy studies, ultrasonography studies, and hospital discharge and national mortality data.[25] The observed difference in the reported prevalence between surgical series and those from other sources may reflect gender bias in the selection of women for surgery. Alternatively, the prevalence of aneurysms may be greatest among elderly women, but they are diagnosed at a time in life when surgery is not considered because of advanced age or coexistent medical problems. This latter hypothesis is supported by the findings of Bickerstaff and associates,[29] who reported that the median age of their patients at diagnosis was 69 years for men and 78 years for women. It has also been suggested that the observed gender difference is not significant for men and women with a family history of abdominal aortic aneurysm.[30]

Katz and colleagues[31] reported gender differences in a population-based statewide study in Michigan that included 11,512 women and 29,846 men with intact or ruptured abdominal aneurysms. The investigators concluded that men were more likely to have intact (1.8 times) and ruptured (1.4 times) aneurysms treated surgically than women.[31] It is essential that further epidemiologic studies be conducted to resolve these issues.

Age

The normal infrarenal aortic diameter is larger in men than women and increases in size with age in both sexes. Ouriel and colleagues[32] reviewed the CT scans of 100 patients with normal aortas and found that the average infrarenal diameter was 2.1 cm. The size, however, depended on gender (ie, average of 2.3 cm in men and 1.9 cm in women) and age (ie, enlargement of 0.1 mm/year in either sex). The extremes were an average diameter of 1.71 cm in women younger than 40 years of age and 2.85 cm in men older than 70 years.[32] The prevalence of abdominal aneurysms also appears to be related to age, as demonstrated in screening of large populations.[8, 33, 34] The age-related changes in the aortic wall may result from elastin destruction in the elderly.[35]

The indication for elective aneurysm repair in the elderly should generally follow the same guidelines as those for repair in younger persons. Patient selection should be individualized, and the final decision for management should be based on physiologic rather than chronologic age. Numerous reports have claimed that aneurysm repair can be conducted with an acceptable operative mortality and morbidity in the octogenarian, but these cases are usually highly selected.[36, 37]

Family History

The clustering of abdominal aneurysms in families has been cited in several studies and has raised the possibility that genetic factors may be involved through X-linked and autosomal dominant inheritance patterns. Although no founder or common mutation has been identified,[38] this familial association has an estimated incidence of approximately 15% to 20%.[30, 39–41] Powell and associates[42] identified an abnormality on the long arm of chromosome 16 that was associated with familial aneurysms. Molecular defects of type III procollagen have been identified in Ehlers-Danlos syndrome (type IV).[43] Type III procollagen is a structural component of arterial walls, and it has been postulated that the defect is related to aneurysm formation.[43] Advances in molecular biology have provided evidence that altered gene expression may cause abnormalities in the elastin and collagen contents of aneurysms.[44]

Because it is difficult to determine the populations at risk for development of significant abdominal aneurysms, identification of familial or genetic tendencies would be invaluable for initiating cost-effective screening programs. In the future, comprehensive genetic analysis may help identify persons at significant risk for aneurysm development.

Conclusions

All abdominal aneurysms are potentially lethal and have been estimated to be responsible for about 15,000 deaths annually in the United States.[29] Standard surgical repair and endoluminal repair are the only methods known to be effective in preventing these deaths. Although most vascular surgeons adhere to the 5-cm cutoff as an indication for elective repair in patients with an acceptable operative risk, the true natural history of asymptomatic abdominal aneurysms is unknown. Focusing on size alone is insufficient to predict the risk for an individual patient, because other factors such as sex, age, and family history also have a significant influence on operative indications and prognosis.

References

1. Johansen K, Kohler TR, Nicholls SC, et al. Ruptured abdominal aortic aneurysm: the Harborview experience. J Vasc Surg 1991;13:240–247.
2. Hannon EL, Kilburn H, O'Donnell JF, et al. A longitudinal analysis of the relationship between in-hospital mortality in New York State and volume of abdominal aortic aneurysm surgeries performed. Health Serv Res 1992;27:517–542.
3. Laroy LL, Cormier PJ, Matalon TAS, et al. Imaging of abdominal aortic aneurysms. AJR Am J Roentgenol 1989;152:785–792.
4. Dubost C, Allary M, Oeconomos N. Resection of an aneurysm of the abdominal aorta: re-establishment of the continuity by a preserved arterial graft, with results after five months. Arch Surg 1952;64:405.
5. Hollier LH, Taylor LM, Ochsner J. Report of a subcommittee of the Joint Council of the Society for Vascular Surgery and the North American Chapter of the International Society for Cardiovascular Surgery. J Vasc Surg 1992;15:1046–1056.
6. Szilagyi DE, Smith RF, DeRusso FJ, et al. Contribution of abdominal aortic aneurysmectomy to prolongation of life. Ann Surg 1966;164:678–699.
7. Darling RC, Messina CR, Brewster DC, Ottinger LW. Autopsy study of unoperated abdominal aortic aneurysms. Circulation 1977;56(suppl II):II161–164.
8. Scott RAP, Ashton HA, Kay DN. Abdominal aortic aneurysm in 4237 screened patients: prevalence, development and management over 6 years. Br J Surg 1991;78:1122–1125.

9. Katz DA, Littenberg B, Cronenwett JL. Management of small abdominal aortic aneurysms: early surgery vs watchful waiting. JAMA 1992;268:2678–2686.
10. Katz AK, Cronenwett JL. The cost-effectiveness of early surgery versus watchful waiting in the management of small abdominal aortic aneurysms. J Vasc Surg 1994;19:980–991.
11. Sterpetti AV, Cavallaro A, Cavallari N, et al. Factors influencing the rupture of abdominal aortic aneurysms. Surg Gynecol Obstet 1991;173:175.
12. Nevitt MP, Ballard DJ, Hallett JW. Prognosis of abdominal aortic aneurysms: a population based study. N Engl J Med 1989;321:1009–1014.
13. Guirguis EM, Barber CG. The natural history of abdominal aortic aneurysms. Am J Surg 1991;162:481–483.
14. Brown PM, Pattenden R, Vernooy C, et al. Selective management of abdominal aortic aneurysms in a prospective measurement program. J Vasc Surg 1996;23:213–222.
15. Glimaker H, Holmberg L, Elvin A, et al. Natural history of patients with abdominal aortic aneurysm. Eur J Vasc Surg 1991;5:125–130.
16. Hallett JW, Naessens JM, Ballard DJ. Early and late outcome of surgical repair for small abdominal aortic aneurysms: a population based analysis. J Vasc Surg 1993;18:684–691.
17. Johnston KW. Multicenter prospective study of nonruptured abdominal aortic aneurysm. Part II. Variables predicting morbidity and mortality. J Vasc Surg 1989;9:437–447.
18. Bernstein EF, Chan EL. Abdominal aortic aneurysm in high-risk patients. Outcome of selective management based on size and expansion rate. Ann Surg 1984;200:255–263.
19. Cronenwett JL, Murphy TF, Zelenock GB, et al. Actuarial analysis of variables associated with rupture of small abdominal aortic aneurysms. Surgery 1985;98:472–483.
20. Sterpetti AV, Schultz RD, Feldhaus RJ, et al. Factors influencing enlargement rate of small abdominal aortic aneurysms. J Surg Res 1987;43;211–219.
21. Delin A, Ohlsen AD, Swedenborg J. Growth rate of abdominal aortic aneurysms as measured by computed tomography. Br J Surg 1985;72:530.
22. Tilson MD. Surgery versus no surgery for 4 to 5 cm abdominal aortic aneurysm. J Vasc Surg 1992;15:871–872.
23. Lederle FA. Management of small abdominal aortic aneurysms [editorial]. Ann Intern Med 1990;113:731–732.
24. Cole CS. Highlights of an international workshop on abdominal aortic aneurysms. Can Med Assoc J 1989;141:393–395.
25. Johnston KW. Influence of sex on the results of abdominal aortic aneurysm repair. J Vasc Surg 1994;20:914–926.
26. Chiriboga DE, Yarzebski J, Goldberg RJ, et al. A community-wide perspective of gender differences and temporal trends in the use of diagnostic and revascularization procedures for acute myocardial infarction. Am J Cardiol 1993;71:268–273.
27. Petticrew M, McKee M, Jones J. Coronary artery surgery: are women discriminated against? Br Med J 1993;306:1164–1166.
28. Steingart RM, Packer M, Hamm P, et al. Sex differences in the management of coronary artery disease: survival and ventricular enlargement investigators. N Engl J Med 1991;325:226–230.
29. Bickerstaff LK, Hollier LH, Van Peenen HJ, et al. Abdominal aortic aneurysms: the changing natural history. J Vasc Surg 1984;1:6–12.
30. Webster MW, St. Jean PL, Steed DL, et al. Abdominal aortic aneurysm: results of a family study. J Vasc Surg 1991;13:366–372.
31. Katz DJ, Stanley JC, Zelenock GB. Gender differences in abdominal aortic aneurysm prevalence, treatment, and outcome. J Vasc Surg 1997;25:561–568.
32. Ouriel K, Green RM, Donayre C, et al. An evaluation of new methods of expressing aortic aneurysm size: relationship to rupture. J Vasc Surg 1992;15:12–20.
33. Castleden WM, Mercer JC. Abdominal aortic aneurysms in Western Australia: descriptive epidemiology and patterns of rupture. Br J Surg 1985;72:109–112.
34. Collin J, Heather B, Walton J. Growth rates of subclinical abdominal aortic aneurysms: implications for review and rescreening programmes. Eur J Vasc Surg 1991;5:141–144.
35. MacSweeney ST, Powell JT, Greenhalgh RM. Pathogenesis of abdominal aortic aneurysms. Br J Surg 1994;81:935–941.
36. Sterpetti AV, Schultz RD, Feldhaus RJ, et al. Abdominal aortic aneurysm in elderly patients: selective management based on clinical status and aneurysmal expansion rate. Am J Surg 1985;150;772–776.
37. Ernst CB. Abdominal aortic aneurysms. N Engl J Med 1993;328:1167–1172.
38. van der Vliet JA, Boll AP. Abdominal aortic aneurysm. Lancet 1997;349:863–866.
39. Collin J, Walton J. Is abdominal aortic aneurysm familial? BMJ 1989;299:493.
40. Powell JT, Greenhalgh RM. Multifactorial inheritance of abdominal aortic aneurysm. Eur J Vasc Surg 1987;1:29.
41. Adamson J, Powell JT, Greenhalgh RM. Selection for screening for familial aortic aneurysms. Br J Surg 1992;79:897–898.
42. Powell JT, Bashir A, Dawson S, et al. Genetic variation on chromosome 16 is associated with abdominal aortic aneurysm. Clin Sci 1990;78:13.
43. Superti-Furga A, Steinmann B, Ramirez F, et al. Molecular defects of type III procollagen in Ehlers-Danlos syndrome type IV. Hum Genet 1989;82:104.
44. Mesh CL, Baxter BT, Pearce WH, et al. Collagen and elastin gene expression in aortic aneurysms. Surgery 1992;112:256.

Preoperative Imaging Studies of Abdominal Aortic Aneurysms: When Are Computed Tomography, Arteriography, or New Modalities Indicated?

William H. Pearce, M.D., and Paul Finn, M.D.

After an abdominal aortic aneurysm has been discovered and the decision has been made to proceed with operative repair, the surgeon can use a variety of imaging modalities to further characterize the morphology of the aneurysm. Although abdominal aortic aneurysms have been repaired with good results based on ultrasonographic information, new imaging modalities provide data that shorten the operative procedure and leave few questions unanswered before surgery.[1] Having detailed knowledge about the anatomy of the aneurysm, associated arterial pathology, and existence of nonarterial pathology enhances the operative procedure by minimizing the chance of dissection, assists in planning the appropriate incision, and helps to identify associated malignancies in some instances.[2, 3] Knowing the aortic dimensions is important for aneurysm repair by endovascular grafting. The diameter and length of the aneurysm must be carefully determined to prevent perigraft leaks caused by poor arterial apposition or by foreshortening of the endovascular graft.[4, 5]

Selection of the appropriate imaging modality often is based on local experience. Because the technology is rapidly changing, image quality at one center may be vastly different from that obtained at a different center using the same modality. Table 3–1 lists imaging techniques and the need for contrast. Standard arteriography requires 100 to 200 mL of contrast and an arterial puncture. An infused computed tomography (CT) scan, though not invasive, requires an equal amount of contrast for images of the abdomen

Table 3–1.
Imaging Modalities

Contrast Studies	Noncontrast Studies
Angiography (100–200 mL)	Magnetic resonance imaging
Computed tomography of abdomen or pelvis (150 mL)	Magnetic resonance angiography
	Ultrasonography
	Intravenous ultrasonography
	Noninfused computed tomography

and pelvis. However, aneurysm size can be determined with a noninfused CT scan. Only occasionally is it necessary to use contrast to define extravasation or enhancement of the arterial wall in patients with inflammatory abdominal aortic aneurysms. Spiral CT (ie, computed tomography angiography [CTA]) relies on contrast and produces excellent images, similar to those of catheter arteriography.

Specialized centers using intravascular ultrasound (IVUS) have reported excellent results in characterizing aortic morphology. This technique, similar to that of arteriography, requires an arterial puncture with the passage of an ultrasonographic catheter through the aneurysm. Accurate measurements of aortic dimensions can be obtained using IVUS,[6] but determining the patency of visceral vessels beyond their orifices is not possible.

Magnetic resonance imaging (MRI) and magnetic resonance angiography (MRA) provide excellent images of the arterial tree and aneurysm morphology without contrast, but gadolinium has dramatically improved image quality over the original "time-of-flight" technique. Multiplanar reconstruction is also possible with MR technology.

Selection of the appropriate preoperative imaging modality depends on the information the surgeon thinks important for planning the operative repair, such as the anatomy of the aneurysm, associated arterial pathology, and nonarterial pathology or abnormalities. This chapter briefly describes CT and MRI and important clinical applications of each.

Imaging Studies

Computed Tomography

Standard CT scans provide important data with and without contrast enhancement. Vascular CT examinations have specific protocols that vary according to the indication for the study. Contrast-enhanced studies provide important information about inflammation and intraluminal flow.[3, 7] Unlike CT scans of solid organs, for which it is desirable for the contrast material to be within the extravascular spaces, vascular CT scans require scanning during the intravascular phase of contrast administration. Important considerations for vascular CT scans include the area of clinical interest and the rate and type of contrast used. Parameters such as slice thickness and the rate of scan acquisition are modified for vascular studies. Standard CT scans are performed using 5-mm slice thicknesses, an interscan delay, and dynamic table incrementation.

Noncontrast CT scans are performed to obtain a diagnosis and provide useful information on hemorrhages and adjacent hematomas. The serious limitation of noncontrast CT scans is the inability to assess vessel patency. Noncontrast CT scans are most often used for patients with renal insufficiency, iodine contrast allergy, or cardiac failure. Noncontrast CT scans are especially important for detection of calcium, which is crucial in patients with aortic dissection. Noncontrast CT scan is also useful for identifying associated abnormalities of the renal parenchyma (Fig. 3–1), hepatic metastasis, or bowel disorders.

Infused CT scans are essential for identifying intraluminal thrombus. In patients who present with peripheral embolism, it is important to obtain a CT scan before any intraluminal manipulation of a catheter. The CT scan in such instances may provide information regarding intraluminal thrombus,

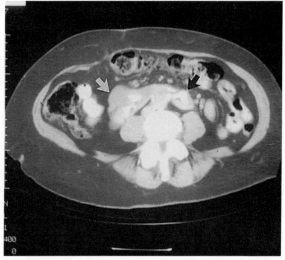

Figure 3–1. Axial computed tomography (CT) image of a patient with an infrarenal abdominal aortic aneurysm. In this image, obtained below the level of the aneurysm, a horseshoe kidney is demonstrated *(white and black arrows).* An advantage of CT scanning over angiography is the superb detail of significant anatomic or pathologic conditions in the surrounding tissues.

particularly in the region of the neck. CT scans of patients with inflammatory aneurysms are also useful for identifying thick, enhancing rims.

Typical contrast protocols for these studies include an initial bolus of 500 mL administered by a power injector at a rate of 2 to 5 mL/sec. A maintenance infusion is then performed using 0.8 to 1.5 mL/sec for administering an additional 100 to 150 mL of contrast.

Computed Tomographic Angiography

Significant technologic advances have been made in the hardware and software used for CT.[8] Conventional CT scans provide transaxial images of the aorta, which are important in determining aortic pathology. With the introduction of fast CT scans and a continuously moving gantry, volume data could be obtained.

Modern spiral CT scanners provide high-quality transaxial images and three-dimensional reconstructions as maximum intensity projections or shaded surface displays (Figs. 3–2 through 3–5). These images are obtained using contrast infusion through the peripheral vein. The contrast is first introduced as a test dose to determine the injection bolus arrival time in the area of interest. A larger contrast bolus is then injected at a rate of 4 to 5 mL/sec during a single breath-hold. The entire examination of the abdomen and the pelvis usually requires less than 2 minutes. Transaxial images obtained from the spiral CT represent 3- to 5-mm slices. These images are notable for their high-contrast definition. As with conventional CT scans, the cross-sectional images provide data on associated venous abnormalities and other intraabdominal pathology. The three-dimensional reconstructions become important when considering associate side branch pathology and aneurysm morphology.

Maximum intensity projections display the images by determining the maximal pixel value encountered along an imaginary ray (Fig. 3–6 and see Figs. 3–4 and 3–5). Calcification appears as islands of bright spots separated from the arterial wall. CTA provides excellent definition of major arterial branches. Compared with standard angiography, renal artery stenosis is accurately identified with CTA (see Fig. 3–4).[9, 10] CTA is also useful in determining visceral vessel stenosis in patients with suprarenal aneurysms (see Fig. 3–5).

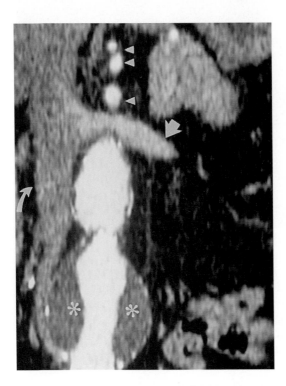

Figure 3–2. Coronal planar reconstruction of an abdominal aortic aneurysm. The patent lumen of the aneurysm is surrounded by thrombus *(asterisks)*. Portions of the celiac and superior mesenteric arteries *(arrowheads)*, the inferior vena cava *(curved arrow)*, and the left renal vein *(arrow)* also can be seen.

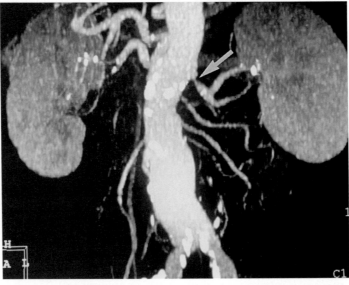

Figure 3–3. Maximum intensity projection of an abdominal aorta shows an infrarenal aneurysm. Notice the stenosis of the left renal artery origin *(arrow)*.

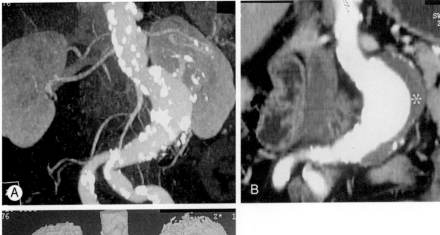

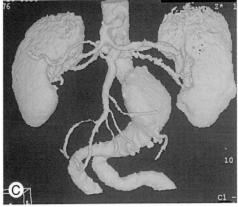

Figure 3–4. *A,* Maximum intensity projection of an abdominal aorta shows an infrarenal aneurysm. Notice the patchy calcification of the wall of the aorta. *B,* In a coronal planar reconstruction of the same aneurysm, visualization of the thrombus lining the lumen of the aneurysm *(asterisk)* is better. *C,* Shaded surface display of the same aneurysm.

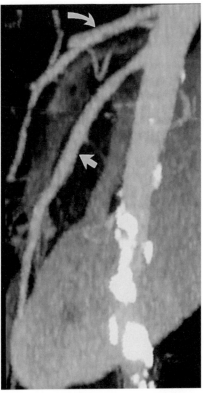

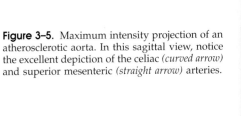

Figure 3–5. Maximum intensity projection of an atherosclerotic aorta. In this sagittal view, notice the excellent depiction of the celiac *(curved arrow)* and superior mesenteric *(straight arrow)* arteries.

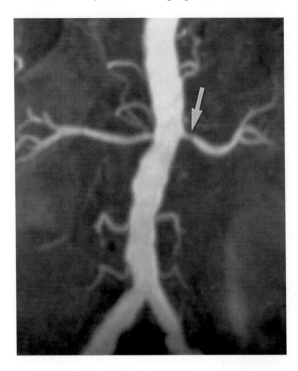

Figure 3–6. Contrast-enhanced, projection magnetic resonance angiogram of the renal arteries was acquired in 17 seconds and directly in the coronal plane during breath holding. A low-grade stenosis *(arrow)* is located near the origin of the left renal artery. The abdominal aorta and proximal iliac arteries are irregular because of atheromatous disease, and several paired lumbar arteries are depicted.

Contrast-Enhanced Magnetic Resonance Angiography

MRA is a noninvasive diagnostic tool that is well established for the diagnosis of venous disease. Because of technical factors, MRA has been less reliable for diagnosing arterial disease. However, the use of intravenous contrast agents has greatly improved the quality of MRA and has stimulated the development of fast MR techniques to exploit the short-lived intravascular peak concentration of these agents.[11]

The most widely used MRA techniques are based on so-called time-of-flight effects, whereby the signal from blood is highlighted by virtue of its flow. If flow is sluggish, visualization of blood vessels may be compromised on many of the more popular MRA techniques. The mechanism whereby the signal from slowly flowing blood is suppressed is called *saturation*, and it has severely limited direct three-dimensional, or "thick-slab," imaging of blood vessels in the body. Saturation results from the repeated application of radio-wave pulses, essential for most MRI applications. If these pulses are applied at very short intervals, some tissues become refractory, or saturated, and cannot generate sufficient signal for detection.

The tendency for tissues to become saturated is described by their *T1 relaxation time*. This is somewhat analogous to the refractory period in muscle and nerve, whereby some time must pass between stimuli for the tissues to be excitable. Tissues with long T1 values (eg, blood, most other biologic fluids) need more time to relax between radio-wave pulses than do tissues with short T1 values (eg, fat). MRA techniques generally use short intervals between pulses and rely on high-flow velocity to offset the tendency toward saturation of the blood. Although this approach often works well for normal blood vessels, diseased vessels commonly are not seen well because of slow flow. If a pharmaceutical agent were available that could selectively shorten the refractory period (T1) of blood, images of the vascular lumen could be acquired independently of flow velocity, and normal and diseased vessels would be well visualized.

One such MR contrast agent, Gd-DTPA, is available for clinical use, and several others are being developed. Gd-DTPA is a chelate of the rare earth element gadolinium (Gd) and the compound diethylenetriamine pentaacetic acid (DTPA). It has been in widespread clinical use for more than 10 years. Gadolinium is one of a class of paramagnetic agents that interact with water in biologic tissues and greatly shorten the T1 of the water. In the bloodstream, the agent shortens the T1 of the blood and therefore acts as a signal-enhancing agent for MRA. The pharmacokinetics of the compound are determined by the DTPA and are identical to those of the radiographic contrast agents. After bolus injection of Gd-DTPA, the blood concentration peaks immediately and then undergoes a rapid fall because of distribution in the extracellular space, followed by a more gradual fall because of elimination in the urine. Like creatinine, DTPA is filtered by the kidneys and subsequently neither secreted nor resorbed. Unlike the iodinated radiographic contrast agents, Gd-DTPA is not nephrotoxic and has been used safely in renally impaired patients.

When used for MRA, Gd-DTPA is injected intravenously as a bolus, usually over 10 to 15 seconds. With modern, high-performance scanners, a three-dimensional angiogram can be acquired in a comparable length of time. The MR images are acquired in a timed fashion to coincide with the arrival of the agent in the vessels of interest (Figs. 3–7 through 3–9 and see Fig. 3–6). The transit time from injection site to target organ depends on what vascular territory is being examined and on the patient's cardiovascular status.

A timing run usually is performed using a small dose of Gd-DTPA to fine-tune the acquisition of the subsequent MR angiogram. If the peak concentration of the agent in the blood is short lived, it is important to time the acquisition accurately relative to the injection. As a first approximation, it takes about 15 seconds for a bolus to reach the abdominal aorta after injection

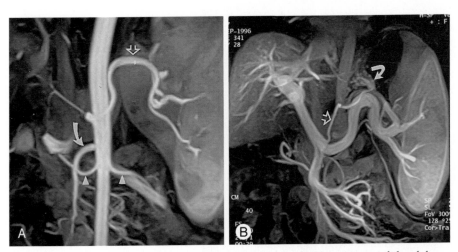

Figure 3–7. *A,* Arterial-phase, projection magnetic resonance (MR) angiogram of the abdomen of a patient with portal hypertension. Notice the tortuous splenic artery *(open arrow)* and the grossly enlarged spleen. The superior mesenteric artery *(curved arrow)* and renal arteries *(arrowheads)* also can be seen. *B,* Venous-phase, projection MR angiogram in the same patient. The entire portal venous tree and the hepatic veins can be seen. Notice the prominent left gastric vein *(open arrow)* and gastric varices *(curved arrow).* (Courtesy of Dr. Jochen Gaa, Klinikum Mannheim, Germany.)

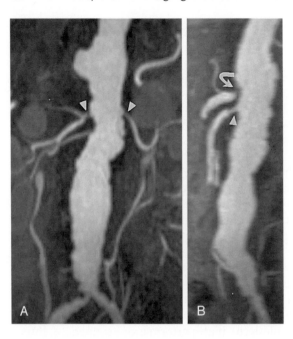

Figure 3–8. *A,* Projection magnetic resonance angiogram of the renal arteries shows bilateral stenosis near the origins *(arrowheads).* Severe atheromatous disease exists throughout the abdominal aorta and extends into the iliac arteries. Notice filling of the ureters bilaterally, caused by renal excretion of the test dose of Gd-DTPA. *B,* Sagittal, thin-slab projection in the same patient. Focal stenosis is located near the origins of the celiac *(curved arrow)* and superior mesenteric *(arrowhead)* arteries. The patient has symptoms of mesenteric ischemia.

into an antecubital vein. However, there is much variation from patient to patient.

MR angiograms are generally displayed as projections, and these projections may contain information from all or only part of the volume examined. For example, if a volume of tissue 10 cm thick and covering a 40 cm² field of view is acquired, information is potentially available about all the vessels contained in that $40 \times 40 \times 10$ cm³ volume. However, if a full-thickness

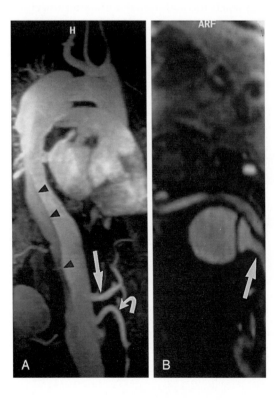

Figure 3–9. *A,* Aortic dissection. Oblique sagittal projection magnetic resonance angiogram shows dissection extending from the thoracic to the abdominal aorta *(arrowheads).* The celiac *(straight arrow)* and superior mesenteric *(curved arrow)* arteries originate from the true lumen. *B,* Transverse reconstruction at the level of the left renal artery *(arrow),* which appears to originate from the false lumen. (Courtesy of Dr. Jochen Gaa, Klinikum Mannheim, Germany.)

projection is collapsed and displayed, some vascular detail may be obscured by vessel overlap. In that case, it may be desirable to collapse only a sub-volume, showing specific vessels of interest in greater detail. One caveat of this type of postprocessing is that some vessels may appear attenuated or absent because they are excluded from the displayed volume.

Magnetic Resonance Angiography Compared With Computed Tomographic Angiography

The technique of contrast-enhanced MRA bears a strong resemblance to CTA, which probably inspired its development. There are, however, several differences between the two techniques. CT images are always acquired in the transverse plane and may be reconstructed into other planes with postprocessing methods. MR angiograms may be acquired in arbitrary planes and reconstructed into other planes; this may be advantageous to optimize specific vascular territories and may increase the useful coverage. The total volume of contrast agent injected is lower with MRI, and Gd-DTPA is not nephrotoxic. MRA and CTA are prone to different artifacts, but both techniques are improved by breath holding. Breath holding is important in examining the chest and abdomen, less crucial for the pelvis, and unnecessary for the extremities. Certain artifacts on MRA depend on the pattern of blood flow, and these can be complex. CTA is relatively independent of the blood flow pattern.

Anatomy of the Aneurysm

In planning the operative procedure it is important to know the extent (ie, suprarenal or iliac) of the aneurysm. Table 3–2 lists the information that can be obtained from current imaging studies. Although these findings can be made intraoperatively, the procedure is aided by prior knowledge.

The length and quality of the aneurysm neck is important in planning placement of the aortic crossclamp and the use of the retroperitoneal or transperitoneal approach. Standard infused CT images can roughly define the length of the aneurysm neck and detect intraluminal thrombus. Depending on the thickness of the transaxial slice, it may be difficult to accurately define the length of the aortic neck. Thin-slice (3-mm) images improve the ability to determine aortic length. In most standard operative repairs, the length of the aorta below the renal arteries can be adjusted by clamping above the renal or

Table 3–2.
Information Obtainable From Imaging Studies

Aortic aneurysm morphology	Nonvascular pathology
Neck: length and diameter	Unsuspected cancer
Body: inflammation, clot, and contained	Renal abnormalities (eg, ectopia, horseshoe
rupture	kidney)
Distal portion: extent, length, and	Venous abnormalities
diameter	
Associated arterial pathology	
Mesenteric or renal artery stenosis	
Abnormal renal arteries	
Associated aneurysms	
Occlusive disease	

celiac vessels. However, when one is using endovascular grafting, it is essential to know precisely the length of the aorta just below the renal vessels.

Spiral CT reconstruction or standard angiography in combination with CT, MRI with MRA, or IVUS is an accurate method for determining the aortic neck length. The length of the aneurysm, which is required only for endovascular grafting, can be accurately determined by IVUS and spiral CT.

Associated Arterial Pathology

The most important argument made for the routine use of arteriography is detection of asymptomatic mesenteric renal artery stenosis, abnormal renal arteries, associated aneurysms, or distal occlusive disease.[12] Gaspar examined this issue in a prospective study of 98 patients.[1] Renal artery stenosis was detected in 13 patients, and 10 patients had accessory renal arteries. Celiac or superior mesenteric artery stenosis was found in three patients, and occlusion of the inferior mesenteric artery was found in 40 patients. For only 3 of 13 patients with renal artery stenosis was the operative repair changed based on the preoperative arteriogram, and for only 2 of 10 with accessory renal arteries were operations similarly modified based on the new findings. Of the newer imaging techniques available, CTA and MRA are able to detect these lesions.[8, 9, 10] Not all asymptomatic stenotic lesions of the renal artery may need repair.

Other Nonarterial Pathology and Abnormalities

In addition to clarifying aortic morphology, these imaging modalities provide information about other vascular and nonvascular intraabdominal structures. Important nonvascular abnormalities that may affect the decision to operate include diverticular disease, certain malignancies, and cholelithiasis. Vascular abnormalities that may have an impact on repair include congenital abnormalities of the vena cava such as left-sided vena cava, venous vessel duplications, retroaortic left renal veins, and venous collars.[13] Prior knowledge of these structures decreases the risk of inadvertent injury.

Conclusions

Abdominal aortic aneurysms can be safely treated using ultrasonography or angiography as the sole preoperative study. However, surgical misadventures, operative duration, and discovery of unexpected abnormalities and disorders can be minimized by selective use of newer imaging modalities. Because of its inability to detect suprarenal extension or associated iliac aneurysms, ultrasonography is used only as a diagnostic screening tool. Preoperative assessment requires clear images of the aneurysm morphology and associated intraabdominal pathology. In the past, we predominantly used standard CT, and arteriography was performed selectively based on the clinical and CT criteria in Table 3–3.

CTA is gradually replacing arteriography in most cases. As MRA technology improves, CT also may be replaced. The ideal test is one that is noninvasive and that provides the surgeon with the arterial anatomy and aneurysm morphology without contrast toxicity. For most patients with normal renal function, the images obtained with three-dimensional spiral reconstruction and CTA are outstanding. Acquisition time and patient discomfort are minimal. MRA with gadolinium enhancement provides excellent images, but the

Table 3–3.
Basis for Selection of Patients for Arteriography

Clinical criteria	Computed tomography criteria

Hypertension
    Two or more medications
Elevated creatinine level
Positive noninvasive blood flow studies
    for aortoiliac or femoropopliteal
    stenosis
Vasculogenic impotence (ankle-brachial
    index <57)
Caval or left renal vein fistulae
	Suprarenal or juxtarenal abdominal aortic
	    aneurysm
	Significant aneurysms of common or internal iliac
	    arteries
	Renal abnormalities
	    Ectopic kidney
	    Horseshoe kidney
	    Partial fusions
	    Lack of nephrogram for normal-size kidney
	Retroperitoneal fibrosis or inflammatory
	    aneurysm

Galt SW, Pearce WH. Preoperative assessment of abdominal aortic aneurysms: noninvasive imaging versus routine arteriography. Semin Vasc Surg 1995;8:103–107.

desire for patient comfort and the presence of metallic implants may limit its usefulness.

References

1. Gaspar MR. Role of arteriography in the evaluation of aortic aneurysms: the case against. *In* Bergan JJ, Yao JST (eds). Aneurysms: Diagnosis and Treatment. New York: Grune & Stratton, 1982:243–254.
2. Galt SW, Pearce WH. Preoperative assessment of abdominal aortic aneurysms: noninvasive imaging versus routine arteriography. Semin Vasc Surg 1995;8:103–107.
3. Papanicolaou N, Wittenberg J, Ferrucci JT Jr, et al. Preoperative evaluation of abdominal aortic aneurysms by computed tomography. AJR 1986;146:711–715.
4. Fox AD, Whiteley MS, Murphy P, et al. Comparison of magnetic resonance imaging measurements of abdominal aortic aneurysms with measurements obtained by other imaging techniques and intraoperative measurements: possible implications for endovascular grafting. J Vasc Surg 1996;24:632–638.
5. Beebe HG. Limitations of conventional imaging methods in planning endovascular stented aortic grafts. Presented at the Twenty-first Annual Symposium of Current Critical Problems in Vascular Surgery; New York, NY, November 15–18, 1994.
6. White RA, Tabbara M, Cavaye D, Kopchok G. Clinical applications of intravascular ultrasound. *In* Yao JST, Pearce WH (eds). Technologies in Vascular Surgery. Philadelphia: WB Saunders, 1992:242–257.
7. Baxter BT, McGee GS, Flinn WR, et al. Distal embolization as a presenting symptom of aortic aneurysms. Am J Surg 1990;160:197–201.
8. Zarins CK, Krievins DK, Rubin GD. Spiral computed tomography and three-dimensional reconstruction in the evaluation of aortic aneurysm. *In* Yao JST, Pearce WH (eds). Progress in Vascular Surgery. Norwalk, CT: Appleton & Lange, 1997:117–128.
9. Galanski M, Prokop M, Chavan A, et al. Renal arterial stenoses: spiral CT angiography. Radiology 1993;189:185–192.
10. Rubin GD, Dake MD, Napel S, et al. Spiral CT of renal artery stenosis: comparison of three-dimensional rendering techniques. Radiology 1994;190:181–189.
11. Kaufman JA, Yucel EK, Waltman AC, et al. MR angiography in the preoperative evaluation of abdominal aortic aneurysms: a preliminary study. J Vasc Interv Radiol 1994;5:489–496.
12. Rich NM, Clagett GP, Salander JM, et al. Role of arteriography in the evaluation of aortic aneurysms. *In* Bergan JJ, Yao JST (eds). Aneurysms: Diagnosis and Treatment. New York: Grune & Stratton, 1982:233–241.
13. Bartle EJ, Pearce WH, Sun JH, et al. Infrarenal venous anomalies and aortic surgery: avoiding vascular injury. J Vasc Surg 1987;6:590–593.

Preoperative Cardiac Evaluation for Aortic Aneurysm Surgery

Gregory J. Landry, M.D., W. Kent Williamson, M.D., Richard A. Yeager, M.D., and John M. Porter, M.D.

The most frequent cause of perioperative morbidity and mortality of patients undergoing abdominal aortic aneurysm (AAA) surgery is coronary artery disease (CAD). The pooled incidence of myocardial infarction (MI) is 6.4%, and the overall fatal MI incidence is 2.2%.[68] Cardiologists and vascular surgeons remain enthusiastic about detecting CAD and prophylactically treating at-risk patients before AAA surgery.[8] The assumption underlying this enthusiasm is that prophylactic treatment of CAD with coronary artery bypass grafting (CABG) or percutaneous transluminal coronary angioplasty (PTCA) can produce significant improvements in morbidity and survival of these patients. We challenge this assumption based on our assessment of a critical lack of data demonstrating any benefit of prophylactic CAD intervention before AAA surgery. In this chapter, we review the available information on preoperative cardiac screening and intervention in patients preparing to undergo AAA repair.

Preoperative Screening Algorithms

In an attempt to identify patients at risk for perioperative myocardial events, several clinical screening systems have been devised. Goldman and colleagues[29] addressed the issue of preoperative screening in a classic article in 1977. Multivariate regression analysis was used to identify factors that significantly correlated with postoperative cardiac death: myocardial infarction in the previous 6 months, a third heart sound or jugular venous distention identified immediately postoperatively, more than five premature ventricular contractions per minute at any time preoperatively, any rhythm other than sinus on the preoperative electrocardiogram, age older than 70 years, significant aortic stenosis, emergency operations, and significant intraoperative hypotension. Others, including Detsky[14] and Eagle,[15] have devised similar clinical scoring systems using the patient's history and screening test results.

Unfortunately, none of these scoring systems appears particularly accurate. Lette and associates[46] reviewed 125 consecutive vascular patients and found that none of the scoring systems reliably predicted major adverse perioperative cardiac outcomes.

A joint commission of the American College of Cardiology and the American Heart Association published guidelines for the preoperative screening of noncardiac surgical patients.[1] The proposed algorithm stratified patients into risk groups based on history and symptoms with the intent of identifying patients who might benefit from coronary revascularization before surgery. Major clinical predictors of perioperative cardiac morbidity included unstable coronary syndromes, such as unstable angina, decompensated congestive heart failure, significant arrhythmias, and severe valvular disease. Mild angina pectoris, prior myocardial infarction, compensated congestive heart failure, and diabetes mellitus were identified as intermediate clinical predictors. Several minor clinical predictors were also identified. After a review of the proposed algorithm and screening tests, the investigators concluded that intervention was rarely necessary to lower the risk of AAA surgery, and patients who ultimately received CABG usually were those who received it on the merits of their cardiac symptoms alone, regardless of future plans for noncardiac surgery.

The registry of the Coronary Artery Surgery Study (CASS) was reviewed by Rihal and coworkers[56] to determine the benefit of CABG before peripheral vascular surgery. Perioperative mortality was lower and long-term survival better for the group of patients who had undergone CABG; however, this study was flawed by obvious selection bias. Those who had undergone CABG had done so at a younger age for severe symptomatic CAD, not for prophylactic revascularization. Because this was not a prospective end point of the study, such analysis constitutes a flagrant example of post hoc analysis (ie, data dredging) and must be rejected.

Screening Tests

Because of a general dissatisfaction with clinical assessment, multiple techniques have been developed to detect patients at risk for perioperative cardiac events. Detecting and quantifying CAD in preoperative AAA patients has proven difficult, especially in patients with diabetes. Silent myocardial ischemia occurs in 2.5% to 10% of middle-aged men with no previous diagnosis, signs, or symptoms of CAD.[9] Resting electrocardiography has notoriously poor predictive value in preoperative assessment, although ischemic changes in the exercising patient that are seen on electrocardiography seem to predict a higher perioperative MI rate.[42] False-positive rates as high as 40% and false-negative rates as high as 15% have been associated with exercise treadmill testing.[23, 26] The positive predictive value from multiple series ranges from 5% to 25%.[31, 36, 43, 50, 65]

Other tests that have been advocated by some surgeons include Holter monitoring, radionuclide ventriculography with dipyridamole-thallium or adenosine-thallium scanning to detect fixed and reperfusion filling defects, ejection fraction determination with radioactive multigated blood pool scanning, and detection of wall motion abnormalities with dobutamine stress echocardiography. Using these tests, it has been estimated that 30% to 50% of patients with vascular disease are at significant risk for perioperative cardiac events; however, fewer than 25% of those identified ever experience adverse cardiac events.[69] As shown by Yeager and others, these tests have a disturbingly low positive predictive value.[68]

Ambulatory electrocardiographic (ECG) monitoring (ie, Holter monitoring) has proven to be an insufficient method of preoperative cardiac screening, in part because of inconsistencies between examiners regarding the length of monitoring (24 or 48 hours) and criteria for an abnormal examination (>1 or >2 mm ST-segment depression). These discrepancies have resulted in reporting a wide range (9% to 39%) of abnormal test results for various series and extremely low positive predictive values (4% to 15%).[38, 49, 51, 54]

Radionuclide ventriculography using pharmacologic vasodilators such as dipyridamole and adenosine is increasingly used for preoperative cardiac evaluation. Unfortunately, this enthusiasm is not supported by data from multiple studies.[4-6, 12, 15, 32, 40, 44, 48, 70] Overall, dipyridamole-thallium scanning identified patients at risk based on redistribution in 33% to 69%. Patients with fixed defects are at significantly lower risk than patients who exhibit redistribution. Most importantly, the positive predictive value is low, ranging from 4% to 20%, which is not significantly better than clinical predictors of risk. L'Italien and colleagues[47] demonstrated no difference in prognostic accuracy between simple clinical markers and dipyridamole-thallium testing, obviating the need for the more expensive testing.

Dobutamine echocardiography relies on pharmacologically increased myocardial oxygen demand to identify patients at cardiac risk based on abnormalities of wall motion, ejection fraction, or both. This relatively new technique has few published studies available to assess its efficacy, and the published studies are difficult to compare because of differences in defining what constitutes a positive or negative test result. Overall, 23% to 50% of patients studied were determined to be at risk.[13, 17, 41, 55] Positive predictive values ranged from 7% to 23%.

Several groups have suggested that preoperative cardiac testing can be limited only to patients with clinical markers for CAD.[6, 16, 59] However, others have shown that a significant subset of patients with advanced CAD but without the clinical markers of CAD are also at risk for adverse events.[12, 40, 45, 49, 54] This controversy indicates to us that surgeons favoring detailed preoperative cardiac evaluation must do so for all patients, not just those with clinical CAD markers. Such extensive cardiac screening programs are extremely expensive, an important consideration in the current environment of health care cost containment.

An additional weakness of preoperative screening tests is demonstrated by evidence that most MIs are caused by cap erosion and thrombosis in plaques that are only moderately stenotic.[21, 24, 25] Larger lesions with greater percentages of stenosis tend to be more highly calcified and stable. Small to medium lesions have a thinner calcified layer overlying soft, lipid-rich, atheromatous debris. These lesions are more prone to plaque disruption and erosion, with resultant ischemic embolization. Because these lesions also tend to be younger than larger, calcified lesions, collateralization of myocardial flow is less developed, thereby increasing the susceptibility of the affected myocardium to ischemic damage.

None of the current methods of cardiac screening is able to accurately identify vulnerable small or medium-sized plaques. This requires visualization of the vessel wall and plaque, rather than merely characterizing the degree of luminal stenosis or identifying areas of underperfused myocardium. In the future, techniques such as intravascular ultrasonography, angioscopy, magnetic resonance imaging, and scintigraphy may hold promise for identifying these lesions, but the current application of these imaging modalities is experimental, and they should not be accepted as routine screening methods.

Coronary Artery Bypass Grafting

Prophylactic CABG before AAA surgery has two goals: to reduce the perioperative morbidity and mortality of the aortic operation and to improve the long-term survival of these patients. A review of the critical data relevant to each of these end points indicates that prophylactic CABG fails on both accounts.

No randomized trial has demonstrated reduced perioperative mortality after vascular surgery preceded by CABG. Our vascular group definitively demonstrated remarkably low perioperative cardiac morbidity and mortality with minimal or no preoperative cardiac workup.[61] Over a 1-year period, 491 patients were prospectively evaluated for perioperative MI based on postoperative cardiac enzyme levels and ECG results. These patients underwent 534 procedures (aortic bypass, 105; carotid endarterectomy, 87; infrainguinal bypass, 207; amputation, 44; extraanatomic bypass, 51; and others, 40). The overall incidence of MI was 3.9%; a rate of 1% was found for asymptomatic MIs detected by screening alone, and a rate of 2.9% was observed for symptomatic MIs. The overall 30-day operative mortality rate was 2.2%. The death rate attributable to MI was 0.7% (Table 4–1). Only 5.8% of patients underwent any type of preoperative cardiac workup other than routine history, physical examination, and ECG. A 0.7% incidence of cardiac death is statistically very close to zero and cannot significantly be improved on with any amount of preoperative intervention.

This position is corroborated by findings from several other studies that have evaluated prophylactic CABG before vascular surgery. Hertzer and colleagues[33] performed 1000 coronary angiograms in patients undergoing vascular procedures, 266 of whom underwent prophylactic CABG. An overall mortality rate of 4.5% (12 patients) was associated with CABG. In contrast, the mortality rate associated with 1066 subsequent vascular procedures was 3.3% (21 patients). Cutler and associates[12] screened 116 patients scheduled to undergo AAA repair with dipyridamole-thallium scanning and referred seven patients (6%) for CABG. One patient died after CABG, and another patient died of a ruptured AAA awaiting CABG. No deaths occurred as a result of AAA repair performed in 106 patients. The overall mortality rate (1.7%) of this series was directly referable to the cardiac screening program. Golden and coworkers[28] screened 240 of 500 patients before performing elective aortic surgery, and of the total, 5.6% (28 patients) underwent prophylactic CABG with no operative deaths. The overall death rate after elective surgery was 1.6% (eight patients). These data are no different from those of the Oregon Health Sciences University (OHSU) experience with minimal preoperative cardiac screening.

Prophylactic CABG in elderly patients is associated with considerable risk. Multiple series examining CABG in the elderly (age >70 years) report

Table 4–1.
Incidence of Myocardial Infarction for Different Operations

Operation Type (n)	Asymptomatic MI	Symptomatic MI	Fatal MI	Total MI
Aortic bypass (105)	1 (1.0%)	3 (2.9%)	1 (1.0%)	5 (4.8%)
Carotid endarterectomy (87)	1 (1.1%)	4 (4.6%)	0	5 (5.7%)
Infraing bypass (207)	2 (1.0%)	3 (1.4%)	2 (1.0%)	7 (3.4%)
Amputation (44)	0	0	0	0
Ax-fem, fem-fem (51)	1 (2.0%)	2 (3.9%)	0	3 (5.9%)
Other* (40)	0	0	1 (2.5%)	1 (2.5%)
Total (534)	5 (1.0%)	12 (2.2%)	4 (0.7%)	21 (3.9%)

MI, myocardial infarction; infraing, infrainguinal; ax-fem, fem-fem, extra-anatomic bypass.
*Includes visceral or renal, multilevel lower extremity, and brachiocephalic operation.
From Taylor LM Jr, Yeager RA, Moneta GL, et al. The incidence of perioperative myocardial infarction in general vascular surgery. J Vasc Surg 1992;15:52–56.

perioperative mortality rates of at least 5% to 10%.[3, 18, 27, 58, 67] Roach and colleagues[57] evaluated adverse cerebral outcomes for patients undergoing CABG and found that a total of 6.1% of patients suffered adverse neurologic sequelae, including stroke, deterioration of intellectual function, coma, seizure, or memory deficit. The anticipated combined perioperative morbidity and mortality from CABG in the elderly exceeds 10%, and in the older groups, it may approach 15%.

The second important end point concerning the impact of preoperative cardiac screening of vascular patients is long-term survival. The best data examining long-term outcomes after CABG come from the Veterans Administration Cooperative Study (VACS),[60, 63, 64] the European Coronary Surgery Study (ECSS),[19, 20, 62] and the Coronary Artery Surgery Study (CASS).[2, 10, 11] These were large, multicenter, randomized trials comparing CABG with medical therapy in patients with symptomatic CAD. Entry criteria included stable angina, angiographic stenosis (50% in VACS and ECSS, 70% in CASS) of one or more major coronary arteries, and an ejection fraction of greater than 25%.

Long-term survival data are available for up to 18 years in the VACS, 12 years in the ECSS, and 10 years in the CASS; however, survival data are incomplete and inconsistent between studies, with 63% follow-up at 18 years in the VACS, 40% and 10% follow-up at 5 and 7 years in the CASS, and 100% and 25% follow-up at 5 and 7 years in the ECSS. The applicability of these data to the general vascular surgery population is also confounded by a number of important factors, including the enrollment of symptomatic patients only, limited female representation, and a minority of patients older than 65 years. In contrast, the vascular surgery patient population is older, has more women, and includes patients without active cardiac symptoms but with advanced arterial disease and multiple medical problems. Statistical analysis in these studies was performed on an intention-to-treat basis, and this was confounded by a very large crossover to surgery, including 38% of the patients in the VACS, 24% in the CASS, and 36% in the ECSS initially assigned to the medical arm.

Even with these limitations, the long-term survival benefit of CABG is in question. With the exception of the ECSS, which showed improved survival at 5 years in the surgery group ($P = 0.0001$), no overall survival benefit was detected for CABG over medical therapy. Subgroup stratification in the VACS and CASS according to degree of ventricular impairment and extent of angiographically demonstrated stenosis did reveal some significant differences. In the VACS trial, surgically treated patients with left main disease (13% of all patients enrolled) exhibited survival benefits at 5 and 7 years ($P = 0.001$), and patients with three-vessel disease and an ejection fraction less than 50% (24% of all patients enrolled) exhibited survival benefits at 5, 7, and 11 years ($P < 0.05$). In the CASS trial, surgically treated patients with ejection fractions less than 50% (20% of all patients enrolled) demonstrated survival benefits at 7 and 10 years compared with the medically treated group ($P < 0.01$). CABG has been shown to benefit only a small number of patients (13% to 24%) in the studies cited, and the actuarial survival benefit at each time interval was modest ($\approx$15%). This finding, along with the previously mentioned differences between the CABG study group patients and the general population of vascular surgery patients, casts a serious doubt on the ability of CABG to prolong life in patients with vasculopathy.

A study by Hertzer and associates[33] claimed to demonstrate a survival benefit for patients undergoing CABG before aortic surgery. CABG was offered to 251 patients with "severe correctable CAD" based on coronary angiograms. Of the 251 patients, 216 underwent CABG, and 35 declined. The 5-year survival rate was 72% for the CABG group and 43% for the control group. Unfortunately, this study is fatally flawed because the groups were not randomized and the control group was small. No valid data indicate that CABG before aortic surgery confers any survival benefit.

Angioplasty

The data supporting PTCA are even less convincing than those for CABG. No randomized trials examining patient survival after PTCA exist. Impressive procedural mortality (0.5% to 1%) and 5-year survival (90% to 95%) rates have been reported for multiple series.[7, 22, 30, 34, 37, 39, 53, 66] However, these patients are in general younger (50 to 60 years old) and have excellent baseline cardiac function (ejection fraction >60%).

The applicability of these data to the general population of vascular surgery patients is suspect. Between 20% and 50% require repeat PTCA, CABG, or both during follow-up. Huber and colleagues[35] reviewed PTCA before noncardiac surgery and reported a postoperative MI rate of 5.4% and mortality rate of 1.9%. These findings suggest PTCA offers no better risk reduction than found in studies in which no preoperative interventions were undertaken. The National Institutes of Health issued a clinical alert[52] suggesting that PTCA should not be the initial coronary therapy for diabetics, an important consideration because 30% to 50% of vascular surgical patients are diabetics.

Conclusions

No reliable evidence has demonstrated decreased perioperative mortality or increased long-term survival for patients undergoing prophylactic CABG or PTCA before AAA repair. Moreover, CABG in elderly vascular patients has significant risks of morbidity and mortality. Nonetheless, unwarranted enthusiasm for extensive preoperative cardiac screening, including CABG and PTCA, persists. In our opinion, vascular surgeons need to critically reevaluate the benefits of these seemingly ineffective and costly interventions. Extensive screening and CABG should be limited only to patients who deserve these procedures on their own merits for the treatment of severe, correctable, symptomatic CAD, without consideration of the need for associated vascular surgery.

References

1. American College of Cardiology and American Heart Association Guidelines Committee. ACC/AHA guidelines for perioperative cardiovascular evaluation for noncardiac surgery. Circulation 1996;93:1280–1317.
2. Alderman EL, Bourassa MG, Cohen LS, et al. Ten-year follow-up of survival and myocardial infarction in the randomized Coronary Artery Surgery Study. Circulation 1990;82:1629–1646.
3. Azariades M, Fessler CL, Floten HS, et al. Five-year results of coronary bypass grafting for patients older than 70 years: role of internal mammary artery. Ann Thorac Surg 1990;50:940–945.
4. Baron JF, Mundler O, Bertrand M, et al. Dipyridamole-thallium scintigraphy and gated radionuclide angiography to assess cardiac risk before abdominal aortic surgery. N Engl J Med 1994;330:663–669.
5. Brown KA, Rowen M. Extent of jeopardized viable myocardium determined by myocardial perfusion imaging best predicts perioperative cardiac events in patients undergoing noncardiac surgery. J Am Coll Cardiol 1993;21:325–330.
6. Bry JD, Belkin M, O'Donnell TF Jr, et al. An assessment of the positive predictive value and cost-effectiveness of dipyridamole myocardial scintigraphy in patients undergoing vascular surgery. J Vasc Surg 1994;19:112–121.
7. Buffet P, Danchin N, Juilliere Y, et al. Percutaneous transluminal coronary angioplasty in patients more than 75 years old: early and long-term results. Int J Cardiol 1992;37:33–39.

8. Bunt TJ. The role of a defined protocol for cardiac risk assessment in decreasing perioperative myocardial infarction in vascular surgery. J Vasc Surg 1992;15:626–634.
9. Cohn PF. Silent myocardial ischemia: dimensions of the problem in patients with and without angina. Am J Med 1986;80:3–8.
10. Coronary Artery Surgery Study Group. Myocardial infarction and mortality in the Coronary Artery Surgery Study (CASS) randomized trial. N Engl J Med 1984;310:750–758.
11. Coronary Artery Surgery Study Group. Coronary Artery Surgery Study (CASS): a randomized trial of coronary artery bypass surgery—survival data. Circulation 1983;68:939–950.
12. Cutler BS, Leppo JA. Dipyridamole-thallium 201 scintigraphy to detect coronary artery disease before abdominal aortic surgery. J Vasc Surg 1987;5:91–100.
13. Davila-Roman VG, Waggoner AD, Sicard GA, et al. Dobutamine stress echocardiography predicts surgical outcome in patients with an aortic aneurysm and peripheral vascular disease. J Am Coll Cardiol 1993;21:957–963.
14. Detsky AS, Abrams HB, Forbath N, et al. Cardiac risk assessment for patients undergoing noncardiac surgery: a multifactorial clinical risk index. Arch Intern Med 1986;146:2131–2134.
15. Eagle KA, Coley CM, Newell JB, et al. Combining clinical and thallium data optimizes preoperative assessment of cardiac risk before major vascular surgery. Ann Intern Med 1989;110:859–866.
16. Eagle KA, Singer DE, Brewster DC, et al. Dipyridamole-thallium scanning in patients undergoing vascular surgery: optimizing preoperative evaluation of cardiac risk. JAMA 1987;257:2185–2189.
17. Eichelberger JP, Schwarz KO, Black ER, et al. Predictive value of dobutamine echocardiography just before non-cardiac vascular surgery. Am J Cardiol 1993;72:602–607.
18. Elayda MA, Hall RJ, Gray AG, et al. Coronary revascularization in the elderly patient. J Am Coll Cardiol 1984;3:1398–1402.
19. European Coronary Surgery Group. Prospective randomized study of coronary artery bypass surgery in stable angina pectoris. Lancet 1980;2:491–495.
20. European Coronary Study Group. Prospective randomized study of coronary artery bypass surgery in stable angina pectoris: a progress report on survival. Circulation 1982;65(pt 2):67–71.
21. Falk E, Sha PK, Fuster V. Coronary plaque disruption. Circulation 1995;92:657–671.
22. Faxon DP, Ruocco N, Jacobs AK. Long-term outcome of patients after percutaneous transluminal coronary angioplasty. Circulation 1990;81(suppl IV):IV9–13.
23. Foster ED, Davis KB, Carpenter JA, et al. Risk of noncardiac operation in patients with defined coronary disease: the Coronary Artery Surgery Study (CASS) registry experience. Ann Thorac Surg 1986;419:42–50.
24. Fuster V. Elucidation of the role of plaque instability and rupture in acute coronary events. Am J Cardiol 1995;76:24C–33C.
25. Fuster V, Badimon L, Badimon JJ, et al. The pathogenesis of coronary artery disease and the acute coronary syndromes. N Engl J Med 1992;326:242–250.
26. Gage AA, Bhayana JN, Balu V, et al. Assessment of cardiac risk in surgical patient. Arch Surg 1977;112:1488–1492.
27. Gardner TJ, Greene PS, Rykiel MF, et al. Routine use of the left internal mammary artery graft in the elderly. Ann Thorac Surg 1990;49:188–194.
28. Golden MA, Whittemore AD, Donaldson MC, et al. Selective evaluation and management of coronary artery disease in patients undergoing repair of abdominal aortic aneurysms. Ann Surg 1990;212:415–423.
29. Goldman L, Caldera DL, Nussbaum SR, et al. Multifactorial index of cardiac risk in noncardiac surgical procedures. N Engl J Med 1977;297:845–850.
30. Gruentzig AR, King SB 3d, Schlumpf M, et al. Long-term follow-up after percutaneous transluminal coronary angioplasty: the early Zurich experience. N Engl J Med 1987;316:1127–1132.
31. Hanson P, Pease M, Berkoff H, et al. Arm exercise testing for coronary artery disease in patients with peripheral vascular disease. Clin Cardiol 1988;11:70–74.
32. Hendel RC, Whitfield SS, Villegas BJ, et al. Prediction of late cardiac events by dipyridamole thallium imaging in patients undergoing elective vascular surgery. Am J Cardiol 1992;70:1243–1249.
33. Hertzer NR, Beven EG, Young JR, et al. Coronary artery disease in peripheral vascular patients: a classification of 1000 coronary angiograms and results of surgical management. Ann Surg 1984;199:223–233.
34. Hollman J, Simpfendorfer C, Franco I, et al. Multivessel and single-vessel coronary angioplasty: a comparative study. Am Heart J 1992;124:9–12.
35. Huber KC, Evans MA, Breshnahan JF, et al. Outcome of noncardiac operations in patients with severe coronary artery disease successfully treated preoperatively with coronary angioplasty. Mayo Clin Proc 1992;67:15–21.
36. Kaaja R, Sell H, Erkola O, et al. Predictive value of manual ECG-monitored exercise test before abdominal aortic or peripheral vascular surgery. Angiology 1993;44:11–15.
37. Kadel C, Vallbracht C, Buss F, et al. Long-term follow-up after percutaneous transluminal coronary angioplasty in patients with single-vessel disease. Am Heart J 1992;124:1159–1169.
38. Kirwin JD, Ascer E, Gennaro M, et al. Silent myocardial ischemia is not predictive of myocardial infarction in peripheral vascular surgery patients. Ann Vasc Surg 1993;7:27–32.
39. Kramer JR, Proudfit WL, Loop FD, et al. Late follow-up of 781 patients undergoing percutaneous transluminal coronary angioplasty or coronary artery bypass grafting for an isolated obstruction in the left anterior descending coronary artery. Am Heart J 1989;118:1144–1153.

40. Kresowik TF, Bower TR, Garner SA, et al. Dipyridamole thallium imaging in patients being considered for vascular procedures. Arch Surg 1993;128:299–302.
41. Lalka SG, Sawada SG, Dalsing MC, et al. Dobutamine stress echocardiography as a predictor of cardiac events associated with aortic surgery. J Vasc Surg 1992;15:831–840.
42. Leppo JA. Preoperative cardiac risk assessment for noncardiac surgery. Am J Cardiol 1995;75:42D–51D.
43. Leppo J, Plaja J, Gionet M, et al. Noninvasive evaluation of cardiac risk before elective vascular surgery. J Am Coll Cardiol 1987;9:269–276.
44. Lette J, Waters D, Cerino M, et al. Preoperative coronary artery disease risk stratification based on dipyridamole imaging and a simple three-step, three-segment model for patients undergoing noncardiac vascular surgery or major general surgery. Am J Cardiol 1992;69:1553–1558.
45. Lette J, Waters D, Lassonde J, et al. Postoperative myocardial infarction and cardiac death: predictive value of dipyridamole-thallium imaging and five clinical scoring systems based on multifactorial analysis. Ann Surg 1990;211:84–90.
46. Lette J, Waters D, Lassonde J, et al. Multivariate clinical models and quantitative dipyridamole-thallium imaging to predict cardiac morbidity and death after vascular reconstruction. J Vasc Surg 1991;14:160–169.
47. L'Italien GJ, Paul SD, Hendel RC, et al. Development and validation of a Bayesian model for perioperative cardiac risk assessment in a cohort of 1,081 vascular surgical candidates. J Am Coll Cardiol 1996;27:779–786.
48. Madsen PV, Vissing M, Munck O, et al. A comparison of dipyridamole thallium 201 scintigraphy and clinical examination in the determination of cardiac risk before arterial reconstruction. Angiology 1992;43:306–311.
49. Mangano DT, Browner WS, Hollenberg M, et al. Association of perioperative myocardial ischemia with cardiac morbidity and mortality in men undergoing noncardiac surgery: the Study of the Perioperative Ischemia Study Group. N Engl J Med 1990;323:1781–1788.
50. McPhail N, Calvin JE, Shariatmadar A, et al. The use of preoperative exercise testing to predict cardiac complications after arterial reconstruction. J Vasc Surg 1988;7:60–68.
51. McPhail NV, Ruddy TD, Barber GG, et al. Cardiac risk stratification using dipyridamole myocardial perfusion imaging and ambulatory ECG monitoring before vascular surgery. Eur J Vasc Surg 1993;7:151–156.
52. National Heart, Lung, and Blood Institute. Bypass over angioplasty for patients with diabetes. Bethesda: National Institutes of Health Clinical Alert; September 21, 1995.
53. O'Keefe JH Jr, Rutherford BD, McConahay DR, et al. Multivessel coronary angioplasty from 1980 to 1989: procedural results and long-term outcome. J Am Coll Cardiol 1990;16:1097–1102.
54. Pasternack PF, Grossi EA, Baumann FG, et al. The value of silent myocardial ischemia monitoring in the prediction of perioperative myocardial infarction in patients undergoing peripheral vascular surgery. J Vasc Surg 1989;10:617–625.
55. Poldermans D, Fioretti PM, Forster T, et al. Dobutamine stress echocardiography for assessment of perioperative cardiac risk in patients undergoing major vascular surgery. Circulation 1993;7:1506–1512.
56. Rihal CS, Eagle KA, Mickel MC, et al. Surgical therapy for coronary artery disease among patients with combined coronary artery and peripheral vascular disease. Circulation 1995;91:46–53.
57. Roach GW, Kanchuger M, Mangano CM, et al. Adverse cerebral outcomes after coronary bypass surgery: multicenter study of Perioperative Ischemia Research Group and the Ischemia Research and Education Foundation Investigators. N Engl J Med 1996;335:1857–1863.
58. Rose DM, Gelbfish J, Jacobowitz IJ, et al. Analysis of morbidity and mortality in patients 70 years of age and over undergoing isolated coronary artery bypass surgery. Am Heart J 1985;110:341–346.
59. Shaw L, Miller DD, Kong BA, et al. Determination of perioperative cardiac risk by adenosine thallium-201 myocardial imaging. Am Heart J 1992;124:861–869.
60. Takaro T, Hultgren HN, Detre KM, et al. The Veterans Administration Cooperative Study of stable angina: current status. Circulation 1982;65(pt 2):60–67.
61. Taylor LM Jr, Yeager RA, Moneta GL, et al. The incidence of perioperative myocardial infarction in general vascular surgery. J Vasc Surg 1992;15:52–61.
62. Varnauskas E and the European Coronary Surgery Study Group. Twelve-year follow-up of survival in the randomized European Coronary Surgery Study Group. N Engl J Med 1988;319:332–337.
63. The Veterans Administration Coronary Artery Bypass Surgery Cooperative Study Group. Eleven-year survival in the Veterans Administration randomized trial of coronary artery bypass surgery for stable angina. N Engl J Med 1984;311:1333–1339.
64. The Veterans Administration Coronary Artery Cooperative Study Group. Eighteen-year follow-up in the Veterans Affairs Cooperative Study of Coronary Artery Bypass Surgery for stable angina. Circulation 1992;86:121–130.
65. Von Knorring J, Lepantalo M. Prediction of perioperative cardiac complications by electrocardiographic monitoring during treadmill exercise testing before peripheral vascular surgery. Surgery 1986;99:610–613.
66. Warner MF, DiSciascio G, Kohli RS, et al. Long-term efficacy of triple-vessel angioplasty in patients with severe three-vessel coronary artery disease. Am Heart J 1992;124:1169–1174.
67. Weintraub WS, Craver JM, Cohen CL, et al. Influence of age on results of coronary artery surgery. Circulation 1991;84(suppl III):III226–235.
68. Yeager RA. Cardiac testing and cardiac risk associated with vascular surgery. *In* Porter JM, Taylor

LM Jr (eds). Basic Data Underlying Clinical Decision Making in Vascular Surgery, ed 1. St. Louis: Quality Medical Publishing, 1994:5–9.

69. Yeager RA, Weigel RM, Murphy ES, et al. Application of clinically valid cardiac risk factors to aortic aneurysm surgery. Arch Surg 1986;121:278–281.

70. Younis LT, Aguirre F, Byers S, et al. Perioperative and long-term prognostic value of intravenous dipyridamole thallium scintigraphy in patients with peripheral vascular disease. Am Heart J 1990;119:1287–1292.

Preoperative Pulmonary Evaluation for Aortic Aneurysm Surgery

Ignacio Rua, M.D., Keith D. Calligaro, M.D.,
Rahul Dandora, M.D., Matthew J. Dougherty, M.D.,
Carol A. Raviola, M.D., and
Dominic A. DeLaurentis, M.D.

Evaluation of a patient for an elective abdominal aortic aneurysm repair involves many factors. Because of well-documented diffuse atherosclerotic disease in these patients, cardiac evaluation has been considered of primary importance, and much attention has been focused on identifying cardiac risk factors before aortic surgery. Often overlooked is evaluation of a patient's pulmonary status. The reported incidence of major pulmonary complications after elective abdominal aortic surgery ranges from 5% to 29%.[2, 5, 17, 19] Predicting pulmonary risk factors for patients undergoing elective abdominal aortic surgery may help minimize the morbidity and mortality associated with these operations.

Anesthesia

Anesthetic techniques can affect pulmonary complications.[20] Successful aortic surgery requires a cooperative effort between the vascular surgeon and anesthesiologist. The surgeon should inform the anesthesiologist before aortic clamping and unclamping to allow optimal fluid loading and unloading to be accomplished. The vascular surgeon must understand the physiologic consequences of different anesthetic techniques.

General Anesthesia

The agents typically used for general anesthesia are classified as inhalational anesthetics, intravenous anesthetics, and neuromuscular blocking agents (Table 5–1). Various agents have different potencies, and to allow comparison between agents, the term *minimum alveolar concentration* (MAC) is used. One MAC is the alveolar concentration at which 50% of patients do not move with a surgical incision.[15] Because the MAC of various agents is additive,[16] using lower doses of different agents together can minimize the side effects of each particular agent.

Nitrous oxide (N_2O) is often used as part of the anesthesia strategy. It has strong analgesic properties, provides some amnesia (ie, unconsciousness), and has little cardiorespiratory depressant effect. Unfortunately, it has a low potency, with a MAC of 104%. N_2O usually is used in combination to lower the dose of other agents that may have adverse effects.

Table 5–1.
Commonly Used Anesthetic Agents

Inhalational Agents	Intravenous Agents	Neuromuscular Blocking Agents
Nitrous oxide	Narcotics	Succinylcholine
Halogenated agents	Barbiturates	
Halothane	Benzodiazepines	
Enflurane		
Isoflurane		

All halogenated or volatile agents provide analgesia, amnesia, and some muscle relaxation. They are potent, with MAC values between 0.75% and 1.7%. They are commonly used in concentrations of 0.5% to 2.0% together with 50% to 70% N_2O.

All three of the volatile agents are significant respiratory depressants. The arterial partial pressure of carbon dioxide (P_{CO_2}) increases with increasing concentrations of the agents. The agents depress the response to hypercarbia to different degrees (halothane < isoflurane < enflurane).[25]

All inhaled anesthetics, including N_2O, reduce the ventilatory response to hypoxemia. This effect is observed even at low concentrations of the agents.

Many patients who undergo aortic reconstructions have chronic obstructive pulmonary disease (COPD). These patients are more sensitive to the ventilatory depressant effect of inhalational anesthetics. This risk continues into the postoperative period, because the hypoxic drive is depressed even at low concentrations of the volatile agents. In the postoperative period, these low concentrations often exist, especially after long anesthetic times, because a portion of the agent is stored in muscle and fat and is slowly eliminated through the lungs. The volatile agents undergo little metabolism in the body.

Narcotics have excellent analgesic properties but provide less amnesia. They are frequently used with a volatile agent and N_2O. They demonstrate a well-known dose-dependent ventilatory depression.

The barbiturates produce amnesia, but no analgesia or muscle relaxation. The ultrashort-acting thiopental, for example, has a rapid onset and short duration of action. Barbiturates commonly are used for induction of anesthesia.

Benzodiazepines produce amnesia but no analgesia or muscle relaxation. They typically are used in combination with intravenous narcotics. Other intravenous agents such as ketamine, etomidate, and propofol have rapid onsets and short durations of action. All three produce amnesia and primarily are used for induction of anesthesia. Propofol administered as a continuous infusion has been used for procedures of short duration.

More important than the particular agents used are the postoperative effects of general anesthesia. Figure 5–1 shows the pathophysiologic mechanisms leading to postoperative pulmonary complications after abdominal surgery. The loss of diaphragm tone is thought to promote atelectasis.[8] General anesthesia also increases the alveolar-arterial oxygen tension gradient, in part because of the shunting that occurs under general anesthesia. This effect is of little consequence to healthy individuals, but patients who are obese or elderly and those with COPD have a greater risk of shunt development.[12]

Another well-known adverse effect of general anesthesia is depression of mucociliary transport. This adverse effect has been observed for 2 to 6 days

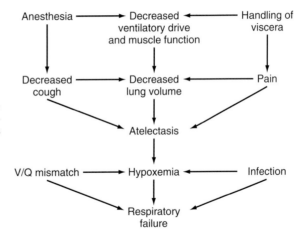

Figure 5-1. Pathophysiologic mechanisms leading to postoperative pulmonary complications after abdominal surgery.

after anesthesia and has been implicated in causing postoperative pulmonary complications.[13]

Regional Anesthesia

Epidural anesthetics may reduce the pulmonary complication rate for patients undergoing abdominal aortic surgery.[1, 3] Epidural analgesia theoretically decreases postoperative pain more effectively and potentially allows better respiratory dynamics. However, we and others have not documented a clear benefit of epidural analgesia in this regard, although we continue to use this adjunct routinely.[2, 20]

Preoperative Factors Predicting Pulmonary Complications

The American Society of Anesthesiologists (ASA) developed a classification system that quantified the physical status of a patient to examine anesthetic morbidity and mortality (Table 5–2).[6] In our review of 181 consecutive patients who underwent abdominal aortic surgery, the ASA class was shown to be the most statistically significant factor associated with major pulmonary complications.[2] This is not surprising considering some of the variables, such as hypertension, obesity, age, diabetes mellitus, and COPD, that are included in the ASA classification. These factors are thought to increase the risk of postoperative pulmonary problems. In a prospective study by Latimer and colleagues,[10] obesity, defined by a weight 10% above the Metropolitan Life Insurance Tables, was the most important risk factor associated with clinically significant atelectasis after upper abdominal surgery and occurred in 53% of his patients. Our study confirmed the importance of weight for patients undergoing aortic surgery.[2] We also documented that advancing age (especially >70 years) significantly increased the rate of major respiratory complications.[2] Other investigators have not confirmed this relationship.[11,21]

Tobacco use was variably linked to the risk of postoperative pulmonary complications. Warner and associates[23] performed a large, retrospective study of patients undergoing coronary artery bypass. The risk for postoperative pulmonary complications statistically decreased for patients who had quit smoking at least 8 weeks before surgery. However, we were unable to confirm

Table 5–2.
American Society of Anesthesiologists Classification of Physical Status

Class 1: The patient has no organic, physiologic, biochemical, or psychiatric disturbance. The pathologic process for which the operation is to be performed is localized and does not entail a systemic disturbance. Examples: a fit patient with inguinal hernia, fibroid uterus in an otherwise healthy woman.

Class 2: Mild to moderate systemic disturbance caused by the condition to be treated surgically or caused by other pathophysiologic processes. Examples: nonlimiting or only slightly limiting organic heart disease, mild diabetes, essential hypertension, anemia. Some may include the extremes of age, the neonate or octogenarian, even though no discernible systemic disease is present. Extreme obesity and chronic bronchitis may be included in this category.

Class 3: Severe systemic disturbance or disease from whatever cause, even though it may not be possible to define the degree of disability with finality. Examples: severely limiting organic heart disease, severe diabetes with vascular complications, moderate to severe degrees of pulmonary insufficiency, angina pectoris, or healed myocardial infarction.

Class 4: Indicative of the patient with severe systemic disorders that are already life threatening and not always correctable by operation. Examples: organic heart disease with marked signs of cardiac insufficiency, persistent anginal syndrome, or active myocarditis; advanced degrees of pulmonary, hepatic, renal, or endocrine insufficiency.

Class 5: The moribund patient who has little chance of survival but undergoes an operation in desperation. Examples: burst abdominal aneurysm with profound shock, major cerebral trauma with rapidly increasing intracranial pressure, massive pulmonary embolus. Most of these patients require operation as a resuscitative measure with little if any anesthesia.

Emergency Operation: Any patient in one of the classes listed previously who is operated on in an emergency is considered to be in poorer physical condition. The letter E is placed beside the numeric classification. The patient with hitherto uncomplicated hernia that becomes incarcerated and associated with nausea and vomiting is classified IE.

that current smoking or a history of smoking predicted major pulmonary complications in our retrospective analysis.[2]

We and others found that a prolonged operative time (>3.5 to 5.0 hours) was associated with increased pulmonary complications.[2, 10] Prolonged operative times, aortic clamp times, and ischemia of the lower extremities may be related to pulmonary complications.

Reperfusion of the lower extremities after prolonged aortic clamping may lead to a pulmonary capillary defect. This mechanism may be mediated by inflammatory agents such as cytokines, complement, mast cells, and leukotrienes that become activated during aortic surgery.[7, 14]

The role of preoperative pulmonary function tests in identifying high-risk patients is controversial. Many of the studies performed were retrospective, and the definition of a pulmonary complication varied among studies. In our review of patients undergoing aortic surgery, we documented that forced vital capacity (FVC) of less than 80% and forced expiratory flow between 25 and 75 mL of FVC (FEF_{25-75}) of less than 60% were associated with major pulmonary complications.[2] No prospective study of comparable groups of patients has shown that pulmonary function tests can reliably detect abdominal surgery patients at increased risk for pulmonary complications. Many clinicians think pulmonary function tests should be recommended only for patients who smoke heavily or have respiratory complaints that have not been previously evaluated.[26]

Evaluation for Pulmonary Thromboembolic Disease

Preoperative screening for the potential risk of pulmonary emboli in patients undergoing aortic reconstructions is part of the complete pulmonary evaluation. Because deep venous thromboses (DVTs) are the precursors of most clinically significant emboli, patients should be evaluated for DVTs. Anesthesia time longer than 30 minutes is a risk factor for patients undergoing a major surgical procedure. Risk factors are cumulative in their effect, and patients with deep venous thrombosis usually have more than one factor.[14, 24] Other risks are advanced age, cancer, sepsis, obesity, and the use of estrogen-containing medications. Deficiencies of antithrombin III, protein S, and protein C can also increase the risk of DVTs (Table 5–3).

To avoid these complications, intermittent pneumatic compression of the calves should be started before the induction of anesthesia and continued into the postoperative period until the patient has regained mobility. Encouragement of early mobilization cannot be overemphasized. Mobilization helps prevent DVTs and reduce atelectasis.

If a venous thrombosis in the iliac, femoral, or popliteal veins is diagnosed in the immediate postoperative period (<7 days), the safest course of action is insertion of a caval interruption device. Full anticoagulation involves a significant risk of hemorrhage with aortic reconstruction.

Perioperative Respiratory Care

As for any surgical patient, the preoperative pulmonary evaluation for aortic surgery begins with a thorough history and physical examination, the findings of which should alert the physician about clinical or subclinical lung disease. Smokers or overweight patients should be counseled, because these two pulmonary risk factors are potentially reversible. However, we have found that admonitions to stop smoking and lose weight are largely unheeded.

If the clinical history reveals COPD or asthma and these conditions have not been fully evaluated, pulmonary function tests are indicated. Patients with COPD benefit from a course of preoperative antibiotics. Chest physical therapy and postural drainage may help patients to mobilize secretions, and

Table 5–3.
Classification of the Risk of Postoperative DVT/PE

Risk Categories	Calf DVT (%)	Prox. DVT (%)	PE (%)

I. High risk
  A. Age >40 y
  B. Surgery >30 min
    1. Orthopedic surgery
    2. Pelvic or abdominal cancer surgery
  C. Previous DVT or PE
  D. Secondary risk factors*
  E. Hereditary or acquired
    coagulopathies†
	40–80	10–20	1–5

II. Moderate risk
  A. Age >40 y
  B. Surgery >30 min
  C. Secondary risk factors*
	10–40	2–10	0.1–7

III. Low risk
  A. Age < or > 40 y
  B. Minor surgery (<30 min)
  C. No secondary risk factors
	<10	<1	<0.01

DVT, deep vein thrombosis; PE, pulmonary embolism; Prox., proximal.
*Obesity, immobilization, malignancy, varicose veins, estrogen use, and paralysis.
†Protein C, protein S, antithrombin III, anticardiolipin antibodies.

deep breathing exercises are taught in the preoperative period. Patients are counseled on how to inhale and maximally expand their rib cage. Deep breathing exercises are effective in recruiting the diaphragm.[4] Patients with asthma may benefit from the use of bronchodilators and antiinflammatory agents. COPD and asthma often necessitate treatment before, during, and after surgery.

Stein and Cassara[18] illustrated the benefits of the described modalities. Fifteen (60%) of 25 patients in a control group who did not receive preoperative treatment developed postoperative pulmonary complications. In contrast, of 23 patients who were treated as described, only 5 (21%) had pulmonary complications. Thorens[22] studied 392 patients who underwent gallbladder surgery and divided them into three groups. One group did not receive physiotherapy and served as the control; one group received deep breathing exercises, assisted cough, and postural drainage postoperatively only; and the third group received this treatment preoperatively and postoperatively. The incidence of postoperative pulmonary complications was highest for the untreated control group (47%), intermediate for the group treated only after surgery (27%), and lowest for the group in which therapy was begun before surgery and continued postoperatively (12%).

Conclusions

Preoperative pulmonary evaluation is important in deciding which patients can safely undergo major abdominal aortic reconstruction. In our experience, the ASA classification has been an important preoperative predictive factor for postoperative pulmonary complications, along with age older than 70 years, body weight greater than 150% of ideal, FVC less than 80%, FEF less than 60%, crystalloid replacement of more than 6 L, and operative time longer than 5 hours.[2] When the preoperative evaluation reveals reversible risk factors such as smoking or obesity, patients should be counseled to stop smoking or lose weight. Existing conditions such as COPD and asthma should be medically optimized before, during, and after surgery.

All patients scheduled for major aortic reconstruction should undergo preoperative coaching, including instructed deep breathing exercises. As soon as possible after surgery, the patient should be encouraged to ambulate, breath deeply, and cough. An intensive and aggressive physiotherapy regimen can help reduce postoperative pulmonary complications, even in higher-risk patients.

References

1. Baron JF, Bertrand M, Barre E, et al. Combined epidural and general anesthesia versus general anesthesia for abdominal aortic surgery. Anesthesiology 1991;75:611–618.
2. Calligaro KD, Azurin DJ, Dougherty MJ, et al. Pulmonary risk factors of elective abdominal aortic surgery. J Vasc Surg 1993;18:914–921.
3. Cambria RP, Brewster DC, Abbott WM, et al. Transperitoneal versus retroperitoneal approach for aortic reconstruction: a randomized prospective study. J Vasc Surg 1990;11:314–325.
4. Celli BR. Perioperative respiratory care of the patient undergoing upper abdominal surgery. Clin Chest Med 1993;14:253–261.
5. Diehl JT, Cali RF, Hertzer NR, Beven EG. Complications of abdominal aortic reconstruction: an analysis of perioperative risk factors in 557 patients. Ann Surg 1982;197:49–56.
6. Dripps RD. Physical status and risk. *In* Dripps RD, Eckenhoff JF, Vandam LD (eds). Introduction to Anesthesia: the Principles of Safe Practice. Philadelphia: WB Saunders, 1977:13–15.
7. Goldman G, Welbourn R, Klausner JM, et al. Mast cells and leukotrienes mediate neutrophil sequestration and lung edema after remote ischemia in rodents. Surgery 1992;112:578–586.

8. Hedenstierna G. New aspects on atelectasis formation and gas exchange impairment during anesthesia. Clin Physiol 1989;9:407–417.
9. Hull R, Raskob G, Hirsh J. Prophylaxis of venous thromboembolism: an overview. Chest 1986;85:379–383.
10. Latimer RG, Dickman M, Day WC, et al. Ventilatory patterns and pulmonary complications after upper abdominal surgery determined by preoperative and postoperative computerized spirometry and blood gas analysis. Am J Surg 1971;122:622–32.
11. Mitchell C, Garrahy P, Peake P. Postoperative respiratory morbidity: identification and risk factors. Aust N Z J Surg 1982;52:203–209.
12. Nunn JF. Respiratory effects of anesthesia. *In* Applied Respirator Physiology, ed 3. London: Butterworth, 1987:350–378.
13. Pizov R, Takahashi M, et al. Halothane inhibition of ion transport of tracheal epithelium. Anesthesiology 1992;76:985–989.
14. Rodriguez JL. Hospital-acquired gram-negative pneumonia in critically ill, injured patients. Am J Surg 1993;165(suppl IIA):34S–42S.
15. Saidman LJ, Eger EI II. Effects of nitrous oxide and narcotic premedication on the alveolar concentration of halothane required for anesthesia. Anesthesiology 1964;25:302–306.
16. Saidman LJ, Wahrenbrock EA, Schroeder CF, et al. Ethylene-halothane anesthesia: addition or synergism? Anesthesiology 1969;21:301–304.
17. Smith PK, Fuchs JCA, Sabiston DC. Surgical management of aortic abdominal aneurysms in patients with severe pulmonary insufficiency. Surg Gynecol Obstet 1980;151:407–411.
18. Stein M, Cassara EL. Preoperative pulmonary evaluation and therapy for surgery patients. JAMA 1970;211:787–790.
19. Svensson LG, Hess KR, Coselli JS, et al. A prospective study of respiratory failure after high-risk surgery on the thoraco-abdominal aorta. J Vasc Surg 1991;14:271–282.
20. Sykes LA, Bowe EA. Cardiorespiratory effects of anesthesia. Clin Chest Med 1993;June:211–226.
21. Tarhan S, Mofitt EA, Sessler AD, et al. Risk of anesthesia and surgery in patients with chronic bronchitis and chronic obstructive pulmonary disease. Surgery 1973;4:720–726.
22. Thorens L. Postoperative pulmonary complications: observations on their prevention by means of physiotherapy. Acta Chir Scand 1954;107:194–205.
23. Warner MA, Divertie MB, Tinker JH. Preoperative cessation of smoking and pulmonary complications in coronary artery bypass patients. Anesthesiology 1984;60:380–383.
24. Wheeler HB, Anderson FH, Cardullo PA, et al. Suspected deep vein thrombosis: management by impedance plethysmography. Arch Surg 1986;117:1206–1209.
25. Wren WS, Allen P, Synnott A, et al. Effects of halothane, isoflurane, and enflurane on ventilation in children. Br J Anaesth 1987;59:399–409.
26. Zibak JD, O'Donnell CR. Indications for preoperative pulmonary function testing. Clin Chest Med 1993;June:227–236.

Thoracoabdominal Aortic Aneurysms and Aortic Stented Grafts

Optimal Repair Methods for Thoracoabdominal Aortic Aneurysms: Spinal Drainage, Bypass, and Intraoperative Drugs

Ian N. Hamilton, Jr., M.D., and Larry H. Hollier, M.D.

Thoracoabdominal aortic aneurysm (TAAA) repair continues to be a formidable procedure associated with complication rates exceeded by few other surgical procedures despite significant improvements since the first successful TAAA repair in 1955.[23] Advancements in risk assessment, diagnostic capabilities, anesthetic support, and surgical techniques have provided the foundation for improvements in perioperative morbidity and mortality rates associated with TAAA repair. However, intraoperative and 30-day mortality rates remain as high as 5% and 10%, respectively, in collected series.[62] Incorporation of a multimodality approach to the prevention of perioperative complications can provide the mechanism for even further reductions in morbidity and mortality rates. Our multimodality approach to TAAA repair includes spinal fluid drainage, distal aortic perfusion, and administration of intraoperative medications.

Etiology and Classification of Disease

Atherosclerotic medial degenerative disease (82%) and aortic dissection (17%) account for 99% of all reported cases of TAAA.[62] Nondissecting (eg, degenerative, Marfan's, Ehlers-Danlos, mycotic, Takayasu's) and dissecting TAAAs are associated with risk factors that significantly influence a patient's treatment and long-term survival. Nondissecting and dissecting TAAAs are associated with a high incidence of hypertension. However, degenerative aneurysms are associated with a higher incidence of coronary artery disease, chronic renal insufficiency, cerebrovascular disease, and peripheral vascular disease than dissecting aneurysms (Table 6–1).

In addition to cause, aneurysms of the thoracoabdominal aorta may be classified by the extent of aortic involvement. Type I aneurysms involve all or most of the descending thoracic aorta and the upper abdominal aorta but do not involve the aorta below the level of the renal arteries. Type II aneurysms involve all or most of the descending thoracic aorta and all or most of the abdominal aorta. Type III aneurysms involve the distal one half or less of the descending thoracic aorta and various segments of the abdominal aorta. Type IV aneurysms involve all or most of the abdominal aorta, including the

The authors thank Mr. James Green for the original artwork appearing in this chapter.

Table 6–1.
Incidence of Risk Factors Associated With Thoracoabdominal Aortic Aneurysms

Risk Factor	Median Nondissecting TAAA (%)*	Average Dissecting TAAA (%)
Smoking	80	
Hypertension	70	83
Coronary artery disease	35	19
Chronic obstructive pulmonary disease	35	25
Visceral occlusive disease	25	
Chronic renal failure	20	9
Marfan's syndrome		6
Congestive heart failure		5
Cerebrovascular disease	15	
Stroke		4
Peripheral vascular disease	15	
Diabetes mellitus	5	3

*Median data has been used because of the wide variance in reporting nondissecting thoracoabdominal aortic aneurysms (TAAA) data.
Adapted from Panneton JM, Hollier LH. Nondissecting thoracoabdominal aortic aneurysms: part I. Ann Vasc Surg 1995;9:503–514 and from Panneton JM, Hollier LH. Dissecting descending thoracic and thoracoabdominal aortic aneurysms: part II. Ann Vasc Surg 1995;9:596–605.

segment from which the visceral vessels arise.[16] This classification proposed by Crawford[16] applies to aortic aneurysms of all etiologies (Fig. 6–1). The Crawford Classification of TAAA has allowed evaluation and comparison of the specific treatment modalities incorporated in TAAA repair.

Aortic dissection, whether responsible for aortic aneurysmal development or not, has also been classified by the extent of aortic involvement. The original classification system was that proposed by DeBakey and coworkers.[21] Subsequent classification systems of aortic dissection have included the Najafi,[53] University of Alabama,[1] Massachusetts General Hospital,[22] and Stanford

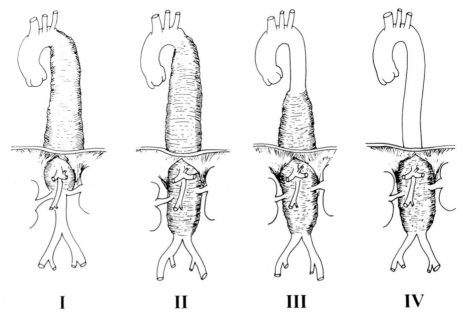

I   **II**   **III**   **IV**

Figure 6–1. Crawford classification of thoracoabdominal aortic aneurysms, types I through IV. (From Hamilton IN, Hollier LH. Thoracoabdominal aortic aneurysms. *In* Moore W (ed). Vascular Surgery: a Comprehensive Review. Philadelphia: WB Saunders 1998:417–434.)

systems[19] (Fig. 6–2). The Stanford type A designates an aortic dissection that involves the ascending aorta. The Stanford type B aortic dissection is used to classify dissections in which the ascending aorta is not involved. Ascending aortic dissections (Stanford type A) may be associated with complications (eg, cardiac tamponade, acute aortic insufficiency, coronary artery dissection, coronary artery occlusion) that require cardiac surgical procedures (eg, aortic arch replacement, ascending aorta replacement, aortic valve replacement or suspension, coronary artery reimplantation), which are beyond the scope of this chapter.

Although aortic dissection may require intervention or surgical treatment for reasons other than aneurysmal degeneration, we have limited our discussion of aortic dissection to those that are aneurysmal and involve the descending thoracic aorta, abdominal aorta, or both, qualifying as Crawford TAAA types I through IV, all of which fall within the realm and responsibility of the vascular surgeon.

Diagnostic Methods

Chest roentgenography, angiography, computed tomography (CT), magnetic resonance imaging (MRI), and transesophageal echocardiography (TEE) may be used alone or in combination to establish the diagnosis of TAAA.

Chest roentgenogram readings associated with TAAA may include aortic tortuosity, aortic dilation, mediastinal widening, pleural effusion, or pleural hematoma (Fig. 6–3). Chest roentgenograms alone are insufficient for operative planning and must be coupled with additional studies.

Aortography remains the single best study for the evaluation of aortic branch vessel anatomy, including aneurysm, dissection, or stenosis. However, aortography is invasive and requires nephrotoxic contrast agents. It cannot evaluate nonperfused nor thrombosed areas of aortic aneurysms. Aortography therefore is frequently coupled with an additional modality that provides better determination of TAAA size and extent.

CT and CT with angiography provide excellent delineation of aortic aneu-

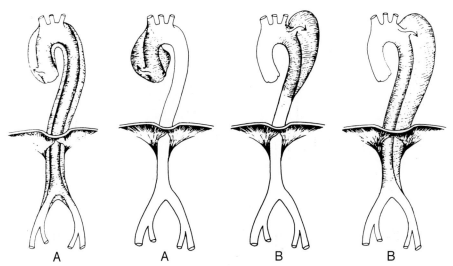

Figure 6–2. Stanford (types A and B) classification of aortic dissection. (From Hamilton IN, Hollier LH. Thoracoabdominal aortic aneurysms. *In* Moore W (ed). Vascular Surgery: a Comprehensive Review. Philadelphia: WB Saunders 1998:417–434.)

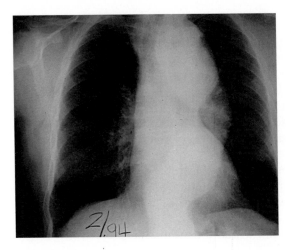

Figure 6–3. Chest radiograph demonstrates the distal aortic arch and a thoracoabdominal aortic aneurysm.

rysm diameter, type and extent of dissection, thrombus location, evidence of leak, branch vessel anatomy, and the anatomy of adjacent venous, mediastinal, retroperitoneal, and abdominal organs (Fig. 6–4). Spiral CT with three-dimensional reconstruction may provide detailed aortic branch vessel anatomy.

MRI of TAAA provides many of the advantages associated with spiral CT while avoiding nephrotoxic contrast agents (Fig. 6–5). Magnetic resonance angiography and cine magnetic resonance angiography have multiplane and three-dimensional reconstruction capability, lack ionizing radiation, and do not require critical timing of contrast infusion or image acquisition. Evaluation of aortic branch vessel anatomy with MRI techniques is generally equal to that of spiral CT angiography, but it is slightly inferior to conventional aortography. MRI cannot be offered to patients with implanted metallic devices and cannot be performed on unstable patients.

TEE provides information on myocardial performance, cardiac valvular function, and the presence of pericardial effusion or tamponade. It may be performed safely and quickly at the patient's bedside or in the operating room. It provides excellent anatomic information about the ascending and descending thoracic aorta and does not require nephrotoxic contrast agents.

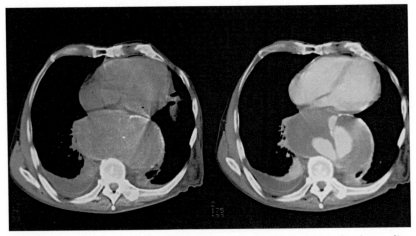

Figure 6–4. Computed tomography scans, with and without contrast, of a large, dissected thoracoabdominal aortic aneurysm demonstrate multiple, perfused lumens and an extensive aneurysm thrombus.

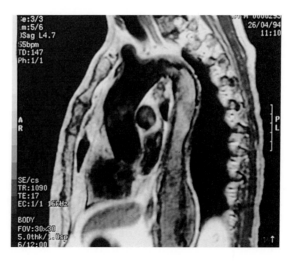

Figure 6–5. Sagittal magnetic resonance image demonstrates a type III thoracoabdominal aortic aneurysm.

However, TEE is limited in its ability to visualize the aortic arch and proximal brachiocephalic vessels compared with CT and MRI, and it is unable to evaluate the infradiaphragmatic aorta.

Preoperative Preparation

A complete history and physical examination should uncover each patient's concomitant risk factors, which may influence the success of TAAA repair. Routine preoperative studies include chest roentgenogram, electrocardiogram, arterial blood gas determination, complete blood cell count, Sequential Multiple Analyzer-6 (SMA-6) and SMA-12 tests, urinalysis, prothrombin time, partial thromboplastin time, and fibrinogen levels. All patients considered for TAAA repair undergo cardiac stress testing and echocardiography to assess coronary artery disease and aortic valvular competency. If significant coronary disease or aortic valvular insufficiency is determined by preoperative testing, coronary angiography and ventriculography are performed.

In elective circumstances, high-risk patients should first undergo indicated myocardial revascularization with percutaneous transluminal coronary angioplasty or coronary artery bypass grafting. For patients who cannot safely undergo indicated preoperative myocardial revascularization, a modified multigraft technique may be employed to minimize myocardial risk and reduce early death rates.[38]

Preoperative optimization of myocardial performance using antianginal and inotropic medications occasionally may be indicated. Cardiovascular anesthesiology, intraoperative TEE, placement of a Swan-Ganz catheter and arterial line, and high thoracic epidural analgesia are recommended intraoperative measures used to decrease perioperative cardiac morbidity.[36, 49] Distal aortic pump perfusion, nitroglycerine, and sodium nitroprusside infusions provide additional myocardial protection.[9, 28, 65, 71]

Pulmonary complications, including pulmonary insufficiency, need for tracheostomy, or prolonged ventilator dependency, are the most common postoperative complications associated with TAAA repair. The prevalence of chronic obstructive pulmonary disease, degree of tobacco use, thoracophrenolaparotomy, lung manipulation, barotrauma, and increased pulmonary microvascular permeability after ischemia and reperfusion[50, 63] account for the high incidence of respiratory morbidity after TAAA repair. Pulmonary morbidity may be modified through the cessation of smoking, antibiotic treatment for bronchitis, bronchodilator treatment, pulmonary physiotherapy, and epidural analgesia. Double-lumen tracheal intubation with left lung collapse provides appropriate surgical exposure of the descending thoracic aorta and minimizes pulmonary trauma, lung manipulation, compression, and barotrauma.

Local and remote organ systems may be injured as a result of the ischemia-reperfusion phenomenon associated with TAAA repair.[57, 63, 75] This neutrophil-dependent increase in microvascular permeability[67, 68] causes a rise in mean pulmonary artery pressure and noncardiogenic pulmonary edema after aortic aneurysmectomy.[63] Ischemia-reperfusion injuries may be preventable through the use of free radical scavengers[63] and by minimizing the ischemic interval through the use of distal aortic pump perfusion and selective visceral perfusion techniques.[11, 12, 37, 46]

Preoperative renal insufficiency is associated with higher rates of operative mortality, postoperative renal dysfunction, neurologic deficits, and late death after TAAA repair.[61, 62] The major determinants of postoperative renal failure after TAAA repair include the degree of preexisting renal dysfunction and the duration of renal ischemia. Minimizing nephrotoxic contrast agents, adjusting or replacing nephrotoxic medications, preoperative hydration, and complete renal artery revascularization at the time of TAAA repair help to preserve existing renal function and minimize the incidence of postoperative renal insufficiency. Distal aortic pump perfusion with selective renal perfusion[48] and renal perfusion using cold (4°C) Collin's solution[31] are also associated with decreased rates of postoperative renal insufficiency.

Carotid artery duplex ultrasonography should be routinely performed as part of the preoperative assessment. Severe carotid stenosis should be treated by carotid endarterectomy before elective TAAA repair. Attempts are made to place patients in a positive nitrogen balance preceding TAAA repair if this does not inappropriately delay surgery. Patients found to be candidates for TAAA repair undergo preoperative hydration, mechanical bowel preparation, bathing with antimicrobial soap, type and crossmatching for 6 units of packed red blood cells, 6 units of fresh-frozen plasma, and 12 units of platelets.

Of patients with large aortic aneurysms (including TAAA), 39% may have a significant elevation of fibrin split products preoperatively, and 4% have a clinical presentation of disseminated intravascular coagulation with extensive bruising, petechiae, and ecchymoses found on physical examination.[25] Treatment for this preoperative coagulopathy is aneurysmectomy; however, the coagulopathy and increased risk of intraoperative bleeding should be appreciated and treated with antifibrinolytics and infusion of platelets and fresh-frozen plasma before and during TAAA repair.

Treatment

Surgical Repair

At surgery, a double-lumen endotracheal tube, Swan-Ganz catheter, radial arterial line, two large-bore central venous catheters, a high thoracic epidural catheter, and an intrathecal catheter are placed. TEE is used to determine cardiac volume status, evaluate intraoperative cardiac valvular function, and detect early signs of myocardial ischemia.

The patient is placed in a right lateral decubitus position with an axillary roll. Access to the left iliofemoral region is necessary for anticipated distal aortic pump perfusion. The skin is widely prepared with povidone-iodine solution and adhesive iodinated plastic drapes. A thoracophrenolaparotomy incision is made based on the level of aortic involvement. The dissection is carried into the left retroperitoneal plane posterior to the left kidney. The inferior pulmonary ligament is divided, and the proximal portions of the visceral and renal arteries are controlled with vessel loops.

The mediastinal pleura overlying the normal aortic segment proximal to the aneurysm is carefully dissected in anticipation of proximal aortic control. For a type I or type II TAAA, obtaining proximal control between the left common carotid and left subclavian arteries may be necessary. The left phrenic, vagus, and recurrent laryngeal nerves and the left pulmonary artery should be protected at this level. Staged aortic clamping and sequential anastomoses with distal aortic pump perfusion during the performance of the proximal aortic and intercostal artery anastomoses require exposure of an additional segment of descending thoracic aorta, as the anatomy of the aneurysm permits. The proximal anastomosis is performed with a low-porosity, collagen-impregnated Dacron graft (Hemashield, Meadox, Oakland, NJ) in end-to-end fashion to uninvolved, spatulated aorta using an oblique anastomosis sewn with a running 0 Prolene on a V7 needle, incorporating any large intercostal arteries in the vicinity. After completing the proximal anastomosis, the proximal clamp is moved onto the graft, thereby restoring antegrade flow to any reimplanted intercostal arteries. Additional large intercostal arteries are reimplanted as separate cuffs onto the posterior aspect of the graft using the Carrel patch technique.[6] Each cuff of intercostal arteries is sequentially reperfused by moving the proximal clamp distally on the graft, restoring flow to the spinal cord as soon as possible.

Next, an infrarenal portion of aorta or, alternatively, the common iliac arteries are clamped for distal control. The remaining section of aneurysmal aorta is opened longitudinally posterior to the orifice of the left renal artery. The ostia of the celiac, superior mesenteric, and renal arteries are inspected. Significant atherosclerotic osteal lesions are treated by endarterectomy. Perfusion catheters are attached to the divided arterial line from the distal aortic pump perfusion system (Fig. 6–6). The superior mesenteric and one or both renal arteries are selectively cannulated and perfused with oxygenated blood

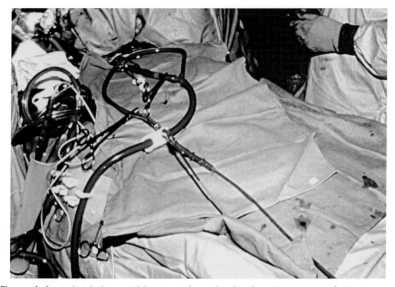

Figure 6–6. A divided arterial line runs from the distal aortic pump perfusion system.

from the centrifugal pump (Fig. 6–7). The visceral vessels are then reimplanted into the side of the graft using the Carrel patch technique. The celiac, superior mesenteric, and right renal arteries are frequently reimplanted as a single cuff. If the origin of the left renal artery is closely approximated to the visceral vessels, all four may be reimplanted as a single cuff. Separate grafts may be used to revascularize renal or mesenteric vessels in an end-to-end fashion beyond the point of intimal disruption in the setting of aortic dissection.[38]

The distal anastomosis is performed to the common iliac arteries or the distal abdominal aorta, as dictated by aneurysm anatomy. Internal iliac artery perfusion should be ensured after completion of the distal anastomosis to decrease the risk of lower spinal cord or lumbosacral nerve root ischemic injury.[30]

After ensuring adequate perfusion to all branch vessels, the wall of the aneurysm is closed tightly over the entire length of the graft. This provides tamponade against oozing and prevents graft erosion into adjacent viscera and lung. After achieving hemostasis, the diaphragm is reapproximated with interrupted mattress sutures. Two chest tubes are used to drain the costophrenic sulcus and the apex of the left chest. The chest and abdomen are closed in multiple layers, and the patient is transferred directly to the surgical intensive care unit.

Postoperative maintenance of hemodynamic stability, adequate oxygenation, normothermia, and urine output decreases the risk of myocardial ischemia, tachycardia, stroke, renal insufficiency, paraplegia, and coagulopathy. Inotropic support may be required in the first few hours postoperatively; however, it is discontinued as soon as adequate volume loading restores hemodynamic stability. The patient is maintained on a low-dose dopamine infusion (2 to 3 μg/kg/min) to enhance renal vasodilatation for the first 24 to 48 hours. Lactated Ringer's solution is infused at a rate to replace urine output on a milliliter per milliliter basis for the first 12 to 24 hours.

Ventilator weaning is initiated on postoperative day 1, as dictated by the arterial blood gas determination and evidence of appropriate pulmonary function and mental status. Furosemide may be given at this point to assist with fluid mobilization and to enhance ventilator weaning. Chest tubes are removed when drainage is less than 100 mL/day. Cephalosporin antibiotics are continued until the intrathecal lumbar catheter is removed around the third postoperative day. Cytoprotective agents are used for ulcer prophylaxis

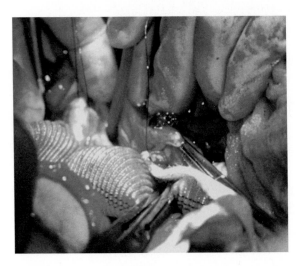

Figure 6–7. Operative photograph demonstrates a visceral perfusion catheter in place during thoracoabdominal aortic aneurysm repair.

until the resolution of postoperative ileus, at which time enteral feedings may be started.

Spinal Fluid Drainage

In 1988, studies using dogs demonstrated that cerebral spinal fluid drainage before thoracic aortic occlusion decreased the incidence of paraplegia compared with control animals without cerebral spinal fluid drainage.[52] Spinal cord perfusion pressure was significantly higher in neurologically normal animals than those that experienced paraplegia or paraparesis. That same year, isotope-tagged microsphere blood flow studies were performed in animals undergoing aortic crossclamping with and without cerebral spinal fluid drainage.[5] Cerebral spinal fluid drainage significantly improved spinal blood flow during aortic crossclamping. Spinal cord blood flow more than tripled from baseline after aortic unclamping in animals without cerebral spinal fluid drainage, whereas animals with cerebral spinal fluid drainage were protected from this reperfusion hyperemia. Cerebral spinal fluid drainage provided statistically significant protection from neurologic deficit by increasing spinal cord blood flow during aortic crossclamping and through the attenuation of a reperfusion hyperemia after aortic unclamping.

Based on this research, cerebral spinal fluid drainage was clinically incorporated as part of a multimodality approach to spinal cord protection during TAAA repair. Initially, this clinical experience emphasized complete intercostal artery reimplantation whenever possible, cerebral spinal fluid drainage, and maintenance of proximal arterial hypertension during aortic crossclamping.[41] The spinal cord metabolic rate also was reduced by moderate hypothermia and intravenous high-dose barbiturates. The reperfusion injury was minimized by the use of mannitol, steroids, calcium channel blockers, and avoidance of hyperglycemia. The protocol for spinal cord protection evolved to include distal aortic pump perfusion with selective visceral artery perfusion and substitution of the intravenous anesthetic agent propofol (Diprivan) for the previously used barbiturate, thiopental[37] (Fig. 6–8).

Spinal cord perfusion pressure is equivalent to the difference between the anterior spinal artery pressure and cerebral spinal fluid pressure.[40] Maintaining a spinal cord perfusion pressure that minimizes or eliminates ischemia may be achieved by increasing the spinal cord mean arterial pressure, decreasing the cerebral spinal fluid pressure, or both measures. We maximize spinal cord perfusion by maintaining a high proximal aortic blood pressure (150 mm Hg) to maximize collateral blood flow during aortic crossclamping. Distal aortic pump perfusion provides oxygenated blood flow to the distal aorta and its branches, including lower intercostal, lumbar, and pelvic arteries, and the technique of staged clamping and sequential anastomoses is used to perform proximal aortic procedures.

We and others have demonstrated the benefit of cerebral spinal fluid drainage to lower the cerebral spinal fluid pressure, thereby maximizing spinal cord perfusion pressure for any mean arterial blood pressure.[41, 42, 52] An intrathecal catheter is placed at the lumbar level immediately preceding the operation (Fig. 6–9). The lumbar catheter is 80 cm long with a closed tip and 12 side holes. This catheter is connected to the Becker external drainage and monitor system (EDMS II Pudenz Shulte Medical Corp., Golet, CA), which allows automatic overflow drainage of cerebral spinal fluid when the pressure rises above a preset value (Fig. 6–10). A pressure transducer can be connected to the drainage system stopcock, allowing continuous monitoring of cerebral

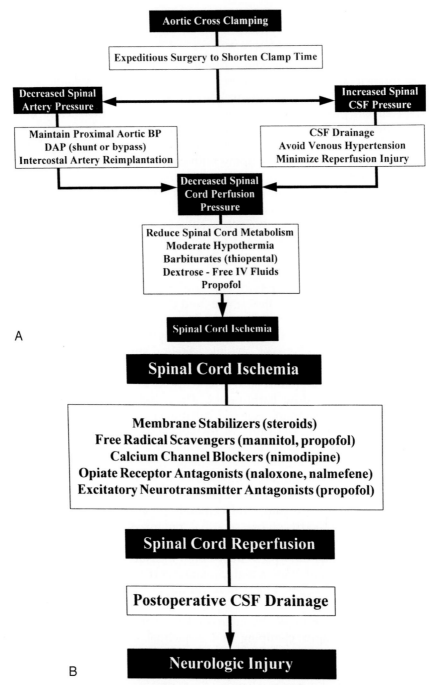

Figure 6–8. *A,* This sequence of events can lead to neurologic injury after aortic crossclamping. The events in *black boxes* represent the natural progression to spinal cord injury. The events in *white boxes* are treatment options used to interrupt the cascade leading to spinal cord injury. *B,* This is another sequence of events that can lead to injury after aortic crossclamping. The events in *black boxes* represent the natural progression to spinal cord injury. The events in *white boxes* are treatment options used to interrupt the cascade leading to spinal cord injury. BP, blood pressure; CSF, cerebrospinal fluid; DAP, distal aortic perfusion. (*A* and *B* from Hamilton IN, Hollier LH. Thoracoabdominal aortic aneurysms. *In* Moore W (ed). Vascular Surgery: a Comprehensive Review. Philadelphia: WB Saunders 1998:417–434.)

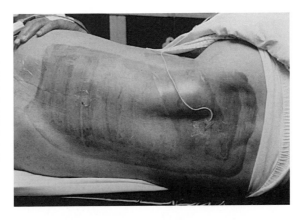

Figure 6–9. Patient in a left lateral decubitus position has thoracic epidural and cerebral spinal fluid drainage catheters in place. (From Hamilton IN, Hollier LH. Adjunctive therapy for spinal cord protection during thoracoabdominal aortic aneurysm repair. Semin Thorac Cardiovasc Surg 1998;10:1–6.)

spinal fluid pressure during and after the operation. The flow chamber on the EDMS II is adjusted to the desired pressure (eg, 10 mm Hg in our clinical experience) by sliding the flow chamber along a graduated scale. Thereafter, cerebral spinal fluid drains automatically into the flow chamber and into the collecting bag when the cerebral spinal fluid pressure exceeds the preset limit. This provides an automatic, closed overflow system that decreases the risk of contamination and meningitis.

Some patients undergoing TAAA repair have been found to awaken with normal neurologic examination findings, only to develop delayed-onset paraplegia several days postoperatively. In 1991, Hollier and colleagues[55] studied the cause of delayed-onset paraplegia after temporary spinal cord ischemia in an awake rabbit model. This study demonstrated a relation between the duration of spinal cord ischemia and delayed-onset paraplegia while controlling for other causes of paraplegia such as spinal artery thrombosis, embolization, and hypotension. Based on this research, cerebral spinal fluid drainage is used during TAAA repair and for up to 3 days postoperatively. We and others have previously reported anecdotal cases of delayed-onset paraplegia occurring in patients after TAAA repair that completely reversed to a normal neurologic state by simple cerebral spinal fluid drainage.[39, 41] A reperfusion injury with secondary spinal cord edema and increased cerebral spinal fluid pressure is thought to be the most likely cause for this delayed-onset paraplegia.

Distal Aortic Perfusion

TAAA repair requires aortic crossclamping for proximal control. The consequences of acute interruption of blood flow through the descending thoracic aorta are proportional to the level of aortic occlusion and include proximal hypertension, increased left ventricular strain, pulmonary congestion, increased cerebral spinal fluid pressure, and spinal cord, mesenteric, and renal ischemia.[28] Proximal hypertension, increases in left ventricular afterload, and pulmonary congestion may be alleviated by the administration of vasodilating agents such as sodium nitroprusside. However, pharmacologic manipulation to lower proximal blood pressure is associated with a reduction in spinal cord perfusion pressure and may increase the incidence of neurologic injury.[4, 18, 69] Moreover, decreasing proximal hypertension and left ventricular afterload does not address the issues of spinal cord, mesenteric, and renal ischemia during aortic occlusion.

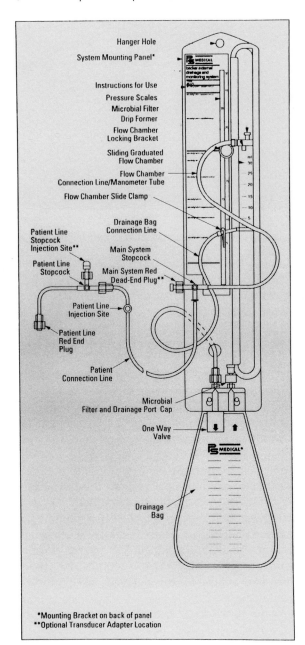

Hanger Hole

System Mounting Panel*

Instructions for Use

Pressure Scales

Microbial Filter

Drip Former

Flow Chamber
Locking Bracket

Sliding Graduated
Flow Chamber

Flow Chamber
Connection Line/Manometer Tube

Flow Chamber Slide Clamp

Drainage Bag
Connection Line

Patient Line
Stopcock
Injection Site**

Main System
Stopcock

Patient Line
Stopcock

Main System Red
Dead-End Plug**

Patient Line
Injection Site

Patient Line
Red End
Plug

Patient
Connection Line

Microbial
Filter and Drainage Port Cap

One Way
Valve

Drainage
Bag

*Mounting Bracket on back of panel
**Optional Transducer Adapter Location

Figure 6–10. The Becker External Drainage and Monitoring System (EDMS) allows a closed system for cerebral fluid drainage and monitoring of cerebral spinal fluid pressure. (From Hamilton IN, Hollier LH. Adjunctive therapy for spinal cord protection during thoracoabdominal aortic aneurysm repair. Semin Thorac Cardiovasc Surg 1998;10:1–6.)

In an attempt to address the pathophysiology on both sides of the proximal aortic clamp, various techniques of retrograde or distal aortic perfusion have been used. These techniques may be broadly categorized as passive shunts or distal aortic pump perfusion. Passive shunts were used experimentally as early as 1910, when Carrel performed intraluminal aorto-aortic shunting and left ventricle to descending thoracic aortic shunting with paraffined rubber tubes and cold-preserved jugular veins.[7] Carrel's concept of passive aortic shunting has been best exemplified clinically as the Gott shunt.[54, 77, 78] Temporary axillary to femoral artery bypass grafting at the time of TAAA repair also has been used as a passive shunt.[14] Passive shunts simplify aortic aneurysmectomy, eliminating the need and risk of systemic anticoagulation. However, even under ideal circumstances, passive shunts are associated with technical problems during placement in atherosclerotic vessels, may not provide adequate perfusion or pressure to meet distal metabolic needs, and may still require vasodilators for treatment of proximal hypertension.[2, 15, 18, 54, 66, 69, 79]

Distal aortic pump perfusion during aortic aneurysmectomy was used experimentally as early as 1955.[17] Although conflicting results have been reported in the past, contemporary studies have shown significant protection from neurologic injury during TAAA repair incorporating a combination of distal aortic pump perfusion and cerebral spinal fluid drainage.[64, 65] Distal aortic pump perfusion is safe during TAAA repair and is associated with some of the lowest morbidity and mortality rates reported in the literature.[18, 64, 65, 74]

Options for distal aortic pump perfusion include bypasses between the left femoral vein and left femoral artery (ie, femoral-femoral bypass) and between the left atrial artery and left femoral artery (ie, atrial-femoral bypass). Femoral-femoral partial cardiopulmonary bypass using a membrane oxygenator and standard uncoated circuitry requires full systemic anticoagulation with heparin: 1 IU/mL in the pump prime and 300 IU/kg intravenously to maintain the activated clotting time (ACT) between 300 to 600 seconds. Advantages of fully heparinized femoral-femoral partial cardiopulmonary bypass include enhanced oxygenation, ease of femoral vein cannulation, absence of circuitry in the operative field, and options for adjunctive equipment, such as cardiotomy suction and a blood reservoir (Fig. 6–11). The disadvantages of this system include the requirement for systemic anticoagulation, protamine reversal, higher costs, and more complex circuitry.

Atrial-femoral distal aortic pump perfusion using a closed system (ie, no oxygenator, cardiotomy suction, or blood reservoir) with a centrifugal pump (Fig. 6–12) is safely performed without anticoagulation.[64] Several types of centrifugal pumps are commercially available, including the Bio-Medicus Bio-pump (Bio-Medicus, Eden Prairie, MN) and the Sarns Delphin (Sarns Incorporated/3M, Ann Arbor, MI). Advantages of this type of system include the elimination of systemic anticoagulation and less complex circuitry. However, disadvantages of atrial-femoral bypass include the need for atriotomy, tubing and cannulas near or in the operative field, and the lack of adjuncts such as cardiotomy suction.

Femoral-femoral partial cardiopulmonary bypass with heparin-coated circuitry can be safely performed with low systemic heparin administration (100 IU/kg bolus and ACT ≥ 180 seconds).[81] The advantages of this system

Figure 6–11. The heparin-coated blood reservoir, membrane oxygenator, and centrifugal pump are the three major components of a femoral-femoral, distal aortic pump perfusion system.

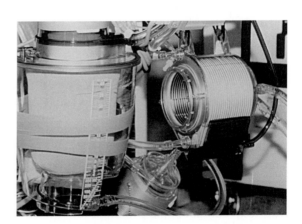

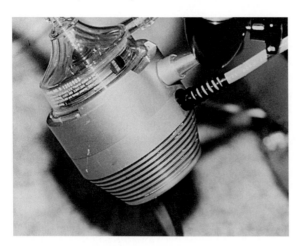

Figure 6–12. Centrifugal pump head.

include those for femoral-femoral bypass plus reduced heparin and protamine administration, reduced bleeding complications, and decreased activation of clotting, complement, and cytokine systems. Disadvantages include the additional expense of heparin-coated circuitry. The choice of distal aortic pump perfusion techniques during TAAA repair is based in large part on local practice patterns, but an additional consideration should be the patient's pulmonary function. Patients with severely compromised pulmonary function may require supplemental oxygenation to allow safe single-lung ventilation that only a circuit with an oxygenator can provide. In the rare circumstance in which hypothermic circulatory arrest may be required for proximal aortic control and anastomoses, a circuit with an oxygenator and blood reservoir is mandatory.

Whether atrial-femoral or femoral-femoral distal aortic pump perfusion techniques are used, constant communication among the surgeon, anesthesiologist, and pump technician is mandatory for the safe performance of distal aortic pump perfusion, especially during the initiation and weaning stages. During distal aortic pump perfusion, several flow and pressure parameters should be kept in mind. Flow should be initiated slowly with the application of aortic clamping. We attempt to balance a right radial blood pressure of 150 mm Hg with pulmonary artery or left ventricular end-diastolic pressures that approximate those of baseline or preclamping values. Increasing pump flow rates effectively lower pulmonary artery and left ventricular end-diastolic pressures, but this may also decrease proximal arterial pressures. We attempt to balance these proximal hemodynamic parameters with a distal aortic (right femoral artery) pressure of 60 mm Hg or greater, which we have found to be associated with adequate lower extremity and visceral perfusion. Pump flow rates generally are dictated by first balancing the proximal and distal hemodynamic values, resulting in flow rates between 1.5 and 3.0 L/min. On opening the visceral abdominal aortic segment, distal aortic perfusion through the femoral artery cannula must be suspended when the iliac arteries are clamped for distal control.

At this point in the procedure, we transition from femoral artery perfusion to selective visceral perfusion through a divided arterial line from the perfusion system (see Fig. 6–6). During this transition period, the centrifugal pump is briefly turned off. Whenever the centrifugal pump is not running, the arterial line must be clamped to avoid the backward flow of blood through the pump and out of the patient, leading to exsanguination. After the selective visceral perfusion catheters have been flushed and placed into the celiac, superior mesenteric, or renal arteries, the arterial line may be unclamped and flow reinitiated slowly for visceral perfusion (see Fig. 6–7).

Systemic anticoagulation for extracorporeal circulation prevents clotting of blood on contact with the artificial surfaces of the circuitry. If the foreign surfaces are rendered nonthrombogenic, systemic anticoagulation may become unnecessary. Heparin's strong acidity allows it to bind to polymer surfaces.[60] Heparin-coated extracorporeal circulation circuitry is available as Duraflow II heparin-coated equipment (Baxter-Bentley Laboratories, Irvine, CA) and Carmeda Bioactive Surface (Medtronic Cardiopulmonary, Anaheim, CA). Clinically, the use of heparin-coated circuitry with low-dose heparin is associated with significantly less bleeding, decreased hemolysis, and reduced transfusion requirements.[26, 35, 80, 81, 83, 84] The reduction in blood loss associated with the use of heparin-coated circuits is attributable to increased biocompatibility and to an 80% reduction in heparin and a 70% reduction in protamine sulfate dose requirements.[82] Heparin-coated circuitry used in conjunction with low levels of systemic heparin (100 IU/kg and ACT $\geq$ 180 seconds) has been successfully used to provide left atrial-femoral and femoral-femoral distal aortic pump perfusion during descending thoracic aortic aneurysm and TAAA repair.[3, 81]

Aneurysmectomy with heparin-coated circuits was performed in these studies with fewer revisions because of bleeding, better postoperative renal function, lower hospital and 30-day mortality, and higher 1-year survival compared with historical controls who underwent simple aortic crossclamping and rapid reanastomosis.[81] These uncontrolled aneurysmectomy data provide strong preliminary evidence that TAAA repair with distal aortic pump perfusion using heparin-coated circuitry is associated with fewer anticoagulation-related complications, less bleeding and hemolysis, and reduced transfusion requirements compared with uncoated circuitry.

Potential arterial (outflow) cannulation sites for distal aortic pump perfusion include the femoral artery, iliac artery, and aorta. Potential venous (inflow) cannulation sites include the right atrium through the femoral vein, left atrium, pulmonary vein, and pulmonary artery. Left atrial cannulation is performed after thoracotomy or thoracophrenolaparotomy and aortic dissection in preparation for aortic crossclamping. The pericardium is incised longitudinally and parallel to the phrenic nerve. The left atrium is cannulated with a straight or angulated cannula (26 to 36 Fr) inserted through one or two purse-string sutures in the left atrial appendage or the left superior or inferior pulmonary vein. Great care must be taken to avoid complications associated with left atrial cannulation, including atrial arrhythmias, atrial lacerations, mitral valve injury, bleeding, air embolization, and cannula malpositioning. Cannulation of the femoral artery is performed through a vertical groin incision over the common femoral artery. After achieving proximal and distal control, a transverse common femoral arteriotomy allows retrograde placement of a straight arterial cannula (16 to 24 Fr) into the iliac artery. Complications associated with femoral artery cannulation include iliofemoral artery injury, thrombosis, bleeding, distal embolization, catheter dislodgment, and retrograde arterial dissection.

For femoral-femoral distal aortic pump perfusion, cannulation of the femoral vein is performed through the same vertical groin incision used for the femoral artery. Proper placement of a single-staged, straight venous cannula (28 to 36 Fr) into the right atrium through the femoral vein provides excellent venous return. Occasionally, the venous cannula may not be appropriately positioned within the right atrium, impairing sufficient venous return. In these circumstances, an additional venous cannula may be placed in the superior vena cava through the internal jugular vein or into the right ventricle through the right pulmonary artery. The femoral venous cannula sometimes is advanced over a J-tipped guide wire after initially meeting resistance offered by the crossing iliac artery.

Complications associated with left atrial cannulation may be avoided through gentle handling of tissues, accurate suture placement, careful cannula positioning, and the use of a side-biting clamp and Valsalva maneuver during atriotomy and cannula placement. Arterial thrombosis and complications of leg ischemia associated with femoral artery cannulation may be reduced with appropriate anticoagulation, shortened operative times, and antegrade limb perfusion using an introducer catheter connected to a side port of the arterial line during prolonged cases.[34] The risk of retrograde arterial dissection is decreased by the use of atraumatic cannulas with tapered ends, appropriately matching cannula and artery size, careful cannula insertion, routinely establishing the presence of good arterial pulsations in the cannula and bypass tubing, placement of the cannula approximately 6 cm proximal to the femoral arteriotomy, and securing the cannula to the artery and the wound edges to avoid dislodgment and motion of the cannula within the artery.[45] Bleeding from groin wounds can be avoided by closing the wounds only after heparin reversal and hemostasis has been achieved.

Distal aortic pump perfusion during TAAA repair ensures perfusion to renal, mesenteric, and spinal cord regions, minimizing ischemic complications compared with clamp and sew or passive shunt techniques.[2, 27, 29, 37, 44, 47, 48, 64, 65, 74, 81] Distal aortic pump perfusion allows TAAA repair to be performed in a staged, segmental fashion while lower intercostal, lumbar, renal, and mesenteric arteries are perfused during the performance of the proximal aortic anastomoses. Distal vessels continue to be perfused from the pump until the respective segment of aneurysmal aorta is clamped and opened. After visceral aortotomy, distal aortic pump perfusion allows selective visceral perfusion. The combination of retrograde aortic perfusion during the proximal aortic and intercostal artery anastomoses and selective visceral perfusion after visceral aortotomy decreases the ischemic period for these critical vascular beds. As a result, distal aortic pump perfusion and selective visceral perfusion decrease the risk and incidence of paraplegia, paraparesis, ischemic renal insufficiency, and coagulopathy resulting from mesenteric ischemia and reperfusion.[11, 12, 37, 48, 64, 65] Distal aortic pump perfusion during TAAA repair maintains lower body perfusion, prevents declamping shock, and avoids systemic acidosis.[8, 29, 81]

Intraoperative Medications

AAA repair requires interruption of blood flow through the descending thoracic, abdominal aorta, or both for various periods. Although distal aortic perfusion reduces or minimizes ischemic time intervals, during periods of aortic crossclamping, some vascular territories are invariably hypoperfused during the reconstruction of aortic segments giving rise to branch arteries subserving these vascular territories. Ischemia followed by reperfusion sets in motion a neutrophil-dependent phenomenon that may cause local and remote organ system injury. Territories most notably affected by ischemia and reperfusion include the spinal cord, gut, kidneys, lungs, and lower extremities.

Medications administered intraoperatively have been helpful in attenuating or eliminating the negative effects of ischemia and reperfusion. Many investigators have demonstrated the ability to modulate the reperfusion injury with free radical scavengers, antioxidants, monoclonal antibodies, excitatory neurotransmitter antagonists, opiate receptor antagonists, and calcium channel blockers.[10, 13, 33, 51, 86, 87] Our protocol, which attempts to reduce reperfusion injury, first tries to minimize the initial ischemic insult by using distal aortic pump perfusion and expeditious surgical technique. Medications administered at the time of surgery are used to minimize the subsequent reperfusion phenomenon. Medications in our protocol aimed at modulating the ischemia-reperfusion phenomenon include propofol, mannitol, steroids, and sodium bicarbonate (Table 6–2).

In the past, we used thiopental sodium to decrease the spinal cord metabolic rate. We have substituted the intravenous anesthetic agent propofol for

Table 6–2.
Intraoperative Medications for Thoracoabdominal Aortic Aneurysm Repair

Agent	Dose	Time or Type of Use
Free radical scavengers		
Propofol	Variable IV dose	Administer as maintenance and/or induction anesthetic
Mannitol	12.5–25 g IV	Before aortic clamping and unclamping
Membrane stabilizers		
Methylprednisolone	30 mg/kg IV	Start of surgery
Hydrocortisone	100 mg IV	Start of surgery
Antiacids		
Sodium bicarbonate	50–100 mEq IV	Before aortic unclamping
Cardiac protective		
Nitroglycerine	Titrated IV drip to keep systolic blood pressure ~150 mm Hg and PAP/LVEDP at preclamping values	Throughout surgery in patients with known coronary artery disease
Sodium nitroprusside	Same as for nitroglycerine	During aortic crossclamping
Renal protective		
Mannitol	12.5–25 g IV	Before aortic clamping and unclamping
Dopamine	2–3 μg/kg/min IV drip	Intraoperatively and postoperatively
Collin's solution (4°C)	Renal artery perfusion	During visceral aortic reconstruction
Anticoagulant or reversal		
Heparin	50–100 IU/kg IV to maintain ACT ≥ 180 sec	Before femoral-femoral DAPP with heparin-coated circuitry
Protamine	1.0–1.3 mg/100 IU heparin IV	After removing arterial and venous DAPP canulas
Hemostatic		
Desmopressin acetate	0.3 μg/kg IV	Preexisting hematologic abnormality (eg, uremia, antiplatelet medications)
Aprotinin	280 mg IV bolus, then 70 mg/h IV drip	Aortic unclamping and/or with fibrinolysis
Fibrin glue		Between graft and native aortic wall or PTFE membrane
Fresh-frozen plasma	6 units IV	Aortic unclamping
Platelets	12 units IV	Aortic unclamping
Cryoprecipitate	10 units IV	Hypofibrinogenemia or fibrinolysis

ACT, activated clotting time; DAPP, distal aortic pump perfusion; LVEDP, left ventricular end diastolic pressure; PAP, pulmonary artery pressure; PTFE, polytetrafluoroethylene.

thiopental because of propofol's ability to reduce central nervous system metabolic requirements for oxygen[72] while maintaining cerebral oxygenation and autoregulation.[59] Propofol also is a free-radical scavenger with excellent central nervous system distribution.[58, 70] This feature may translate into enhanced central nervous system protection from ischemic injury. Propofol is administered as part of a balanced intravenous anesthetic.

Propofol may be used for the induction of anesthesia, but it appears to possess some negative inotropic effects on papillary muscle. Propofol should therefore be used with caution in patients with preexisting cardiac disease.[72] We prefer to use a titrated infusion of propofol for maintenance of anesthesia during TAAA repair. We have not found this method of propofol use to be associated with any increased requirement for inotropic support during or after TAAA repair. The specific dose of propofol during induction and maintenance anesthesia depends on whether it is used as a component of a total intravenous anesthetic technique (in combination with benzodiazepines or opioid analgesics) and the patient's overall cardiac condition.[59]

Oxygen free radicals have been implicated as a cause of local and remote organ damage after ischemia and reperfusion in a number of tissues, including pulmonary, myocardial, intestinal, and renal organ systems. Mannitol has been shown to be an effective scavenger of oxygen-derived free radicals through its inhibition of thromboxane synthesis.[63] It has been recommended as a standard precaution to administer intraoperative mannitol immediately before aortic crossclamping in patients with chronic renal insufficiency undergoing aneurysmectomy.[36] We administer mannitol (12.5 to 25 g) immediately before proximal aortic clamping and again preceding aortic unclamping. We continue to use the intravenous steroids methylprednisolone (30 mg/kg) and hydrocortisone (100 mg) at the start of the operation. However, we have not yet documented the effectiveness of steroids in reducing the reperfusion injury associated with TAAA repair, although experimental studies suggest that they may be beneficial.[13, 40] We also empirically administer sodium bicarbonate (50 to 100 mEq) at the time of aortic unclamping and reperfusion in an attempt to maintain near-normal pH values.

The hemodynamic consequences of proximal thoracic aortic crossclamping include proximal hypertension, increased myocardial wall stress, and decreased cardiac output. Sodium nitroprusside (see Table 6–2) has been used to control proximal aortic hypertension during thoracic aortic crossclamping with or without nitroglycerin. However, sodium nitroprusside may risk a decrease in spinal cord perfusion pressure during proximal aortic crossclamping resulting from a steal phenomenon.[71] We therefore administer sodium nitroprusside titrated to maintain proximal aortic blood pressure at 150 mm Hg during aortic occlusion simultaneously with distal aortic pump perfusion, thereby preventing the steal phenomenon that may result when sodium nitroprusside is given in the absence of distal aortic pump perfusion. The resultant left ventricular protection decreases the risk of perioperative myocardial infarction and pulmonary insufficiency.[28]

The renal protective effects of low-dose, intravenously administered dopamine (2 to 3 μg/kg/min) are not universally agreed on. However, we routinely administer dopamine during the intraoperative and postoperative periods to maximize renal vasodilatation and avoid an oliguric state (see Table 6–2). After the patient begins to mobilize third-space fluid and enters a diuretic phase, dopamine is tapered. When selective renal perfusion with the divided arterial line cannot be instituted, we perform renal perfusion using cold (4°C) Collin's solution.[31]

Our distal aortic pump perfusion technique of choice includes femoral-femoral partial cardiopulmonary bypass with a heparin-coated oxygenator, centrifugal pump, and cardiotomy suction. AAA repair may be performed with such a system using low systemic heparinization and maintaining the ACT at 180 seconds or higher (see Table 6–2). We initially administer heparin at 50 to 100 IU/kg and institute distal aortic pump perfusion with heparin-coated equipment after the ACT is 180 seconds or higher. The ACT is monitored throughout the procedure to maintain its value at 180 seconds or higher.[81] At the conclusion of distal aortic pump perfusion, any residual heparin effect should be reversed with protamine to minimize bleeding complications (see Table 6–2).

Several different dose regimens for protamine reversal of heparin anticoagulation have been employed. Accurate calculation of the protamine dose for reversal is important, because unneutralized heparin can increase postoperative bleeding and overdosages of protamine may paradoxically have an anticoagulant effect when complexed with heparin.[43, 56] The easiest method of calculating the protamine dose is a fixed-dose ratio of protamine to heparin. This method involves administering 1.0 to 1.3 mg of protamine for each 100 IU of heparin administered. The ease of dosage calculation constitutes the main advantage of this method. However, because of the variability of heparin's half-life, the protamine dose is less precise. Additional methods for determining the need for protamine include the ACT/heparin dose-response curve, measurement of serum heparin levels, and protamine titration.[56]

Several pharmacologic agents have been used for the treatment and prophylaxis of bleeding complications associated with TAAA repair and the use of extracorporeal circulation techniques. Of these agents, we selectively use desmopressin acetate and aprotinin (Trasylol) (see Table 6–2).

Desmopressin acetate is modified from arginine vasopressin. Desmopressin acetate releases a variety of hemostatically active substances from vascular endothelium, including factor VIII, prostacyclin, tissue plasminogen activator, and von Willebrand factor. Desmopressin acetate is administered by intravenous, intranasal, or subcutaneous routes at a dose of 0.3 µg/kg. During elective cardiac surgery incorporating extracorporeal circulation, desmopressin acetate provided no hemostatic effect. However, desmopressin acetate has been shown to be effective when administered to patients undergoing extracorporeal circulation who have a preexisting hematologic abnormality such as uremia, hemophilia, or von Willebrand's disease and those on antiplatelet therapy such as aspirin.[76]

Aprotinin is a naturally occurring inhibitor of proteolytic enzymes. As a serine protease inhibitor, aprotinin has been shown to inhibit human trypsin, plasmin, plasma kallikrein, and tissue kallikrein by forming reversible enzyme-inhibitor complexes. Aprotinin also inhibits plasmin- and kallikrein-mediated fibrinolysis.[20] Aprotinin is thought to improve hemostasis during and after extracorporeal circulation by preserving the adhesive receptor glycoprotein 1b on platelet membranes.

In the setting of extracorporeal circulation, two dosage regimens of aprotinin have been evaluated. The high-dose regimen includes aprotinin 280 mg infused over 20 to 30 minutes preceding sternotomy in patients undergoing cardiac surgery. This is followed by a continuous infusion of aprotinin at 70 mg/hour until the surgical procedure is completed. Aprotinin (280 mg) also is added to the priming fluid of the extracorporeal circulation circuitry. A low-dose aprotinin regimen includes 50% of the previously described high dose or a single dose of aprotinin (280 mg) added to the priming fluid of the

Table 6–3.
Mortality

Factor	Type of Thoracoabdominal Aortic Aneurysm				Total
	I	*II*	*III*	*IV*	
Patients (*n*)	52	81	97	77	307
Operating room deaths	5 (9.6%)	2 (2.5%)	2 (2.1%)	0	9 (2.9%)
Death (30 d)	3 (5.8%)	5 (6.2%)	6 (6.2%)	1 (1.3%)	15 (4.9%)
Total	8 (15.4%)	7 (8.6%)	8 (8.2%)	1 (1.3%)	24 (7.8%)

extracorporeal circulation circuit. Aprotinin has also been used in human and animal studies in which heparin-coated extracorporeal circulation circuitry was used.[84] These studies demonstrated significantly less heparin and protamine requirements, no evidence of clot formation on extracorporeal circulation circuitry, and no adverse effects.

Aprotinin inhibits contact activation of the intrinsic clotting system and therefore prolongs the results of coagulation assays that depend on contact activation, including activated partial thromboplastin time and celite-activated clotting time. As a result, the standard method for monitoring heparinization during extracorporeal circulation is not likely to indicate adequate heparinization after aprotinin administration.[20] The effect of aprotinin on celite ACT makes the use of this method for monitoring heparin levels potentially unsafe. However, when kaolin is used as the contact activator, the ACT obtained with aprotinin and concomitant heparin administration were not significantly different from that observed with heparin alone.[20, 85]

In patients undergoing descending thoracic or thoracoabdominal aneurysmectomy using extracorporeal circulation, administration of aprotinin was associated with significant decreases in extracorporeal circulation time, surgical duration, intraoperative blood loss, and transfusions of packed red blood cells, Cell Saver units, fresh-frozen plasma, and platelets.[32] We have incorporated aprotinin into our protocol for TAAA repair by administering a loading dose of 280 mg at the time of aortic declamping in patients demonstrating any evidence of coagulopathy or fibrinolysis. The loading dose is followed by a continuous infusion of aprotinin (70 mg/hour) until the end of the operation and achievement of hemostasis.

The most commonly reported adverse events after aprotinin administration include renal dysfunction (1%) and hypersensitivity reactions (1.6%). Because aprotinin undergoes active reabsorption by the proximal renal tubules, the effect of high-dose aprotinin on renal function has been investigated.[24] In patients undergoing coronary artery bypass grafting, high-dose aprotinin was associated with a selective renal tubular dysfunction lasting approximately 5 days postoperatively that was well tolerated in patients with normal preoper-

Table 6–4.
Neurologic Deficit

Factor	Type of Thoracoabdominal Aortic Aneurysm				Total
	I	*II*	*III*	*IV*	
Patients (*n*)	52	81	97	77	307
Paraplegia or paraparesis	3 (5.8%)	5 (6.2%)	5 (5.2%)	1 (1.3%)	14 (4.6%)
Deficit at discharge	1 (1.9%)	4 (4.9%)	1 (1.0%)	0	6 (2.0%)

ative renal function. However, recommendations resulting from this study included aprotinin dosage reduction in patients with preoperative serum creatinine levels greater than 2 mg/dL. The use of aprotinin in patients undergoing hypothermic circulatory arrest has been associated with an increased incidence of postoperative renal dysfunction and renal failure requiring hemodialysis.[73] It was thought that the adverse effects of aprotinin might be temperature dependent, and the use of aprotinin in the setting of hypothermic perfusion should be adopted very cautiously.

Additional intraoperative hemostatic agents administered during and after TAAA repair include the injection of fibrin glue between the newly placed aortic graft and reapproximated native aortic wall, Gore-Tex membrane, or both. We also administer fresh-frozen plasma, platelets, and cryoprecipitate as dictated by intraoperative partial thromboplastin time, prothrombin time, and fibrinogen levels (see Table 6–2).

Results

Our technique of TAAA repair has evolved over many years, and the various aspects of the procedure have been modified as additional research findings have demonstrated new adjunctive techniques and mechanisms of improvement. During the past 16 years, Hollier has undertaken surgical repair of 307 TAAAs using routine intercostal reimplantation in a major effort to reduce neurologic deficit. During the past 10 years, cerebral spinal fluid drainage has been added to the protocol, and during the past 7 years, use of a shunt or distal aortic pump perfusion has been added for type I and II TAAAs. Since the routine addition of distal aortic pump perfusion, we have seen no case of postoperative paraplegia, though transient paraparesis sometimes occurred. Since institution of selective visceral perfusion, there have been no intraoperative deaths. Table 6–3 summarizes the overall mortality rate associated with our TAAA repairs, and Table 6–4 summarizes the overall neurologic deficit rate.

References

1. Appelbaum A, Karp RB, Kirklin JW. Ascending vs descending aortic dissections. Ann Surg 1976;183:296.
2. Ataka K, Okada M, Yamashita C, et al. Beneficial circulatory support by left heart bypass with a centrifugal (Bio-Medicus) pump for aneurysms of the descending thoracic aorta. Artif Organs 1993;17:300.
3. Bennett J, Hill J, Long W, et al. Biocompatible circuits: an adjunct to non-cardiac extracorporeal cardiopulmonary support. J Extracorpor Technol 1992;24:6.
4. Berendes JN, Bredee MM, Schipperheyn JJ, et al. Mechanisms of spinal cord injury after cross-clamping of the descending thoracic aorta. Circulation 1982;66:I-112.
5. Bower TC, Murray MJ, Gloviczki P, et al. Effects of thoracic aortic occlusion and cerebrospinal fluid drainage on regional spinal cord blood flow in dogs: correlation with neurologic outcome. J Vasc Surg 1989;9:135.
6. Carrel A. The surgery of blood vessels, etc. Johns Hopkins Hosp Bull 1907;190:18.
7. Carrel A. On the experimental surgery of the thoracic aorta and the heart. Ann Surg 1910;52:83.
8. Cartier R, Orszulak TA, Pairolero PC, et al. Circulatory support during cross-clamping of the descending thoracic aorta. J Thorac Cardiovasc Surg 1990;99:1038.
9. Cernaianu AC, Olah A, Cilley JH Jr, et al. Effects of sodium nitroprusside on paraplegia during cross-clamping of the thoracic aorta. Ann Thorac Surg 1993;56:1035.
10. Clark WM, Madden KP, Rothlein R, et al. Reduction of central nervous system ischemic injury by monoclonal antibody to intracellular adhesion molecule. J Neurosurg 1991;75:623.
11. Cohen JR, Angus L, Asher A, et al. Disseminated intravascular coagulation as a result of supraceliac clamping: implications for thoracoabdominal aneurysm repair. Ann Vasc Surg 1987;1:552.
12. Cohen JR, Schroder W, Leal J, et al. Mesenteric shunting during thoracoabdominal aortic clamping to prevent disseminated intravascular coagulation in dogs. Ann Vasc Surg 1988;2:261.

13. Coles JC, Ahmed SN, Mehta HU, et al. Role of free radical scavenger in protection of spinal cord during ischemia. Ann Thorac Surg 1986;41:551.
14. Comerota AJ, White JV. Reducing morbidity of thoracoabdominal aneurysm repair by preliminary axillofemoral bypass. Am J Surg 1995;170:218.
15. Connolly ME, Wakabayashi A, German JC, et al. Clinical experience with pulsatile left heart bypass without anticoagulation for thoracic aneurysms. J Thorac Cardiovasc Surg 1971;62:568.
16. Crawford ES, Crawford JL, Safi HJ, et al. Thoracoabdominal aortic aneurysms: preoperative and intraoperative factors determining immediate and long-term results of operations in 605 patients. J Vasc Surg 1986;3:389.
17. Cross FS, Hirose Y, Jones RD, et al. Evaluation of a mechanical shunt to bypass segments of the thoracic aorta including the arch. Surg Forum 1955;6:166.
18. Cunningham JN, Laschinger JC, Spencer FC. Monitoring of somatosensory evoked potentials during surgical procedures on the thoracoabdominal aorta. J Thorac Cardiovasc Surg 1987;94:275.
19. Daily PO, Trueblood HW, Stinson EB, et al. Management of acute aortic dissections. Ann Thorac Surg 1970;10:237.
20. Davis R, Whittington R. Aprotinin: a review of its pharmacology and therapeutic efficacy in reducing blood loss associated with cardiac surgery. Drugs 1995;49:954.
21. DeBakey ME, Henley WS, Cooley DA, et al. Surgical management of dissecting aneurysms of the aorta. J Cardiovascular Surgery 1965;49:130.
22. Doroghazi RM, Slater EE, DeSanctis RW, et al. Long-term survival of patients with treated aortic dissection. J Am Coll Cardiol 1984;3:1026.
23. Etheredge SN, Yee J, Smith JV, et al. Successful resection of a large aneurysm of the upper abdominal aorta and replacement with homograft. Surgery 1955;38:1171.
24. Feindt PR, Walcher S, Volkmer I, et al. Effects of high-dose aprotinin on renal function in aortocoronary bypass grafting. Ann Thorac Surg 1995;60:1076.
25. Fisher DF, Yawn DH, Crawford ES. Preoperative disseminated intravascular coagulation caused by abdominal aortic aneurysm. Arch Surg 1983;118:1252.
26. Fosse E, Moen O, Johnson E, et al. Reduced complement and granulocyte activation with heparin-coated cardiopulmonary bypass. Ann Thorac Surg 1994;58:472.
27. Frank SM, Parker SD, Rock P, et al. Moderate hypothermia, with partial bypass and segmental sequential repair for thoracoabdominal aortic aneurysm. J Vasc Surg 1994;19:687.
28. Gelman S. The pathophysiology of aortic cross-clamping and unclamping. Anesthesiology 1995;82:1026.
29. Gloviczki P, Bower TC. Visceral and spinal cord protection during thoracoabdominal aortic reconstructions. Semin Vasc Surg 1992;5:163.
30. Gloviczki P, Cross SA, Stanson AW, et al. Ischemic injury to the spinal cord or lumbosacral plexus after aorto-iliac reconstruction. Am J Surg 1991;162:131.
31. Gloviczki P, Toomey BJ, Panneton JM, et al. Visceral and spinal cord protection during repair of thoracoabdominal aortic aneurysms: the Mayo Clinic experience. In Weimann S (ed). Thoracic and Thoracoabdominal Aortic Aneurysms. Bologna, Italy: Monduzzi Editore, 1994:189.
32. Godet G, Bertrand M, Samama C, et al. Aprotinin to decrease bleeding and intraoperative blood transfusion requirements during descending thoracic and thoracoabdominal aortic aneurysmectomy using cardiopulmonary bypass. Ann Vasc Surg 1994;3:452.
33. Granke K, Hollier LH, Zdrahal P, et al. Longitudinal study of cerebral spinal fluid drainage in polyethylene glycol-conjugated superoxide dismutase in paraplegia associated with thoracic aortic cross-clamping. J Vasc Surg 1991;13:615.
34. Greason KL, Hemp JR, Maxwell JM, et al. Prevention of distal limb ischemia during cardiopulmonary support via femoral cannulation. Ann Thorac Surg 1995;60:209.
35. Gu YJ, van Oeveren W, Akkerman C, et al. Heparin-coated circuits reduce the inflammatory response to cardiopulmonary bypass. Ann Thorac Surg 1993;55:917.
36. Hallett JW Jr, Bower TC, Cherry KJ, et al. Selection and preparation of high-risk patients for repair of abdominal aortic aneurysms. Mayo Clin Proc 1994;69:763.
37. Hamilton IN Jr, Hollier LH. Thoracoabdominal aortic aneurysms. In Moore WS (ed). Vascular Surgery: a Comprehensive Review. Philadelphia: WB Saunders, 1998:417.
38. Hamilton IN Jr, Hollier LH. Thoracoabdominal aortic aneurysm repair in high risk cardiac patients: a modified grafting technique. Int J Angiol 1998;118–122.
39. Hill AB, Kalman PG, Johnston KW, et al. Reversal of delayed-onset paraplegia after thoracic aortic surgery with cerebrospinal fluid drainage. J Vasc Surg 1994;20:315.
40. Hollier LH. Protecting the brain and spinal cord. J Vasc Surg 1987;5:524.
41. Hollier LH, Money SR, Naslund TC, et al. Risk of spinal cord dysfunction in patients undergoing thoracoabdominal aortic replacement. Am J Surg 1992;164:210.
42. Hollier LH, Symmonds JB, Pairolero PC, et al. Thoracoabdominal aortic aneurysm repair: analysis of postoperative morbidity. Arch Surg 1988;123:871.
43. Horrow JC. Protamine: a review of its toxicity. Anesth Analg 1985;64:348.
44. Janusz MT. Experience with thoracoabdominal aortic aneurysm resection. Am J Surg 1994;167:501.
45. Jones TW, Vetto RR, Winterscheid LC, et al. Arterial complications incident to cannulation in open-heart surgery. Ann Surg 1960;152:969.
46. Kazui M, Andreoni KA, Williams GM, et al. Visceral lipid peroxidation occurs at reperfusion after supraceliac aortic cross-clamping. J Vasc Surg 1994;19:473.
47. Kazui T, Komatsu S, Sasaki T, Yamada O. Graft inclusion technique for thoracoabdominal aortic

aneurysms involving visceral branches with the aid of a femoro-femoral bypass. Cardiovasc Surg 1987;28:663.

48. Kazui T, Komatsu S, Yokoyama H. Surgical treatment of aneurysms of the thoracic aorta with the aid of partial cardiopulmonary bypass: an analysis of 95 patients. Ann Thorac Surg 1987;43:622.

49. Kirno K, Friberg P, Grzegorczyk A, et al. Thoracic epidural anesthesia during coronary artery bypass surgery: effects on cardiac sympathetic activity, myocardial blood flow and metabolism, and central hemodynamics. Anesth Analg 1994;79:1075.

50. Klausner JM, Paterson IS, Mannick JA, et al. Reperfusion pulmonary edema. JAMA 1989;261:1030.

51. Madden KP, Clark WM, Marcoux FW, et al. Treatment with conotoxin, an "N-type" calcium channel blocker, in neuronal hypoxic-ischemic injury. Brain Res 1990;537:256.

52. McCullough JL, Hollier LH, Nugent M. Paraplegia after thoracic aortic occlusion: influence of cerebrospinal fluid drainage. Experimental and early clinical results. J Vasc Surg 1988;7:153.

53. Meng RL, Najafi H, Javid H, et al. Acute ascending aortic dissection: surgical management. Circulation 1981;64:II-231.

54. Molina JE, Cogordan J, Einzig S, et al. Adequacy of ascending aorta-descending aorta shunt during cross-clamping of the thoracic aorta for prevention of spinal cord injury. J Thorac Cardiovasc Surg 1985;90:126.

55. Moore WM Jr, Hollier LH. The influence of severity of spinal cord ischemia in the etiology of delayed-onset paraplegia. Ann Surg 1991;213:427.

56. Moorman RM, Zapol WM, Lowenstein E. Neutralization of heparin anticoagulation. *In* Gravlee GP, Davis RF, Utley JR (eds). Cardiopulmonary Bypass Principles and Practice. Baltimore: Williams & Wilkins, 1993:381.

57. Murphy ME, Kolvenbach R, Aleksis M, et al. Antioxidant depletion in aortic cross clamping ischemia: increase of the plasma α-tocopheryl quinone/α-tocopherol ratio. Free Radic Biol Med 1992;13:95.

58. Murphy PG, Bennett JR, Myers DS, et al. The effect of propofol anaesthesia on free radical-induced lipid peroxidation in rat liver microsomes. Eur J Anaesthesiol 1993;10:261.

59. Newman MF, Murkin JM, Roach G, et al. Cerebral physiologic effects of burst suppression doses of propofol during nonpulsatile cardiopulmonary bypass: CNS subgroup of McSPI. Anesth Analg 1995;81:452.

60. Ovrum E, Holen EA, Tangen G, et al. Completely heparinized cardiopulmonary bypass and reduced systemic heparin: clinical and hemostatic effects. Ann Thorac Surg 1995;60:365.

61. Panneton JM, Hollier LH. Nondissecting thoracoabdominal aortic aneurysms: part I. Ann Vasc Surg 1995;9:503.

62. Panneton JM, Hollier LH. Dissecting descending thoracic and thoracoabdominal aortic aneurysms: part II. Ann Vasc Surg 1995;9:596.

63. Paterson IS, Klausner JM, Goldman G, et al. Pulmonary edema after aneurysm surgery is modified by mannitol. Ann Surg 1989;210:796.

64. Safi HJ, Bartoli S, Hess KR, et al. Neurologic deficit in patients at high risk with thoracoabdominal aortic aneurysms: the role of cerebral spinal fluid drainage and distal aortic perfusion. J Vasc Surg 1994;20:434.

65. Safi HJ, Hess KR, Randel M, et al. Cerebral spinal fluid drainage and distal aortic perfusion: reducing neurologic complications in repair of thoracoabdominal aortic aneurysm type I and II. J Vasc Surg 1996;23:223.

66. Sasaki S, Matsui Y, Gohda T, et al. Clinical investigation on the adjunctive method in the surgery of thoracic aortic aneurysms—comparison of the temporary bypass and partial extracorporeal bypass. Nippon Kyobu Geka Gakkai Zasshi 1991;39:2006.

67. Seekamp A, Mulligan MS. Role of $\beta 2$ integrins and ICAM-1 in lung injury following ischemia-reperfusion of rat hind limbs. Am J Pathol 1993;143:464.

68. Seekamp A, Mulligan MS, Till GO, et al. Requirements for neutrophil products and L-arginine in ischemia-reperfusion injury. Am J Pathol 1993;142:1217.

69. Shenaq SA, Svensson LG. Paraplegia following aortic surgery [review]. J Cardiothorac Vasc Anesth 1993;7:81.

70. Shyr MH, Tsai TH, Tan PP, et al. Concentration and regional distribution of propofol in brain and spinal cord during propofol anesthesia in the rat. Neurosci Lett 1995;184:212.

71. Simpson JI, Eide TR, Schiff GA, et al. Effect of nitroglycerin on spinal cord ischemia after thoracic aortic cross-clamping. Ann Thorac Surg 1996;61:113.

72. Smith I, White PF, Nathanson M, et al. Propofol: an update on its clinical use. Anesthesiology 1994;81:1005.

73. Sundt TM, Kouchoukos NT, Saffitz JE, et al. Renal dysfunction and intravascular coagulation with aprotinin and hypothermic circulatory arrest. Ann Thorac Surg 1993;55:1418.

74. Svensson LG, Hess KR, Coselli JS, et al. Influence of segmental arteries, extent, and atriofemoral bypass on postoperative paraplegia after thoracoabdominal aortic operations. J Vasc Surg 1994;20:255.

75. Tan S, Gelman S, Wheat JK, et al. Circulating xanthine oxidase in human ischemia reperfusion. South Med J 1995;88:479.

76. Temeck BK, Bachenheimer LC, Katz NM, et al. Desmopressin acetate in cardiac surgery: a double-blind, randomized study. South Med J 1994;87:611.

77. Valiathan MS, Weldon CS, Bender HW Jr, et al. Resection of aneurysms of the descending thoracic aorta using a GBH-coated shunt bypass. J Surg Res 1968;8:197.

78. Verdant A, Page A, Cossette R, et al. Surgery of the descending thoracic aorta: spinal cord protection with the Gott shunt. Ann Thorac Surg 1988;46:147.

79. Verdant A, Page A, Cossette R, et al. Surgery of the descending thoracic aorta: spinal cord protection with the Gott shunt. Ann Thorac Surg 1995;60:1151.
80. Videm V, Svennevig JL, Fosse E, et al. Reduced complement activation with heparin-coated oxygenator and tubings in coronary bypass operations. J Thorac Cardiovasc Surg 1992;103:806.
81. von Segesser LK, Killer I, Jenni R, et al. Improved distal circulatory support for repair of descending thoracic aortic aneurysms. Ann Thorac Surg 1993;56:1373.
82. von Segesser LK, Weiss BM, Garcia E, et al. Reduced blood loss and transfusion requirements with low systemic heparinization: preliminary clinical results in coronary artery revascularization. Eur J Cardiothorac Surg 1990;4:639.
83. von Segesser LK, Weiss BM, Garcia E, et al. Reduction and elimination of systemic heparinization during cardiopulmonary bypass. J Thorac Cardiovasc Surg 1992;103:790.
84. von Segesser LK, Weiss BM, Pasic M, et al. Risk and benefit of low systemic heparinization during open heart operations. Ann Thorac Surg 1994;58:391.
85. Wang JS, Lin CY, Hung WT, et al. Monitoring of heparin-induced anticoagulation with kaolin-activated clotting time in cardiac surgical patients treated with aprotinin. Anesthesiology 1992;77:1080.
86. Wisselink W, Money SR, Crockett DE. Ischemia-reperfusion injury of the spinal cord: protective effect of the hydroxyl radical scavenger dimethylthiourea. J Vasc Surg 1994;20:444.
87. Yum SW, Faden AI. Comparison of the neuroprotective effects of the N-methyl-D-aspartate antagonist MK-801 and the opiate-receptor antagonist nalmefene in experimental spinal cord ischemia. Arch Neurol 1990;47:277.

CHAPTER 7

Thoracoabdominal Aortic Aneurysm Repair

Hazim J. Safi, M.D., Charles C. Miller, III, Ph.D.,
Matthew P. Campbell, M.D., and
Dimitrios C. Iliopoulos, M.D.

When mid-century surgeons considered the feasibility of thoracoabdominal aortic aneurysm (TAAA) repair, their first hurdle was to avoid catastrophic bleeding while supplying adequate blood to the lower extremities and vital organs. Major developments in antibiotics, anticoagulants, and blood transfusions set the stage, and in 1955, Etheredge described the method that "helped give us the courage to operate on the patient we are reporting." In this first successful TAAA operation, blood supply was adequately maintained to the limbs by a temporary shunt.[1, 2]

Training for a second generation of cardiovascular surgeons extends well beyond basic technique and mechanics. To continue the decline in morbidity and mortality rates, research efforts are directed at preservation of the different organ systems involved in TAAA repair, each of which produces its own vascular syndromes. To safeguard the spinal cord, kidneys, liver, and lungs, the surgeon must have a comprehensive understanding of the related hemodynamics, pathophysiology, and drug therapies.

In this chapter, we discuss some of our findings and ideas in regard to research and the ways in which information is collected, analyzed, and communicated. Great strides have been made in some areas of multi-organ protection, but in others, we are only beginning to determine the function and risk factors of the systems involved.

Aneurysm Classification

The surgical community has amassed a large sum of cases, experience is varied, and procedures continue to evolve. As data mount, analysis becomes increasingly complex. A meaningful exchange of ideas and information between investigators requires a standardized system for collecting and reporting data that are readily distributed and easily understood.

In 1986, Crawford, recognizing the correlation between aneurysm extent and patient outcome, defined four significant types of TAAAs.[3] Since then, many investigations, involving groups of 2 to 1500 patients, have considered the relationship of aneurysm extent to patient outcome and organ system dysfunction. The reported data are often difficult to interpret, largely because aneurysm classification has been uneven or sometimes nonexistent. Although repair of any portion of the aorta can result in organ dysfunction, we know that the aneurysm of greatest extent (ie, type II TAAA) places the patient at highest risk (Figs. 7–1 and 7–2). Studies that combine analyses of all patients cannot discern the effectiveness of surgical adjuncts on organ protection. Comparison studies are of great value and need a standardized system of classification.

As data analyses have become further refined, we have found that a modification of the Crawford classification can be useful (Fig. 7–3). Using the original Crawford classification, an aneurysm that occurs within the sixth intercostal space to above the renal arteries is poorly defined. Most of these aneurysms are labeled as type I, but they occasionally are classified as type II. Designating these aneurysms type V and labeling all future TAAAs as types I through V would help to better analyze study results. We suspect that separating type V from type I will shed new light on the cause of neurologic complications and the success or failure rates of surgical adjuncts.

Statistical Analysis

Critical to learning from experience are appropriate data organization and analysis. Standardized protocols are essential for ensuring complete, unbiased data collection on critical variables and in maintaining uniformity of data acquisition for all patients. We have found it extremely useful to collect data prospectively in an electronic database, and statistical theory and practical experience have taught us to be alert to missing data. Ironically, we often find that data are most likely to be absent for the most complex patient. Patients for whom data are difficult to collect are the ones we need to track most closely.

Formal statistical analysis of collected data permits us to summarize experience in ways we can understand and allows us to make inferences about future experience based on past results. Statistics also give us an estimate of

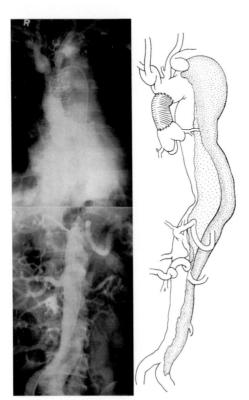

Figure 7–1. Aortogram and illustration of type II thoracoabdominal aortic aneurysm (TAAA) after ascending aorta graft replacement. The type II TAAA extended from distal to the left subclavian artery to the aortic bifurcation with type B aortic dissection.

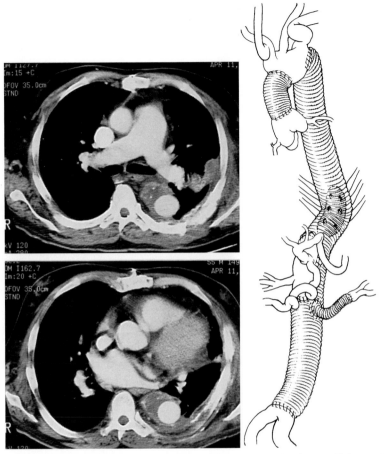

Figure 7–2. Computed tomography scan and illustration of repair for the type II thoracoabdominal aortic aneurysm in Figure 7–1. Intercostal arteries T10 through T12 were reattached, and a bypass was performed to the left renal artery.

how precise our inferences are, so that patients and surgeons can know what to expect. In our research, we start with simple univariate analyses to look for individual risk factors before attempting multivariate analyses. When possible, we also use visual inspection of plotted data to better understand the data properties and to ensure the mathematical descriptions are reasonable. Statistical analysis has been invaluable in helping us to understand complex relationships among patient characteristics, organ preservation techniques, and outcome, and we have adapted our techniques based on our findings.

Protective Measures During Aneurysm Repair

Spinal Cord Protection

A clamp applied to the aorta and halting blood flow for sufficient time to perform TAAA graft replacement aggravates the risk of transient neurologic dysfunction or, at worse, irreversible paraplegia. For the earliest TAAA operations, passive shunts directed the flow of blood around the operative field.[1, 2, 4, 5] Though a passive shunt can maintain distal aortic flow, spinal cord circulation is adequate only if the arterial radicularis magna, or artery of Adamkiewicz, originates beyond the distal clamp. Early TAAA operations were plagued by higher morbidity and mortality from bleeding embolization or

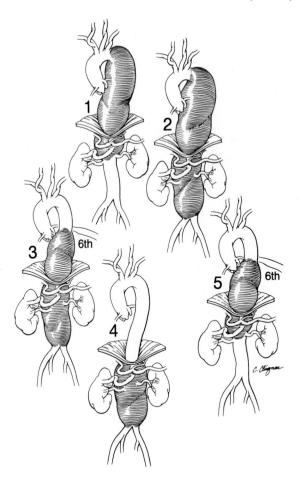

Figure 7–3. Thoracoabdominal aortic aneurysm classification. Type I: from below the left subclavian to above the celiac axis or opposite the superior mesenteric and above the renal arteries. Type II: from below the left subclavian and including the infrarenal abdominal aorta to the level of the aortic bifurcation. Type III: from the sixth intercostal space, tapering to just above the infrarenal abdominal aorta to the iliac bifurcation. Type IV: from the 12th intercostal space, tapering to above the iliac bifurcation. Type V: from the sixth intercostal space, tapering to just above the renal arteries.

aortic disruption at the site of shunt implantation.[6] The next logical step was the pump. Pump bypass provides a controlled flow rate and proximal and distal aortic pressure and somewhat reduces the risk of neurologic deficit.[7–11]

At the same time that cardiovascular surgeons probed the efficacy of shunts and bypasses, many other ways to lower the incidence of neurologic deficit were examined. Hypothermic circulatory arrest, spinal cord cooling, cerebrospinal fluid drainage, and pharmacologic agents demonstrated limited success.[12–20] Many of these methods, including shunts, remain in use, but no standardized technique is considered clearly superior in the prevention of neurologic deficits. Our group found that distal aortic perfusion combined with cerebrospinal fluid drainage provided the best protection.[21–23]

Cerebrospinal Fluid Drainage and Distal Aortic Perfusion

The rationale for combining cerebrospinal fluid drainage and distal aortic perfusion is illustrated in Figure 7–4. During aortic crossclamping, distal aortic pressure decreases markedly, causing a reduction in spinal artery perfusion pressure and a subsequent rise in cerebrospinal fluid pressure. Left atrial to left femoral bypass, or distal aortic perfusion, increases distal aortic pressure, leading to an increase in the spinal artery perfusion pressure and increasing blood flow to the spinal cord. Cerebrospinal fluid drainage further decreases cerebrospinal fluid pressure and augments perfusion of the spinal cord.[14, 15] These modalities have significantly reduced the incidence of neurologic deficit in our experience.

Figure 7–5 shows the cannulation and perfusion route delivered by a Bio-Medicus pump throughout TAAA repair. Figure 7–6 illustrates catheter insertion for cerebrospinal fluid drainage. These modalities are implemented in all instances, except when patient anatomy or emergency procedures make cannulation or catheter insertion impossible. Cerebrospinal fluid drainage is continuous, applied intraoperatively and until 3 days postoperatively. The drainage catheter is immediately reinserted if there is neurologic deficit after the regular postoperative period.

Our first series to explore the effectiveness of these adjuncts was limited solely to highest-risk type I and type II TAAAs.[21] We investigated the results of 94 patients who underwent TAAA repair with cerebrospinal fluid drainage and distal aortic perfusion, and we compared these data with those for 42 patients who underwent similar repair, although without adjuncts. Neurologic complications occurred in 8 (9%) of 94 patients in the first group and in 8 (19%) of 42 in the second ($p = .090$). We later studied the outcome of 343 patients operated for TAAA and descending thoracic aortic aneurysm (DTAA) between January 1991 and March 1996.[22] The outcome of these patients was similar to that found in our previous study, with the incidence of neurologic complications for types I and II remaining at 9%. In 1993, Svensson and colleagues reported the incidence of neurologic deficit for crossclamped patients: 16% overall, 15% for types I and II, and 31% for type II.[24]

Before the adjuncts of distal aortic perfusion and cerebrospinal fluid drainage were used, speed of the operation was linked to probability of a good outcome. With clamp time as the critical variable, the value of reimplanting intercostal arteries—which requires additional time—has been controversial. We investigated the role of intercostal artery management in the occurrence

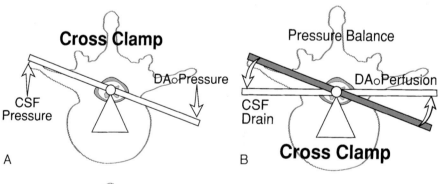

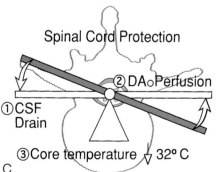

Figure 7–4. *A,* Aortic crossclamping decreases distal aortic pressure and elevates cerebrospinal fluid pressure. *B,* Distal aortic perfusion increases distal aortic pressure, leading to an increase in the spinal artery perfusion pressure, thereby increasing blood flow to the spinal cord. *C,* The addition of cerebrospinal fluid drainage further decreases cerebrospinal fluid pressure and augments the perfusion of the spinal cord. Moderated hypothermia, lowering the core temperature to 32°C, provides additional protection.

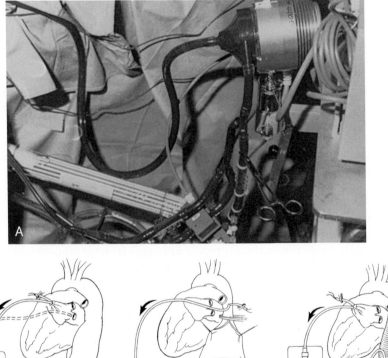

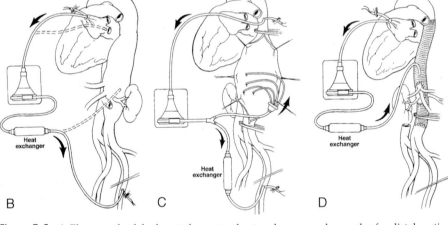

Figure 7–5. *A,* Photograph of the layout for pump, heat exchanger, and cannulas for distal aortic perfusion. (Courtesy of BioMedicus, Minneapolis, MN.) *B,* Initial cannulation of the left atrial appendage and left femoral artery for distal aortic perfusion. Alternatively, in cases of occlusion or previous aortobifemoral bypass, the upper or lower pulmonary vein and the distal thoracic or proximal abdominal aorta are used. *C,* Perfusion of the visceral vessels. *D,* After graft replacement and reattachment of visceral arteries, the heat exchanger is used to rewarm the patient.

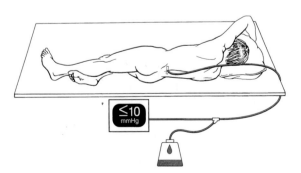

Figure 7–6. Catheter insertion for cerebrospinal fluid drainage. Pressure is maintained at or below 10 mm Hg.

of neurologic deficit. Management of arteries from T6 to T12 was reviewed to determine whether patterns of ligation, reimplantation, or occlusion due to long-standing thromboembolism or atrophy were associated with variations in outcome. We determined that ligation of patent arteries below the level of T9 was associated with large increases in the prevalence of neurologic deficit (Fig. 7–7). Patients whose vessels were occluded below this level had the best neurologic outcome, presumably because of well-established collateralization. When technically feasible, we recommend that all patent intercostal arteries from T9 to T12 be reimplanted.

Cerebrospinal fluid drainage and distal aortic perfusion decrease the incidence of neurologic deficit and are particularly effective for patients at highest risk with type II TAAAs. Moderate hypothermia appears to further extend the tolerance of the spinal cord to ischemia and should be studied at length in the future. Neurologic complications, although diminished, continue to pose a great risk to the patient. Ongoing research is critical for continued improvement that will be best communicated by carefully analyzed data and a universal system of aneurysm classification.

Renal Protection

The incidence of acute renal failure in TAAA or DTAA repair varies between 4% and 29%, depending on the series.[25-28] Studies have linked the incidence of renal failure to age, male sex, renal occlusive disease, preoperative renal failure, stroke, elevated preoperative creatinine, and visceral ischemia.[25, 28] Surgical adjuncts to decrease renal failure have included various methods of renal perfusion, intraoperative treatment with agents such as mannitol and dopamine, free radical scavengers, and angiotensin antagonists.[25, 28-32] Loop diuretics and free radical scavengers have not proved effective.[33] Inhibition of endothelial-derived relaxing factor aggravated ischemic renal failure.[34] Another study suggested that endothelin antagonists might provide a protective effect against the development of postischemic renal failure.[35]

A profound increase in angiotensin II was found in dogs undergoing nonpulsatile cardiopulmonary bypass with pulsatile perfusion attenuating this response.[36] Normalization of renal cortical blood flow was demonstrated after infusion of a converting enzyme inhibitor in dogs undergoing thoracic aortic crossclamping.[37]

We evaluated the outcome of 234 patients who underwent TAAA and

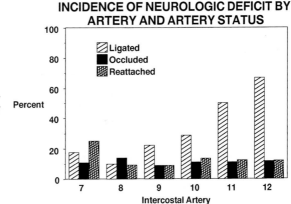

Figure 7–7. Incidence of neurologic deficit by artery and artery status.

DTAA repair with visceral or distal aortic perfusion or both.[38] Perfusion of the distal aorta or visceral arteries was used as an adjunct in most cases, and we used no further adjunctive renal protective modalities such as dopamine or diuretic therapy. Distal aortic perfusion alone (see Fig. 7–5B) was used when the aneurysm did not extend below the renal arteries (ie, DTAA and type I TAAA). Visceral perfusion (see Fig. 7–5C) was used in conjunction with distal perfusion for repair of aneurysms that extended below the renal arteries (ie, type II TAAA). Distal aortic perfusion was protective against renal failure, but visceral perfusion was not.

We found that acute renal failure, defined as an increase in the serum creatinine concentration of 1 mg/dL each day above the preoperative value for 2 consecutive days or defined by required hemodialysis, developed in 41 (17.5%) of 234 patients. Of the patients who developed acute renal failure, 36 (88%) of 41 went on to require hemodialysis, and 20 (49%) of 41 patients died. Age; sex; hypertension; right renal artery reattachment; DTAA; TAAA types I, III, and IV; renal perfusion time; and chronic obstructive pulmonary disease were not associated with an increased risk of renal failure. In univariate analysis, the risk factors were type II TAAA, elevated preoperative creatinine, preoperative renal insufficiency, visceral perfusion, simple aortic clamp technique, and left renal artery reattachment.

The association of direct visceral perfusion with increased risk was unexpected and difficult to explain. A working hypothesis during the exploration of these data was that the increased acute renal failure associated with visceral perfusion in part resulted from confounding aneurysm extent (TAAA type II in particular) with the perfusion technique required to support the kidneys during this type of repair. But multivariate statistical methods did not separate these effects mathematically, indicating that the risk associated with visceral perfusion was not accounted for entirely by the extent of the aneurysm.

These inconclusive results warrant further experimental studies to elucidate the mechanisms of renal failure with direct perfusion. Such studies may include randomized trials of pulsatile compared with nonpulsatile perfusion adjuncts, comparisons of use and nonuse of direct perfusion, and studies of pharmacologic agents with specific renal action that may be useful in further reducing the serious problem of renal failure in TAAA and DTAA surgery.

Liver Protection

Aneurysm rupture, a history of hepatitis, and emergency presentation are significant predictors of liver function abnormalities for all patients. Type II TAAA, of all aneurysm types, is most vulnerable to liver dysfunction after graft replacement. A patient with this type of aneurysm also is most likely to suffer neurologic, renal, and pulmonary complications and diminished long-term survival.[21, 22, 38–40] Liver dysfunction is difficult to study because the diagnosis is made clinically and because definitive criteria for diagnosing liver disease from retrospective data do not exist.

Despite the difficulty of diagnosis, practical measurements of clinical laboratory values can be used to study hepatic insult after surgery. Although nonspecific for hepatic injury, elevated enzyme levels are a well-documented result of ischemic hepatitis.[41–44] In our study of 286 patients operated for TAAA or DTAA between January 1991 and July 1996, we used a variety of laboratory and statistical tests to measure hepatic insult and to identify risk factors for such insult that might be amenable to modification through refinements in surgical technique.[45] A comparison of baseline with postoperative enzyme measurements determined the impact of visceral and distal perfusion on liver function after TAAA and DTAA repair.

Linear regression models were used to evaluate the effects of aneurysm extent and distal and visceral perfusion on postoperative laboratory values expressed as continuous variables. For categorical analyses, an indicator variable for abnormal laboratory values was set to a value of one of any of the laboratory values of alkaline phosphates, lactate dehydrogenase, aspartate aminotransferase, alanine aminotransferase, prothrombin time, or partial thromboplastin time greater than four times the upper limit of the normal range or the total bilirubin value greater than 10.

Univariate analysis of risk factors for all patients revealed type II TAAA, rupture, a history of hepatitis, and emergency presentation to be significant predictors of liver function abnormalities. In multivariate categorical analysis, type II aneurysm, history of hepatitis, and emergency presentation remained significant predictors of abnormal laboratory findings.

In linear regression analysis, predictors of postoperative laboratory values were rupture, preoperative value of each variable, and type II aneurysm. In the frequency analysis, in which only the most severe laboratory abnormalities were counted, visceral perfusion was not shown to be significantly protective, although such a trend was observed. In the linear regression analyses, in which the response variables are continuous rather than dichotomous, the effect of visceral perfusion was significant and scaled almost identically to the deleterious effect of type II aneurysm.

Lung Protection

Not surprisingly, TAAA patients are prone to respiratory complications after surgery. Many of these patients are older and have been smokers, which increases the risk of general anesthesia and may complicate ventilator weaning. The operation requires deflation of one lung and prolonged atelectasis and demands administration of blood and blood products. We have begun to study the incidence of postoperative respiratory problems and are investigating the contributions of preoperative pulmonary function, age, smoking history, and use of blood products intraoperatively. Preliminary results indicate that total clamp time, current cigarette smoking, and blood transfusions increase the risk of postoperative respiratory failure.

Preoperative adjuncts to decrease respiratory failure that must be examined closely include cessation of smoking and preoperative pulmonary treatment, including bronchodilators and chest physiotherapy. Studies of the effect of diaphragm preservation in selected patients may be helpful. Further investigation into this vexing problem is warranted.

Conclusions

In the quest to resolve the complex problems of multi-organ protection for TAAA and DTAA repair, many more questions may be raised than are answered. Spinal cord protection, the most critical issue in the outcome of the patient, has been our main focus. Great progress has been made since the 12% to 31% incidence of neurologic deficit recorded in the early days of TAAA repair.[3, 24] Protection of the lungs, liver, and kidneys, however, has largely shared the type of adjuncts devoted to spinal cord protection.

Using consistent aneurysm classification and sound statistical analysis, we have learned much about the risk factors involved in organ dysfunction. We must now further refine our methods to better safeguard each area of the multi-organ system.

References

1. Etheredge SN, Yee J, Smith JV, et al. Successful resection of a large aneurysm of the upper abdominal aorta and replacement with homograft. Surgery 1955;38:1071–1081.
2. Schafer PW, Hardin CA. The use of temporary polythene shunts to permit occlusion, resection and frozen homologous graft replacement of vital vessel segments. Surgery 1952;31:186–199.
3. Crawford ES, Crawford JL, Safi HJ, et al. Thoracoabdominal aortic aneurysms: preoperative and intraoperative factors determining immediate and long-term results of operations in 605 patients. J Vasc Surg 1986;3:389–404.
4. DeBakey ME, Crawford ES, Garrett HE, et al. Surgical considerations in the treatment of aneurysms of the thoraco-abdominal aorta. Ann Surg 1965;162:650–662.
5. Gott LL, Whiffen JD, Dutlon RC. Heparin binding on colloidal graphite surfaces. Science 1963;142:1297–1298.
6. Hollier LH. Protecting the brain and spinal cord. J Vasc Surg 1987;5:524.
7. Olivier HF, Maher TD, Liebler GA, et al. Use of the Bio-Medicus centrifugal pump in traumatic tears of the thoracic aorta. Ann Thorac Surg 1984;38:586–591.
8. Austen GW, Shaw RS. Experimental studies with extracorporeal circuits as a method to enable surgical attack on thoracic aneurysms. J Thorac Cardiovasc Surg 1960;39:337–356.
9. Connolly JE, Wakabayashi A, German JC, et al. Clinical experience with pulsatile left heart bypass without anti-coagulation for thoracic aneurysms. J Thorac Cardiovasc Surg 1971;62:568–576.
10. Crawford ES, Mizrahi EM, Hess KR, et al. The impact of distal aortic perfusion and somatosensory evoked potential monitoring on prevention of paraplegia after aortic aneurysm operation. J Thorac Cardiovasc Surg 1988;95:357–367.
11. Wadouh F, Lindemann EM, Arndt CF, et al. The arteria radicularis magna anterior as a decisive factor influencing spinal cord damage during aortic occlusion. J Thorac Cardiovasc Surg 1984;88:1–10.
12. Kouchoukos NT, Wareing TH, Izumoto H, et al. Elective hypothermic cardiopulmonary bypass and circulatory arrest for spinal cord protection during operations on the thoracoabdominal aorta. J Thorac Cardiovasc Surg 1990;99:659–664.
13. Davison JK, Cambria RP, Vierra DJ, et al. Epidural cooling for regional spinal cord hypothermia during thoracoabdominal aneurysm repair. J Vasc Surg 1994;20:304–310.
14. Miyamoto K, Ueno A, Wada T, et al. A new and simple method of preventing spinal cord damage following temporary occlusion of the thoracic aorta by draining the cerebrospinal fluid. J Cardiovasc Surg (Torino) 1960;16:188–197.
15. Hollier LH, Money SR, Naslund TC, et al. Risk of spinal cord dysfunction in patients undergoing thoracoabdominal aortic replacement. Am J Surg 1992;164:210–214.
16. Archer CW, Wynn MM, Archibald J. Naloxone and spinal fluid drainage as adjuncts in the surgical treatment of thoracoabdominal and thoracic aneurysms. Surgery 1990;108:755–762.
17. Agge JM, Flanagan T, Blackbourne LH, et al. Reducing postischemic paraplegia using conjugated superoxide dismutase. Ann Thorac Surg 1991;51:911–915.
18. Gerhardt EB, Stewart JR, Morrison JG, et al. Spinal cord protection during ischemia: comparison of mannitol, thiopental, and free radical scavengers. Surg Forum 1987;38:197–199.
19. Svensson LG, Stewart RW, Cosgrove DM, et al. Intrathecal papaverine for the prevention of paraplegia after operation on the thoracic or thoracoabdominal aorta. J Thorac Cardiovasc Surg 1988;96:823–829.
20. Granke K, Hollier LH, Zdrahal P, et al. Longitudinal study of cerebral spinal fluid drainage in polyethylene-glycol-conjugated superoxide dismutase in paraplegia associated with thoracic aortic cross-clamping. J Vasc Surg 1991;13:615–621.
21. Safi HJ, Bartoli S, Hess KR, et al. Neurologic deficit in patients at high risk with thoracoabdominal aortic aneurysms: the role of cerebral spinal fluid drainage and distal aortic perfusion. J Vasc Surg 1994;20:434–443.
22. Safi HJ, Hess KR, Randel M, et al. Cerebrospinal fluid drainage and distal aortic perfusion: reducing neurologic complications in repair of thoracoabdominal aortic aneurysm types I and II. J Vasc Surg 1996;23:223–229.
23. Safi HJ, Campbell MP, Miller CC, et al. Cerebral spinal fluid drainage and distal aortic perfusion decrease the incidence of neurological deficit: the results of 343 descending and thoracoabdominal aortic aneurysm repair. Eur J Endo Vasc Surg 1997;14:118–124.
24. Svensson LG, Crawford ES, Hess KR, et al. Experience with 1509 patients undergoing thoracoabdominal aortic operations. J Vasc Surg 1993;17:357–368.
25. Frank SM, Parker SD, Rock P, et al. Moderate hypothermia with partial bypass and segmental sequential repair for thoracoabdominal aortic aneurysm. J Vasc Surg 1994;19:687–697.
26. Schepens MA, Defauw JJ, Hamerlinjnck MP, Vermeulen FE. Risk assessment of acute renal failure after thoracoabdominal aortic aneurysm surgery. Ann Surg 1994;219:400–407.
27. Golden MA, Donaldson MC, Whittemore AD, Mannick JA. Evolving experience with thoracoabdominal aortic aneurysm repair at a single institution. J Vasc Surg 1986;13:792–797.
28. Svensson LG, Coselli JS, Safi HJ, et al. Appraisal of adjuncts to prevent acute renal failure after surgery on the thoracic or thoracoabdominal aorta. J Vasc Surg 1989;10:230–239.

29. Safi HJ, Cox GS. A new technique for left renal cryopreservation. J Am Coll Surg 1994;178:629–631.
30. Waite RB, White G, Davis JH. Beneficial effects of verapamil on postischemic renal failure. Surgery 1983;94:276–282.
31. Pedraza-Chaverri J, Tapia E, Bobadilla N. Ischemia-reperfusion induced acute renal failure in the rat is ameliorated by the spin-trapping agent α-phenyl-*N*-tert-butyl nitrone (PBN). Ren Fail 1992;14:467–471.
32. Abbott WM, Abel RM, Beck CH. The reversal of renal cortical ischemia during aortic occlusion by mannitol. J Surg Res 1974;16:482–487.
33. Wolgast M, Bayati A, Hellberg O, et al. Osmotic diuretics and hemodilution in postischemic renal failure. Ren Fail 1992;14:297–302.
34. Chintala MS, Chiu PJS, Vemapulli S, et al. Inhibition of endothelial derived relaxing factor (EDRF) aggravates ischemic acute renal failure in anesthetized rats. Naunyn Schmiedebergs Arch Pharmacol 1993;348:305–310.
35. Kusumoto K, Kubo K, Kandori H, et al. Effects of a new endothelin antagonist, TAK-044, on post-ischemic acute renal failure in rats. Life Sci 1994;55:301–310.
36. Watkins L, Lucas SK, Gardner TJ, et al. Angiotensin II levels during cardiopulmonary bypass: a comparison of pulsatile and nonpulsatile flow. Surg Forum 1979;30:229–230.
37. Joob AW, Dunn C, Miller E, et al. Effect of left atrial to left femoral artery bypass and renin-angiotensin system blockade on renal blood flow and function during and after thoracic aortic occlusion. J Vasc Surg 1987;5:329–335.
38. Safi HJ, Harlin S, Joshi A, et al. Predictive factors for renal failure in thoracic and thoracoabdominal aortic aneurysm surgery. J Vasc Surg 1996;24:338–345.
39. Svensson LG, Hess KR, Coselli JS, et al. A prospective study of respiratory failure after high risk surgery on the thoracoabdominal aorta. J Vasc Surg 1991;14:271–272.
40. Safi HJ, Miller CC, Iliopoulos DC, Griffiths G. Long-term results following thoracoabdominal aortic aneurysm repair. *In* Branchereau A (ed). La Chirurgie Vasculaire Actuelle. Marseille: Arnette Blackwell, 1997.
41. Bynum TE, Boitnott JK, Maddrey WC. Ischemic hepatitis. Dig Dis Sci 1979;24:129–135.
42. Cassidy WM, Reynolds TB. Serum lactic dehydrogenase in the differential diagnosis of acute hepato-cellular injury. J Clin Gastroenterol 1994;19:118–121.
43. Gitlin N, Serio KM. Ischemic hepatitis: widening horizons. Am J Gastroenterol 1992;87:831–836.
44. Kamiyama T, Miyakawa H, Tajiri K, et al. Ischemic hepatitis in cirrhosis: clinical features and prognostic implications. J Clin Gastroenterol 1996;22:126–130.
45. Safi HJ, Miller CC, Yawn DH, et al. The impact of distal aortic and visceral perfusion on liver function during thoracoabdominal and descending thoracic aortic repair. J Vasc Surg 1998;27:145–153.

Treatment of Type B Aortic Dissections

David C. Brewster, M.D.

Although the term *aneurysme dissequant* (ie, dissecting aneurysm) was first used by Laennec in 1819 and has continued to be used to describe the disease process since that time, it is a misnomer. During the acute phase of the condition, the aorta is often somewhat dilated but is rarely aneurysmal. The process is more accurately described as an intramural hematoma that dissects between layers of the aortic wall because of arterial pressure. The term *acute aortic dissection* is therefore a more appropriate depiction of the disorder and is more commonly employed today.[1]

Although significant advances in the diagnosis and treatment of aortic dissection have occurred during the past five decades, this condition remains a relatively common and highly morbid clinical event. Acute aortic dissection is the most common lethal catastrophe involving the aorta, with an incidence surpassing that of ruptured abdominal aortic aneurysm (AAA).[2,3] The misconception that ruptured AAA are more common results from the fact that most patients with this condition survive long enough to be seen by physicians, whereas those with acute dissection often die suddenly or are misdiagnosed as having died of a myocardial infarction or another condition.

The initiating mechanism in acute aortic dissection is a tear in the aortic intima through which blood surges into the media, separating aortic intima from adventitia. Dissections usually propagate from the intimal tear distally in the aorta, although retrograde extension can occur. The origin of any arterial trunk arising from the aorta may be compromised or the aortic valve rendered incompetent. Blood in the false channel can reenter the true aortic lumen anywhere along the course of the dissecting process, or external rupture may occur. Rupture of the aorta, the most common cause of death, occurs most frequently into the pericardial space or left pleural cavity. The importance of timely diagnosis lies in the fact that approximately 65% to 75% of patients with untreated acute aortic dissection die within the first 2 weeks after onset.[4,5]

Diagnosis

Although refinement in diagnostic modalities has clearly contributed to improved outcome over the past decade, a high index of suspicion for the condition remains the key to rapid diagnosis. Severe chest or back pain leading to presentation for treatment within hours of onset is reported by more than 90% of patients.[1] Pulse deficits can be a helpful physical examination finding. Because symptoms referable to aortic branch occlusion (eg, abdominal pain from mesenteric ischemia, acute lower extremity ischemia) may rapidly supersede back pain, the vascular surgeon may be the first to see the patient and have the opportunity to establish the diagnosis. We found that about 10% of patients with dissections present with primary complaints of lower extremity ischemia.

Diagnostic confusion with acute coronary syndromes is usually eliminated with appropriate electrocardiography, and plain chest radiographic findings usually are not helpful. Although contrast arteriography was previously the diagnostic procedure of choice, graft replacement of the ascending aorta for dissection is frequently undertaken in contemporary practice without it. Rapid diagnosis in the emergency room can readily be made with transesophageal echocardiography, rapid-sequence dynamic computed tomography (CT), or magnetic resonance imaging.[6] Even after the diagnosis is confirmed by any of these imaging modalities, aortography may be desirable to assess the degree of aortic insufficiency, assess the distal extent of the dissection, and elucidate the presence and mechanism of aortic branch compromise.

Treatment

Influence of Classification on Management

A key component in determining optimal therapy for patients with acute aortic dissection is the anatomic extent of the pathologic process. Patients with involvement of the ascending aorta or aortic arch in the dissection process, regardless of the extent of involvement beyond the left subclavian artery, are considered to have *proximal dissection* (ie, DeBakey classifications I and II, Stanford classification type A). Patients with aortic dissection originating beyond the left subclavian artery and involving variable extents of the descending thoracic or abdominal aorta (or both) and without involvement of the proximal aorta are classified as having *distal dissection* (ie, DeBakey types III A and B, Stanford type B).

The major risk for early death from acute aortic dissection correlates with central complications, including acute rupture of the aorta into the mediastinum or pleural cavity; rupture into the pericardium, causing acute tamponade; acute aortic valvular insufficiency with compromise of left ventricular function; or interference with coronary blood flow, causing myocardial ischemia or infarction. Such potentially lethal events are much more common in dissections involving the proximal aorta and account for the generally accepted approach of immediate direct surgical repair of the ascending aorta, aortic arch, or both in patients with proximal dissections, even if more distal segments of the aorta are involved.

Perhaps because of aortic structural differences and various profiles of changes in pressure over time (dP/dt), distal aortic dissections are considerably less likely to rupture in the acute phase. Optimal therapy for patients with acute type B dissection therefore remains much more controversial.[7-9] Possible management approaches include emergent direct surgical repair, medical management alone, selective surgical repair (ie, direct grafting or peripheral procedures), and endovascular interventions.

Direct Surgical Repair

In some centers, early thoracic aortic repair is thought to provide the best overall outcome.[10, 11] Graft replacement is performed through a left thoracotomy from just distal to the left subclavian origin, presumably just proximal to the site of the initiating intimal tear, to the middle or distal thoracic aorta, including the tear and portion of the distal aorta dilated more than 4 cm in diameter. The aorta is transected circumferentially and the intimal septum sutured to the outer adventitial layers so that the true lumen is reperfused and the false channel obliterated.

Although results of early graft repair of acute distal (type B) dissections have improved in the past decade, operative mortality remains significant, usually 10% to 25%, depending on the individual series reported.[10-13] This high rate frequently reflects the fact that dissection often occurs in older, severely hypertensive patients with multiple comorbid medical problems. Although highly dependent on individual preferences that vary considerably from center to center, immediate direct repair for acute type B dissection is probably best limited to younger, good-risk patients in whom early surgical replacement of the diseased aortic segment may confer the best long-term protection by decreasing the incidence of subsequent aneurysmal dilation, extension of the dissection, or late ischemic complications.[7, 9] It is also generally agreed that acute distal dissections in patients with Marfan's syndrome should be treated surgically.[1]

Medical Management Alone

In most centers, the consensus of opinion is that initial medical management of uncomplicated distal dissection is preferred and can provide better outcome.[1, 8, 12] The rationale for medical management in patients with distal dissections is based on several observations.[1] Proper drug therapy reduces the major forces tending to increase the dissection and its disastrous sequelae,[2] and medical therapy successfully prevents early death of most patients.[3] Even the contemporary operative mortality rate for immediate surgical therapy remains relatively high, because these patients are usually elderly with significant comorbid diseases.[4] Long-term outcomes have been similar for surgically and medically treated patients with distal dissections.

Medical therapy is continued unless indications for surgery develop. As first described by Wheat and colleagues in 1965, the aim of early and long-term medical treatment is to control the blood pressure and the force of ejection of blood from the heart by lowering the dP/dt.[14] Both these goals hope to prevent further extension of dissection and prevent progressive aortic dilatation and rupture. All patients should be managed initially in an intensive care unit setting with full monitoring. Intravenous administration of a fast-acting agent (eg, nitroprusside, Arfonad) is required to reduce cardiac output and blood pressure to the lowest possible level consistent with maintaining cerebral, coronary, and renal perfusion. Simultaneously, to reduce dP/dt quickly, an intravenous β-blocking drug (eg, propranolol, esmolol, metoprolol) is administered until there is evidence of satisfactory β-adrenergic blockade indicated by a pulse rate of less than 70 beats/min. Calcium channel antagonists (eg, diltiazem, nifedipine) can be used if other measures fail, because these agents lower blood pressure and decrease the dP/dt.

Although medical therapy generally suffices in the acute treatment of type B dissections, aortic rupture did occur in 10% of distal dissection cases in our review.[15] An important component of initiating and following the progress of medical therapy is the *size of the proximal descending thoracic aorta*. For patients with significant (>5 cm) aneurysmal dilation at the site of the aortic tear, consideration of early graft replacement is appropriate. When acute dissection occurs in continuity with a preexisting degenerative aortic aneurysm, the risk of rupture is high, and graft replacement is the appropriate therapy.[16]

After patients are stable and pain free, with good blood pressure and pulse rate control, intravenous medications can be gradually withdrawn and oral antihypertensive and negative inotropic medications begun. Careful follow-up is mandatory, and serial chest radiographs and CT scans are required to monitor aortic size and detect progressive chronic aneurysmal formation of the false channel.

Selective Surgical Therapy

If initial medical management of distal aortic dissections proves unsuccessful or complications of the dissection occur, selective surgical therapy by direct graft repair of the aorta or peripheral surgical repair of obstructed aortic branches may be undertaken. With such a selective approach, surgical repair is reserved for patients who experience continuous pain, evidence of bleeding, progressive aneurysmal dilation of the dissected aortic segment of more than 5 cm, or evidence of peripheral vascular complications. The latter is a relatively frequent complication of aortic dissection, with an incidence of approximately 33% of obstruction of major aortic branches, causing malperfusion of the lower extremities, kidneys, or major abdominal visceral organs. Such aortic branch occlusion sometimes constitutes the principal manifestation or becomes the primary focus of treatment in some patients.[2, 15, 17, 18] For this reason, the vascular surgeon may become an important member of the patient care team.[19]

Lower extremity ischemia due to aortic or iliac obstruction is the most common peripheral vascular manifestation of acute dissection.[15, 20] Ischemic complications of aortic branch vessel compromise also include upper extremity ischemia, neurologic events, and visceral (mesenteric and renal) ischemia (Fig. 8–1). The latter two are highly morbid conditions and associated with significantly increased mortality rates.[10, 15]

The most common mechanism of vessel obstruction involves extrinsic compression of the true arterial lumen by the bulging dissected false lumen, thereby compromising or obstructing flow to the vascular territory perfused by the branch vessel.[15, 20] This process may be circumferential at a branch vessel orifice, or it may extend for various distances into the particular branch (Fig. 8–2). On other occasions, the ostium of a branch vessel may be obstructed by disrupted intimal flaps or intussusception of detached intima into the proximal aspect of the branch artery. Rarely, embolic occlusion of vessels remote from the dissection process may occur after discharge of a clot from the false lumen.[18] Such embolic material may originate at the site of the initiating intimal tear or at a more distal point of reentry.

In addition to possible compromise of branch vessel origins by the dissection, in situ thrombus formation distal to the point of occlusion may occur because of stasis if the branch vessel flow obstruction is complete. In these circumstances, branch obstruction may persist despite correction of the dissection by proximal direct thoracic aortic repair. Similarly, continued obstruction of branch orifices by residual intimal flaps or remote embolization may persist despite redirection of flow into the true lumen by initial central repair. These circumstances explain why primary aortic repair may not always relieve the peripheral vascular complications of aortic dissection, and they emphasize that additional methods of revascularization may occasionally be required for a successful outcome.

Distribution of Peripheral Vascular Complications

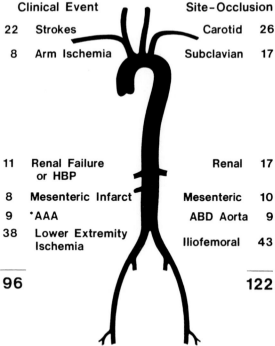

Clinical Event			Site-Occlusion	
22	Strokes		Carotid	26
8	Arm Ischemia		Subclavian	17
11	Renal Failure or HBP		Renal	17
8	Mesenteric Infarct		Mesenteric	10
9	*AAA		ABD Aorta	9
38	Lower Extremity Ischemia		Iliofemoral	43
96				**122**

*Aneurysm of abdominal or thoracoabdominal aorta resulting from dissection

Figure 8–1. Sites and distribution of peripheral vascular complications and related clinical events described in a Massachusetts General Hospital study. Disparity between occlusions and clinical events reflects asymptomatic occlusions. HBP, incidence of hypertension, ABD, abdominal. (From Cambria RP, Brewster DC, Gertler J, et al. Vascular complications associated with spontaneous aortic dissection. J Vasc Surg 1988;7:199–209.)

Spontaneous reentry of the false lumen (Fig. 8–3) may relieve obstruction in the true lumen and account for the fluctuating clinical picture of visceral or peripheral ischemic manifestations often observed in patients with acute dissection.[1] Reentry commonly occurs at points where aortic tributaries are

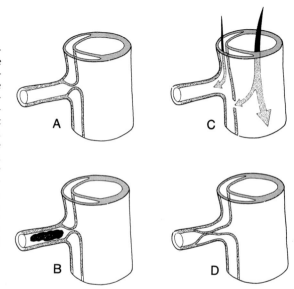

Figure 8–2. Mechanisms of aortic branch obstruction in acute dissection. Bulging of the false lumen can produce occlusion at the branch orifice *(A),* and subsequent thrombosis may occur distally *(B).* Intimal detachment at the branch orifice may occur with perfusion, largely through the false channel *(C).* The dissection process may also extend into the branch, causing obstruction beyond the branch orifice *(D).* (From Cambria RP, Brewster DC, Gertler J, et al. Vascular complications associated with spontaneous aortic dissection. J Vasc Surg 1988;7:199–209.)

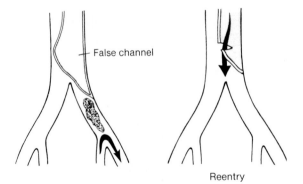

Figure 8–3. Compromise of true lumen by a dissection channel, producing distal aortic obstruction. This may be complicated by distal thrombosis or relieved by spontaneous or surgical reentry. (From Brewster DC, Cambria RP. Role of the vascular surgeon in the management of dissecting aortic aneurysms. *In* Veith FJ (ed). Current Critical Problems in Vascular Surgery. St. Louis: Quality Medical Publishing, 1989:291–302.)

sheared off or may occur spontaneously at one or more points along the dissection. Reentry provides communication between the true and false lumens, and it has the potential for double-channel distal perfusion or continued adequate perfusion of certain aortic branches solely from the false lumen. This concept provides the rationale for the surgical procedure of fenestration.

Although some complications (eg, pain, rupture, progressive dilation) mandate direct surgical repair, management of peripheral vascular complications may sometimes be treated by vascular procedures directed specifically at the obstructed branches. Such procedures include aortic fenestration, extraanatomic bypasses such as femorofemoral or axillofemoral grafts, and revascularization of ischemic renal or visceral arteries by means of bypasses from the infrarenal aorta or iliac vessels. Although most peripheral vascular complications may be successfully relieved with direct graft repair of the thoracic aortic dissection itself, branch obstruction may persist in approximately 10% to 15% of patients,[15, 17, 18] or a patient may be considered to be a high risk for direct graft repair of the thoracic aorta if it is not clearly necessary. These indirect surgical procedures continue to play a potentially useful role in selected patients.

The fenestration procedure as the only treatment modality can effectively restore lower extremity circulation and lead to acceptable long-term survival.[15, 21–24] Similarly, by establishing effective communication between true and false lumens, it often successfully restores perfusion of compromised renal or visceral arteries to treat acute renal or mesenteric or renal ischemia. The principal appeal of fenestration is that it offers potential correction of life- or limb-threatening vascular complications of dissection by means of a procedure that is probably safer and less morbid than others because it does not entail thoracic aortic clamping, require any form of cardiopulmonary bypass, or expose the patient to the possibility of ischemic spinal cord injury.

The procedure is usually carried out in the infrarenal aorta, and a retroperitoneal approach can be used if desired. The aorta is divided, and a portion of the proximal septum between the true and false lumens is excised, providing a reentry point and free communication of flow between the two channels (Fig. 8–4). Most often, segmental graft insertion is carried out, although primary reanastomosis of the divided aorta may be done. Proximally, the suture line involves all three layers of the normal aortic wall in the portion of the aortic circumference uninvolved with dissection (true lumen) and only the aortic adventitia in that portion representing the false lumen. Use of pledgeted sutures may obviate many of the acknowledged problems of anastomosis involving such friable aortic tissue. Distally, the graft anastomosis may reapproximate the true and false lumens by incorporating both layers of the aortic wall in the distal suture line, or a distal anastomosis may be constructed more distally into nondissected portions of the iliac or femoral vessels.

For lower extremity ischemia involving only one limb secondary to unilateral iliac obstruction, femorofemoral grafts offer an expedient and effective treatment, particularly in patients with otherwise uncomplicated distal (type III or B) dissections who may be treated preferentially by medical management.[15, 18] Use of axillobifemoral grafts has been described by Laas and colleagues for patients with bilateral lower extremity ischemia associated with compromise of the aortic lumen by more chronic dissections.[24] Extraanatomic grafts may be extremely useful in other locations, such as correction of persistent upper extremity ischemia after repair of proximal dissection by means of an axilloaxillary bypass.[15] Occasionally, carotid-carotid or subclavian-carotid bypass may be employed for cerebral ischemia persisting after aortic repair. Alternately, the possible existence of an acute neurologic deficit is believed to preclude immediate operation.[15]

Relief of acute mesenteric or renal ischemia, either following initial aortic repair that fails to adequately restore flow to these branches or in selected patients as a primary intervention, may be accomplished by either a fenestration procedure or direct bypass grafting. Grafts to the visceral or renal vessels may originate from the lower aspect of the infrarenal aorta if uninvolved with the dissection or, more commonly, from an uninvolved iliac artery. Alternatively, an aortic graft inserted as part of a fenestration procedure may serve as an origin for such bypass grafts to renal or visceral arteries if the surgeon does not feel confident enough that fenestration alone will adequately restore bowel or kidney perfusion.[25] Renal artery reconstruction may also be readily achieved by hepatorenal or splenorenal bypass grafts if the celiac origin is spared by the dissection.[26] Use of renal autotransplantation has also been reported as a method of renal salvage in aortic dissection.[27]

Endovascular Interventions

The continued high morbidity and mortality of aortic dissection, particularly when associated with peripheral vascular complications, has spawned interest in development of alternative forms of therapy that may perhaps be

Figure 8–4. In the fenestration procedure, the aorta is divided distal to the renal arteries, with true and false lumens evident. An ellipse or "window" of dissected intima is excised, and then the graft is sutured end to end to the composite lumen. (From Hunter JA, Dye WS, Javid H, et al. Abdominal aortic resection in thoracic dissection. Arch Surg 1976;111:1258–1262. Copyright 1976, American Medical Association.)

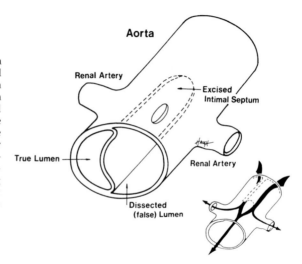

less morbid and more expedient than conventional surgical approaches. This is particularly true of dissections complicated by ischemia of the kidneys or abdominal viscera, in which irreversible and often lethal renal or bowel infarction may occur within hours of onset.

Several reports have described percutaneous catheter-based endovascular approaches and their potential application and appeal in the management of acute and chronic dissections.[28–36] Balloon dilatation catheters may be used percutaneously to enlarge small reentry points that are providing flow to end organs being exclusively perfused from the false channel or, in some instances, to establish de novo a point of reentry when these are absent by fenestrating the septum between the true and false lumens, thereby providing satisfactory flow and alleviating ischemic manifestations. As with surgical fenestration, balloon fenestration can be employed to decompress the false lumen if it is encroaching significantly on the true aortic lumen, thereby improving ante-grade flow to the lower extremities. Similarly, endovascular stents have been employed to treat the site of initiating intimal tear itself, improve a compromised true aortic lumen, or improve flow in compromised major aortic branches.[29, 30, 33, 35]

Such techniques may be applied for vascular complications of subacute or chronic dissections, but perhaps have their greatest appeal as emergent therapies performed at the time of diagnostic angiography.[29, 30, 33] In this fashion, they can serve as valuable adjunctive measures by minimizing critical organ ischemic time and thereby improving the patient's prognosis for definitive thoracic repair, or they can sometimes represent definitive therapy when nonoperative treatment of the dissection is judged preferable. In the largest experience reported, Slonim and colleagues[29] from Stanford reported results of balloon fenestration or endovascular stenting in a series of 22 patients (16 men, 6 women; mean age, 52 years) who had ischemic complications of 15 acute aortic dissections (6 Stanford type A, 9 type B) and 7 chronic aortic dissections (6 type A, 1 type B). Symptoms included renal ischemia in 13 patients, lower extremity ischemia in 10 patients, and mesenteric ischemia in 6 patients. Of these 22 patients, 16 were treated with endovascular stenting, including 11 patients with renal stents, 6 with lower extremity stents, 2 with a superior mesenteric artery stent, and 2 with aortic stents. Four patients were treated with balloon fenestration of the intimal flap, and 2 were treated with a combination of stenting and balloon fenestration.

Technically successful revascularization with initial clinical success was achieved in all 22 patients. Two patients had to be brought back for further endovascular management of persistent ischemic symptoms between 6 days and 2 months after the initial procedure. A third patient required additional intervention when new ischemic symptoms developed after spontaneous recanalization and expansion of his previously thrombosed false lumen. One patient died 3 days after the procedure of peritonitis that probably was related to prolonged bowel ischemia. One patient died of unrelated causes 13.4 months after the procedure. One patient was lost to follow-up. The mean follow-up time is 14.6 months. No patient has required surgical revascularization for an ischemic vascular bed. The only complication has been a guide wire–induced perinephric hematoma, which was treated with endovascular coil embolization. This complication had no long-term sequelae. For 8 patients, the endovascular procedure was the only therapy, because no surgical repair of the dissection was performed.[29]

Conclusions

Peripheral vascular complications occur in approximately one third of aortic dissections as a consequence of compromise of major branch vessel flow by the dissection process. A variety of ischemic manifestations may occur, most often involving lower extremity ischemia but also potentially affecting the upper extremities, central nervous system, or circulation to the kidneys or intestines. Although direct thoracic repair of the dissection itself often corrects or alleviates the peripheral vascular complications, vascular surgical procedures may be necessary if branch vessel obstruction persists after thoracic aortic repair or if the dissection is preferentially treated by nonoperative management. In some patients, critical renal, mesenteric, or advanced lower extremity ischemia may assume treatment priority. A variety of reconstruction options are available. Newer endovascular treatment modalities appear to hold promise in the treatment of some of these complications.

References

1. DeSanctis RW, Doroghazi RM, Austen WG, Buckley MJ. Medical progress: aortic dissection. N Engl J Med 1987;317:1060–1067.
2. Walker PJ, Sarris GE, Miller DC. Peripheral vascular manifestations of acute aortic dissection. *In* Rutherford RB (ed). Vascular Surgery. Philadelphia: WB Saunders, 1995:1087–1102.
3. Wheat MW Jr, Palmer RF. Dissective aneurysms of the aorta. Curr Probl Surg 1971;July:1–43.
4. Hirst AE Jr, Johns VJ Jr, Kime SW Jr. Dissecting aneurysm of the aorta: a review of 505 cases. Medicine (Baltimore) 1958;37:217–279.
5. Miller DC. Surgical management of aortic dissections: indications, perioperative management, and long-term results. *In* Doroghazi RM, Slater EE (eds). Aortic Dissection. New York: McGraw-Hill, 1983:193–243.
6. Nienaber CA, Kodolitsch YV, Nicholas V, et al. The diagnosis of thoracic aortic dissection by noninvasive imaging procedures. N Engl J Med 1993;328:1–9.
7. Miller DC. The continuing dilemma concerning medical versus surgical management of patients with acute type B dissections. Semin Thorac Cardiovasc Surg 1993;5:33–46.
8. Glower DD, Famn JI, Speier RH, et al. Comparison of medical and surgical therapy for uncomplicated descending aortic dissection. Circulation 1990;82(suppl IV):39–46.
9. Roberts CS, Roberts WC. Aortic dissection with the entrance tear in the descending thoracic aorta. Ann Surg 1991;213:356–368.
10. Miller DC, Mitchell RS, Oyer PE, et al. Independent determinants of operative mortality for patients with aortic dissections. Circulation 1984;70(suppl I):153–164.
11. Fann JI, Smith JA, Miller DC, et al. Surgical management of aortic dissection during a 30-year period. Circulation 1995;92(suppl II):113–121.
12. Svensson LG, Crawford ES, Hess KR, et al. Dissection of the aorta and dissecting aortic aneurysms. Circulation 1990;82(suppl IV):24–38.
13. Jex RK, Schaff HV, Piehler JM, et al. Early and late results following repair of dissections of the descending thoracic aorta. J Vasc Surg 1986;3:226–237.
14. Wheat MW, Palmer RF, Bartley TB, et al. Treatment of dissecting aneurysms of the aorta without surgery. J Thorac Cardiovasc Surg 1965;50:364–373.
15. Cambria RP, Brewster DC, Gertler J, et al. Vascular complications associated with spontaneous aortic dissection. J Vasc Surg 1988;7:199–209.
16. Cambria RP, Brewster DC, Moncure AC, et al. Spontaneous aortic dissection in the presence of coexistent or previously repaired atherosclerotic aortic aneurysm. Ann Surg 1988;208:619–624.
17. Fann JI, Sarris GE, Mitchell RS, et al. Treatment of patients with aortic dissection presenting with peripheral vascular complications. Ann Surg 1990;212:705–713.
18. Hughes JD, Bacha EA, Dodson TF, et al. Peripheral vascular complications of aortic dissection. Am J Surg 1995;170:209–212.
19. Brewster DC. Role of the vascular surgeon in the management of dissecting aortic aneurysms. *In* Veith FJ (ed). Current Critical Problems in Vascular Surgery. St. Louis: Quality Medical Publishing, 1989:291–302.
20. Brewster DC. Management of peripheral artery complications in patients with aortic dissection. *In* Yao JST, Pearce WH (eds). Arterial Surgery: Management of Challenging Problems. Stamford, CT: Appleton & Lange, 1996:247–264.
21. Hunter JA, Dye WS, Javid H, et al. Abdominal aortic resection in thoracic dissection. Arch Surg 1976;111:1258–1262.
22. Elefteriades JA, Hartleroad J, Gusberg RJ, et al. Long-term experience with descending aortic dissection: the complications-specific approach. Ann Thorac Surg 1992;53:11–21.

23. Elefteriades JA, Hammond GL, Gusberg RJ, et al. Fenestration revisited: a safe and effective procedure for descending aortic dissection. Arch Surg 1990;125:786–790.
24. Laas J, Heinemann M, Schaefers H-J, et al. Management of thoracoabdominal malperfusion in aortic dissection. Circulation 1991;84(suppl III):20–24.
25. Cogbill TH, Gundersen AE, Travelli F. Mesenteric vascular insufficiency and claudication following acute dissecting thoracic aortic aneurysm. J Vasc Surg 1985;2:472–476.
26. Moncure AC, Brewster DC, Darling RC, et al. Use of splenic and hepatic arteries for renal revascularization. J Vasc Surg 1986;3:196–203.
27. Adib K, Belzer FO. Renal autotransplantation in dissecting aortic aneurysm with renal artery involvement. Surgery 1978;84:686–688.
28. Slonim SM, Miller DC, Dake MD. Endovascular techniques of treatment of complications of aortic dissection. *In* Yao JST, Pearce WH (eds). Arterial Surgery: Management of Challenging Problems. Stamford, CT: Appleton & Lange, 1996:283–289.
29. Slonim SM, Dake MD, Semba CP, et al. Aortic dissection: percutaneous management of ischemic complications with endovascular stents and a balloon fenestration. J Vasc Surg 1996;23:241–253.
30. Slonim SM, Nyman UR, Semba CP, et al. True lumen obliteration in complicated aortic dissection: endovascular treatment. Radiology 1996;201:161–166.
31. Williams DM, Brothers TE, Messina LM. Relief of mesenteric ischemia in type III aortic dissection with percutaneous fenestration of the aortic septum. Radiology 1990;174:450–452.
32. Saito S, Arai H, Kim K, et al. Percutaneous fenestration of dissecting intima with a trans-septal needle: a new therapeutic technique for visceral ischemia complicating acute aortic dissection. Cathet Cardiovasc Diagn 1992;26:130–135.
33. Walker PJ, Dake MD, Mitchell RS, et al. The use of endovascular techniques for the treatment of complications of aortic dissection. J Vasc Surg 1993;18:1042–1051.
34. Akaba N, Ujiie H, Umezawa K, et al. Management of acute aortic dissections with a cylinder-type balloon catheter to close the entry. J Vasc Surg 1986;3:890–894.
35. Trent MS, Parsonnet VP, Schnoenfeld R, et al. A balloon-expandable intravascular stent for obliterating experimental aortic dissection. J Vasc Surg 1990;11:707–717.
36. Shimshak TM, Giorgi LV, Hartzler CO. Successful percutaneous transluminal angioplasty of an obstructed abdominal aorta secondary to a chronic dissection. Am J Cardiol 1988;61:486–487.

Endovascular Treatment of Thoracic Aortic Aneurysms and Dissection

*James I. Fann, M.D., Suzanne M. Slonim, M.D., and
D. Craig Miller, M.D.*

Conventional treatment of patients with descending thoracic aortic aneurysms is surgical replacement of the aorta with a tubular Dacron graft. Despite improved surgical techniques, intraoperative monitoring, and postoperative care, major complications, such as paraplegia, renal failure, and pulmonary insufficiency, persist.[11, 16, 20, 28, 29, 33, 36] In an effort to decrease perioperative morbidity, early operation before rupture, preservation of spinal cord perfusion, and prevention of perioperative hypotension are emphasized. Distal circulatory perfusion, including extracorporeal circulation or temporary extravascular shunting, also has been employed to prevent these complications.[2, 4, 5, 11, 16, 19, 20, 28, 29, 33, 36]

One alternative technique in the treatment of descending thoracic aortic pathology is endovascular stent grafting.[17, 18, 25, 34, 35, 39, 40, 41] This approach is less invasive, is potentially less expensive, and may be associated with lower morbidity than open surgical repair. Endovascular technology has been extended to the treatment of complications of aortic dissections, providing the surgeon with additional therapeutic options for this devastating problem.[17, 18, 34, 35, 39, 40, 41] In this chapter, we review the results of our experience with endovascular stent grafting of descending thoracic aortic aneurysms and developments in the endovascular approach to treating complications of aortic dissection.

Descending Thoracic Aortic Aneurysms

Clinical Evaluation

The estimated annual incidence of thoracic aortic aneurysms is 6 cases per 100,000 persons.[1] The descending thoracic aorta is involved in approximately 40% of these patients, the ascending aorta in 50%, and the aortic arch in the remainder.[1, 30, 31] Descending thoracic aortic aneurysms are primarily caused by atherosclerosis; less common causes include trauma, infection, connective tissue disorders such as Marfan's syndrome, and congenital aortic anomalies.[28, 30, 31] Untreated, thoracic aortic aneurysms progressively enlarge and eventually rupture. Of those followed medically, 40% to 74% developed aneurysm rupture, and more than 90% were fatal.[1, 30, 31] The average survival time was less than 3 years from the time of diagnosis.[31] For patients with thoracic aortic aneurysms not treated surgically, the actuarial survival estimates at 1 and 5 years were 60% and 20%, respectively.[1, 31]

Most patients with descending thoracic aortic aneurysms are asymptomatic; the diagnosis typically is suspected on the basis of an abnormal chest radiograph or during evaluation for other illnesses.[7, 22, 30, 31] In those with symptoms, back or chest pain usually localized to the site of the aneurysm is the most common symptom. Other signs and symptoms include compression or erosion of adjacent structures, such as hoarseness from stretching or compression of the left recurrent laryngeal nerve; respiratory symptoms resulting from tracheal or smaller airway compression; hemoptysis from bronchial or pulmonary erosion; dysphagia from esophageal compression; and superior vena cava syndrome.[7, 11, 22]

Preoperatively, the patient's cerebrovascular, cardiac, pulmonary, and renal conditions are carefully evaluated. Imaging of the descending thoracic aorta includes aortography and computed tomography (CT) or magnetic resonance imaging (MRI). Aortography is useful in imaging adjacent aortic branches and intercostal arteries. CT (particularly spiral CT) or MRI provides additional information regarding the pathoanatomy of the aneurysm and the contiguous structures. Coronary arteriography is obtained for older patients and those clinically suspected of having coronary artery disease.

Surgical Therapy

Because of the risk of rupture, therapeutic intervention is considered for all patients with descending thoracic aortic aneurysm. For those who are symptomatic, operative repair is warranted; in asymptomatic patients, indications for surgery include an aneurysm diameter twice that of a relatively normal contiguous segment of aorta or larger than 6 cm or documented aneurysm enlargement over time.[22, 28] Smaller aneurysms are followed with serial CT or MRI scans every 6 to 12 months.

The operative mortality rate for graft replacement of descending thoracic aortic aneurysms is approximately 11%.[2, 5, 7, 16, 20, 28–30] In the Stanford experience, emergency operation and congestive heart failure were independent risk factors for operative death.[28] Factors that did not correlate significantly with hospital mortality included age, hypertension, chronic lung disease, previous myocardial infarction, angina, cause of the aneurysm, and aneurysm location.[28] Although distal circulatory support has been useful in providing cardiac decompression and reducing distal ischemic injury, it does not necessarily eliminate the risk of paraplegia (which averages 4%) or renal insufficiency (which averages 5%).[2, 4, 7, 16, 20, 28, 29, 33, 38] The actuarial survival estimates for discharged patients were 70% to 79% at 5 years and 40% to 49% at 10 years.[7, 16, 28, 30] Late deaths were caused by cardiovascular and cerebrovascular events in 41% to 59% of cases and rupture of another aortic aneurysm in 20% to 25% of cases.[7, 28]

Endovascular Stent Grafting

An alternative to conventional surgical repair is endovascular stent grafting of descending thoracic aortic pathology. Preoperative diagnostic evaluation of patients for this technique is similar to that for the surgical approach, because conversion to the latter may be necessary if the endovascular approach fails. Spiral CT provides a three-dimensional image of the descending thoracic aorta and distal arch, and aortography is used to evaluate critical side branches, such as the intercostal, renal, and visceral arteries.[6, 32] The size and morphology of the iliofemoral arteries are carefully measured and assessed to determine whether the delivery sheath can be passed safely. The relationships of the proximal aneurysm neck to the origin of the left subclavian artery and the distal neck to the celiac axis are defined.

Patient selection criteria are based on theoretical and anatomic considerations. The origin of major aortic branches, such as the left subclavian or the celiac arteries, must not be involved by the aneurysm; the aneurysm neck is of relatively normal caliber; the aneurysm is localized; the aneurysm is amenable to stent grafting (eg, aneurysmal dilation from chronic dissection is excluded because the true lumen is small and distorted and the false lumen eccentric); and there is adequate arterial or abdominal aortic access for the delivery devices.[6] With increased experience, involvement of the subclavian artery is no longer a contraindication, because a left carotid–subclavian transposition can be performed such that the proximal fixation point of the stent graft is in the distal arch.

Each stent graft is custom constructed of a stainless-steel Z-stent endoskeleton (Cook, Inc., Bloomington, IN) covered with Cooley Verisoft woven Dacron graft (Meadox Medicals, Inc., Oakland, NJ) (Fig. 9–1).[6] The diameter, length, taper, and curvature of the prosthesis are based on the measurements obtained from the patient's spiral CT and aortogram. The length of the stent graft is measured to allow for an additional 1.5 to 2 cm to serve as a friction anchor in the proximal and distal aneurysm necks. The delivery apparatus includes a delivery sheath, a tapered dilator, a loading cartridge, and a solid "pusher" rod. The delivery sheath is constructed of polytetrafluoroethylene (PTFE, Teflon) and has an external diameter of 20 or 24 Fr. A PTFE dilator is placed within the delivery sheath, and the sheath and dilator are advanced over a stiff guide wire. After removal of the dilator and guide wire, a PTFE pusher rod is used to advance the compressed stent graft (within the loading cartridge) into and up the delivery sheath for deployment.

Technique

Endovascular stent grafting of descending thoracic aortic aneurysms is performed in the operating room under general anesthesia.[6] Cardiopulmonary bypass is available on standby. A transesophageal echocardiographic probe is

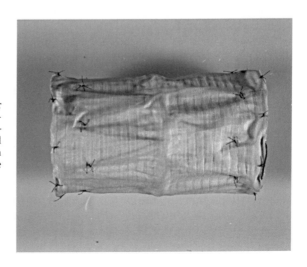

Figure 9–1. The endovascular stent grafts are custom constructed of a stainless-steel endoskeleton consisting of Z-shaped stent elements covered with a woven Dacron graft with the crimps removed.

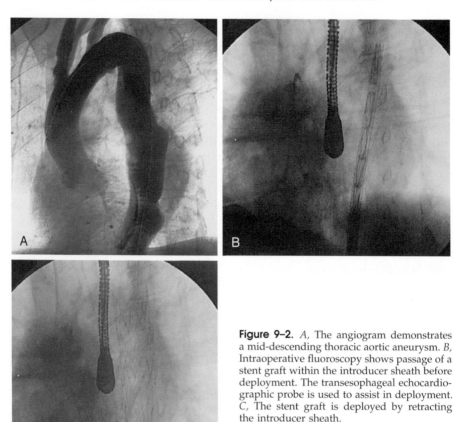

Figure 9–2. *A,* The angiogram demonstrates a mid-descending thoracic aortic aneurysm. *B,* Intraoperative fluoroscopy shows passage of a stent graft within the introducer sheath before deployment. The transesophageal echocardiographic probe is used to assist in deployment. *C,* The stent graft is deployed by retracting the introducer sheath.

used to assess cardiac function and to guide stent graft deployment. The patient is usually placed in a right lateral decubitus position, depending on the fluoroscopic projection that provides the optimal image of the descending thoracic aorta. The chest, abdomen, and femoral regions are prepared and draped in the routine fashion. Potential vascular access sites include the femoral artery, iliac artery, and infrarenal aorta, depending on the anatomy and concomitant procedures.

The access site is surgically exposed and punctured with an 18-gauge needle, followed by passage of a guide wire, sheath, and pigtail angiographic catheter directed into the ascending aorta. Intraoperative aortography is performed using a radiographic image intensifier with digital road-mapping capability. The pigtail angiographic catheter and sheath are removed over a stiff 0.035-inch guide wire, which is advanced into the aortic arch or descending thoracic aorta proximal to the aneurysm. After the patient is fully heparinized, a femoral or iliac arteriotomy or small aortotomy is made. Under fluoroscopic guidance, the dilator is passed over the guide wire and advanced into the descending thoracic aorta; the delivery sheath is advanced with the dilator. The dilator and guide wire are removed, leaving the delivery sheath at the level of the proximal aneurysm neck. The stent graft within the loading cartridge is inserted into the delivery sheath and advanced to the end of the sheath using the pusher rod.

The mean arterial pressure is lowered to between 50 and 60 mm Hg using a combination of intravenous esmolol, sodium nitroprusside, and inhalational isofluorane. The stent graft is deployed by holding the pusher in position and retracting the delivery sheath (Fig. 9–2). After prosthesis deployment, the blood pressure is permitted to rise, and the pusher is removed; the retracted delivery sheath is left in an intravascular position to permit further instrumentation if necessary. The guide wire is reinserted within the delivery sheath, followed by a pigtail catheter; completion aortography is performed to assess adequacy of stent graft fixation. The delivery sheath is removed and the arterial access site repaired. Protamine sulfate is given for heparin reversal.

Follow-up radiologic evaluations are obtained based on an established protocol. Chest radiography, CT, and angiography are obtained before the procedure and before discharge from the hospital (Fig. 9–3). At 2 months after the procedure, a chest radiograph is obtained. At 6 months and 1 year of follow-up, chest radiography, CT, and angiography are repeated. At 2 years after the procedure and annually thereafter, chest radiography and CT are obtained for follow-up assessments.

Special Considerations

For a patient with a proximal descending thoracic aortic aneurysm extending to the origin of the left subclavian artery, a left carotid–subclavian transposition is performed before the endovascular stent graft procedure to create an adequate proximal neck without compromising subclavian artery flow.[6] After the subclavian-to-carotid anastomosis is performed, the patient is repositioned and prepared for the stent graft procedure.

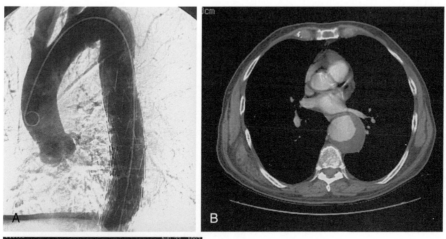

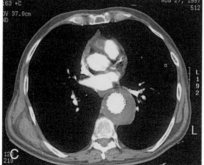

Figure 9–3. *A,* Follow-up angiogram demonstrates exclusion of the descending thoracic aortic aneurysm. *B* and *C,* Preprocedure and postprocedure computed tomography scans with contrast show the stent graft within the descending thoracic aneurysm.

Patients with separate abdominal aortic and thoracic aortic aneurysms have been successfully treated with a conventional open abdominal aortic aneurysm repair coupled with placement of a descending thoracic aortic stent graft.[27] Thoracic aortic stent graft placement is facilitated by sewing a side limb (10-mm Dacron graft) onto the abdominal aortic graft; alternatively, if a bifurcation graft is necessary, one limb of this graft may be used. The side limb is used for delivery sheath access, and the stent graft is deployed in the previously described manner. At the conclusion of the procedure, the auxiliary side limb is oversewn.

In patients with multiple thoracic aortic aneurysms (ie, involving the ascending aorta or arch and the descending thoracic aorta), it is possible to replace the ascending aorta and arch using the "elephant trunk" technique initially; this is followed at a later date, if necessary, with stent grafting of the descending thoracic component of the aneurysm. The proximal end of the stent graft is deployed inside the distal opening of the elephant trunk graft (Fig. 9–4).[3, 9]

Patent intercostal arteries are identified preoperatively by angiography so that attempts can be made to preserve them during stent graft placement. One method is to use a segment of a noncovered stent body attached to the stent graft to anchor the prosthesis within the proximal or distal neck of the aneurysm at the level of a patent branch artery. Deployment of this composite stent graft requires a high degree of precision to achieve an adequate seal of the prosthesis to a portion of the aneurysm neck and at the same time maintain flow into the branch artery.

Results

The most recent update of our experience with endovascular stent grafting of the descending thoracic aorta extends to late 1996 and includes 81 patients

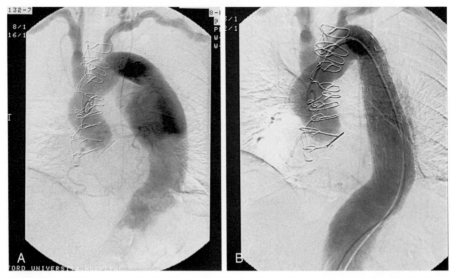

Figure 9–4. *A,* In a patient who had a previous ascending aortic aneurysm repair with placement of an elephant trunk graft, the intraoperative angiogram shows the descending thoracic aortic aneurysm and the transesophageal echocardiographic probe. *B,* Intraoperative angiogram after placement of a stent graft in the descending thoracic component of the aneurysm. The proximal aspect of the stent graft is situated within the previously placed elephant trunk graft. (From Fann JI, Dake MD, Semba CP, et al. Endovascular stent-grafting after arch aneurysm repair using the "elephant trunk." Ann Thorac Surg 1995;60:1102–1105. Reprinted with permission of the Society of Thoracic Surgeons.)

with descending thoracic aortic disease.[6, 12] The mean age of the patients was 66 years, with a male to female ratio of 3 to 1. Seventy-six patients underwent stent graft placement at Stanford University, and five patients underwent stent graft procedures at outside institutions using this technique. Approximately one half of these patients were not considered operative candidates by the referring surgeons because of comorbidities.[25] The predominant pathology was atherosclerotic or degenerative aneurysmal disease, occurring in 67 patients; the remainder included posttraumatic aneurysms, pseudoaneurysms, and aortic dissections (five patients). Fifty-two patients were approached using a femoral arteriotomy, three through an iliac arteriotomy, 25 through the abdominal aorta, and one through the aortic arch (ie, combined aortic arch aneurysm repair and stent grafting using hypothermic circulatory arrest). Among those who required the abdominal aortic approach, seven patients were accessed through a small aortotomy (ie, inadequate distal access), and 18 patients underwent concomitant abdominal aortic aneurysm repair. The mean diameter of the diseased descending thoracic aorta was 6.2 cm; the mean diameter of the stent graft was 3.5 cm, and the average length of the stent graft was 10.2 cm.

Patient follow-up was 100% complete and averaged 13.2 months; a large fraction of patients underwent stent grafting in the latter part of the reported experience.[12] There were seven procedure-related deaths (early mortality rate of 9% ± 3% [± 70% confidence limit]). Paraplegia occurred in three patients (4% ± 2%), and stroke occurred in four patients (5% ± 3%). No patient required conversion to an open surgical approach, and there have been no cases of stent graft infection. In four patients (5% ± 3%), thrombosis of the aneurysm was incomplete after stent graft deployment; three of these subsequently died (two of these deaths were sudden and categorized as possible treatment failures), and one developed a fatal aneurysm rupture into the esophagus. Angiographic manipulation and stent graft instrumentation at the level of the aortic arch were associated with three embolic strokes. Another patient sustained an intracerebral hemorrhage; although this patient was fully heparinized during the procedure, there were no identifiable periods of hypertension intraoperatively or postoperatively. Among the three patients who sustained paraplegia, two had complicated intraoperative and post-procedure courses associated with hypotension; one patient with an extensive aneurysm underwent stent grafting of the entire descending thoracic aorta.

For the 76 patients who underwent endovascular stent grafting at Stanford University, the actuarial survival estimates were 87% ± 4% at 1 year, 81% ± 6% at 2 years, and 81% ± 6% at nearly 4 years.[12] Given the high-risk nature of this patient cohort, these results are satisfactory. This survival curve compares with a 5-year actuarial survival estimate of 70% to 79% for patients who underwent open surgical repair in previous series.[7, 16, 28, 30] Five patients died late. Two deaths were sudden, and one resulted from aneurysm rupture; these three deaths can be categorized as one definite and two possible treatment failures. Five patients developed late recanalization or filling of the aneurysm sac over time; three of these were successfully treated with secondary radiologic embolization procedures, one underwent open surgical repair (with exclusion of the descending thoracic aorta), and one continues to be monitored expectantly. There have been no cases of stent graft infection, distal embolization, or stent graft migration.

Limitations

Despite known and theoretical advantages of endovascular stent grafting of descending thoracic aortic pathology, there are limitations. The advantage of this technique is that the thoracic aorta is not crossclamped during the procedure; however, the risk of spinal cord ischemia and paraplegia still exists, because critical intercostal vessels can be compromised by the prosthesis. Large intercostal arteries cannot be directly evaluated and reimplanted as in the open surgical procedure. The delivery system is relatively large, requiring adequate vascular access. Although one attractive feature of the stent graft system is its simplicity, it can be relatively imprecise in the deployment, and the position of the stent graft cannot be easily adjusted after its expansion.

An important question involves the stability of stent graft fixation and the ultimate fate of the aneurysm. The deployed stent graft is held in place by friction fixation to the proximal and distal necks of the aneurysm; stent graft migration is therefore a possibility, especially if one neck dilates over time.[6] Late aneurysm filling and recanalization of a tract around the stent graft have been observed. In the absence of postmortem evaluations, the described cases of sudden death or aneurysm rupture may be considered to result from progressive aneurysm expansion due to perigraft leak.

Another limitation includes anatomic considerations. Adequate proximal and distal aneurysm necks need to be identified; critical branches in the diseased portion of the aorta must be avoided; and only relatively straight aortic aneurysms can be treated using this technique. Endovascular stent grafting close to the distal arch appears to be associated with a higher incidence of strokes, presumably because of catheter manipulation at the level of the arch.

The long-term efficacy and clinical outcome of endovascular stent grafting of descending thoracic aortic pathology remains unknown. This key question awaits 5- to 10-year follow-up of a large number of patients with serial imaging studies.

Endovascular Interventions for Aortic Dissections

Acute aortic dissection is one of the most common catastrophes involving the aorta, with an estimated incidence of 9000 cases per year in the United States.[1, 8, 10, 24] Although surgical replacement of the ascending aorta is the treatment of choice for patients with acute type A dissection, the optimal mode of therapy (medical or surgical) for patients with acute type B dissection is not fully elucidated.[8, 10, 13–15, 23, 24] Peripheral vascular complications, including limb and visceral ischemia, frequently develop as a result of the acute dissecting process.[13, 34, 35] The variability of dissection flap propagation may result in multiple true and false lumens and a variety of branch vessel involvement. Surgical repair of the dissected aorta usually relieves the peripheral ischemic symptoms, but in some cases, the ischemia is severe at the time of presentation, particularly if the visceral vessels are involved, or persists after the surgical procedure. In such cases, the pathophysiologic findings can be addressed using endovascular techniques directed at stenting open the true lumen or fenestrating the intimal flap to achieve adequate flow to the compromised vascular beds.[17, 18, 34, 35, 39, 41, 42]

Many investigators have evaluated thoracic aortic stenting in surgically created aortic dissections in the canine model.[21, 27, 37, 42] Moon and colleagues[26] employed balloon-expandable intravascular Palmaz stents (Johnson & Johnson Interventional Systems, Warren, NJ) to compress the intimal flap after creation of the dissection. At 6 weeks, postmortem evaluation showed the stented true lumens to be patent without thrombus formation and the stents to be covered by neointima. In those with only proximal obliteration of the false lumen by the stent, the distal false lumen remained patent, analogous to a chronic dissection in the clinical setting. Using the canine model, Yoshida and associates[42] performed endovascular stent grafting of aortic dissection with a spiral nitinol stent covered with a polyurethane tube. The stent graft was compressed inside a 14-Fr catheter at a low temperature; once in contact with body temperature at time of deployment, it regained its original shape, thereby fixing itself to the aortic intima. Conversely, Marty-Ane and coworkers[21] found that nitinol coil grafts resulted in incomplete expansion within the aorta in a canine model of aortic dissection, resulting in aortic thrombosis. Placing balloon-expandable stents at the entry and reentry sites resulted in only partial obliteration of the dissection, whereas stenting the entire length of the dissected aorta led to obliteration of the dissection.

Clinical Experience With Stenting

Peripheral ischemic complications of aortic dissection can be categorized into two pathophysiologic groups.[34] The ischemic complication may be primarily a peripheral problem from extension of the dissection flap into the aortic branch vessel. If there is no distal reentry of the dissection process, the true lumen within the branch vessel can be compressed, resulting in compromised perfusion of the vascular bed. Even with a reentry tear, an intimal flap may compromise distal blood flow. In these cases, endovascular treatment directed at stenting open the true lumen with compression of the false lumen can reestablish adequate perfusion.

In the second group, the ischemia is the consequence of a more generalized hemodynamic problem within the aorta. The ischemia is caused by a pressure gradient between the true and false lumens, sometimes resulting in severe compression of the true lumen and compromised flow to its branches. In this setting, endovascular therapy includes creating fenestrations that simulate reentry tears and allow equalization of pressures between the two lumens. Another potential therapeutic approach to patients with this problem is deployment of stents within the aortic lumen to maintain patency of the true lumen by displacing the intimal flap toward the false lumen.[34] Although intuitively attractive, aortic stenting cannot reliably obliterate the false lumen. The usual process of aortic dissection results in an increase in the overall aortic diameter and stretching of the outer layers of the media and the adventitia; however, the intimal layer that surrounds the true lumen does not dilate and maintains the original aortic dimensions. It is therefore difficult to obliterate the false lumen by stenting the aortic true lumen, and a patent false lumen often persists. In chronic aortic dissection, the intimal flap usually thickens and contracts as it heals, making it less pliable and more resistant to stretching. Depending on the pathophysiology, obliteration of the false lumen may not be necessarily a reasonable goal, because it may be the only blood supply to a given vascular bed.

Various endovascular techniques in the treatment of complications of aortic dissection have been described.[34, 35, 39, 41] At Stanford, the following endovascular approach has been adopted. The pathoanatomy of the aortic dissection is initially determined with a spiral CT scan to decrease cost and contrast requirement during angiography. Angiography of the true and false lumens is performed; intravascular ultrasonography is used to assist evaluation of complex flaps. Endovascular stenting is performed using balloon-expandable Palmaz stents or self-expanding Wallstents (Schneider, Plymouth, MN), both of which may be deployed in the aorta or any of the major branches (Fig. 9–5). High radial strength is important to buttress the true lumen against the compressed false lumen, especially in the aorta. Stent size is based on measurements from angiography or intravascular ultrasonography. Because of the pathophysiology of the dissection and the enlarged vessel caliber, larger stent diameters are often needed in the branch vessels than are used for other indications. The sizes of the vascular access sheaths vary from 7 to 14 Fr.

Endovascular balloon fenestration is performed using intravascular ultrasonographic or fluoroscopic guidance. Intravascular ultrasonography allows the needle used for fenestration to be more precisely directed than with cross-sectional imaging. When the fenestration is being performed just above the aortic bifurcation, however, the intravascular ultrasonographic probe in one iliac artery may not adequately visualize the needle approaching from the other iliac artery. Fluoroscopic guidance is therefore more useful in the region of the aortic bifurcation. Fenestration of the intimal flap is typically performed

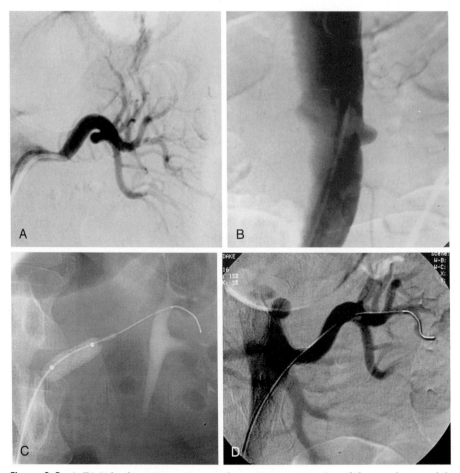

Figure 9–5. *A,* Digital subtraction angiogram demonstrates narrowing of the true lumen of the renal artery. *B,* Angiogram with contrast injection into the false lumen shows a cuff of false lumen at the level of the left renal artery that is causing compression of the true lumen of the renal artery. *C,* Fluoroscopic image shows deployment of a balloon-expandable stent in the true lumen of the left renal artery. *D,* Fluoroscopic image shows a patent renal artery after stenting.

using a Rosch-Uchida set (Cook, Inc.), which contains a long, curved, metallic cannula covered by a 7-Fr PTFE sheath, through which a 0.038-inch needle covered by a 5-Fr angiographic catheter passes coaxially. The Rosch-Uchida set, which requires a 10-Fr sheath, is placed in the smaller (usually true) lumen so that the needle can be advanced across the flap into the larger (usually false) lumen. When using intravascular ultrasonographic guidance, the probe is positioned at the same level as the Rosch-Uchida cannula to allow real-time visualization during fenestration. The needle and 5-Fr catheter combination is passed through the intimal flap into the opposite lumen. Intravascular ultrasonography is continuously monitored to ensure that the puncture is made into the false lumen rather than into an extravascular space. After the fenestration is made with the needle, a guide wire can be passed through the 5-Fr catheter into the opposite lumen. A balloon catheter is then advanced over the guide wire to dilate the fenestration in the intimal flap. When using fluoroscopic guidance, a balloon catheter is inflated in the false lumen to act as a target for the needle puncture (Fig. 9–6). Alignment of the tip of the needle with the inflated balloon is confirmed fluoroscopically. Otherwise, the technique is similar to that with intravascular ultrasonographic guidance.

Slonim and colleagues[34] presented 22 patients who underwent percutaneous treatment of peripheral ischemic complications of 12 type A (five acute, seven chronic) and 10 type B (nine acute, one chronic) aortic dissections from 1991 to 1995 at Stanford University. Ten patients presented with leg ischemia, 13 with renal ischemia, and six with visceral ischemia. Sixteen patients were treated with endovascular stenting, including 11 with renal, six with lower extremity, two with superior mesenteric artery, and two with aortic stents. Three patients had balloon fenestration of the intimal flap, and three had balloon fenestration with endovascular stenting. Successful revascularization was achieved in all 22 patients. One case was complicated by a guide wire–induced perinephric hematoma. Two patients died at 3 days and 13 months after the procedure. At a mean follow-up of nearly 14 months, one was lost to follow-up, and 19 had continued relief of symptoms.

Slonim and coworkers[35] reported a series of 11 patients who underwent endovascular techniques directed at true lumen obliteration in complicated aortic dissections between 1992 and 1995. Two patients had chronic type A dissection, and nine had type B dissection (six acute and three chronic). In these cases, the aortic dissection resulted in compression of the true lumen to a paper-thin sliver. True lumen obliteration was associated with branch vessel ischemia that included renal ($n = 7$), mesenteric ($n = 6$), and lower extremity ($n = 6$) arterial compromise. Two patients were treated with aortic stents, four with balloon fenestration of the intimal flap, and three with stent placement and fenestration. Successful revascularization was achieved in nine patients with true lumen obliteration; in two patients, ischemic complications could not be treated using endovascular techniques. In two patients, endovascular revascularization was unsuccessful; one required surgical revascularization of the superior mesenteric artery, and the other required continued medical therapy for hypertension. One patient developed thrombosis of a renal artery in which a stent had been placed. The early mortality rate was 9%, and the mean follow-up was 10.1 months. Results demonstrated that true lumen obliteration could be safely and effectively treated with endovascular stent placement and balloon fenestration in selected patients.[35]

Williams and colleagues[41] reported 24 patients who underwent endovascular treatment of ischemic complications of aortic dissection. The complications

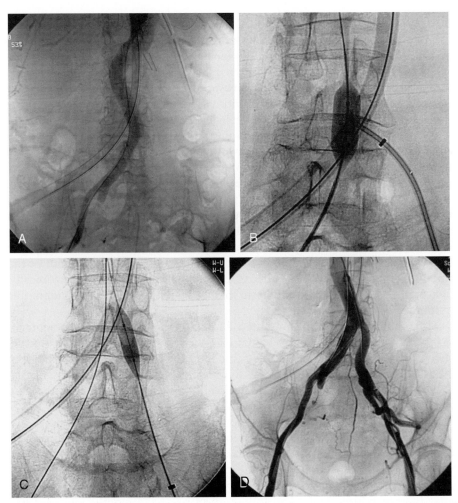

Figure 9–6. *A*, Digital subtraction angiogram with true lumen injection demonstrates absence of flow into the left lower extremity. *B*, Fluoroscopic image shows an inflated balloon catheter in the false lumen, which provides a target for the fenestration needle. The Rosch-Uchida cannula is in the true lumen of the left iliac artery; the needle is later passed through the cannula toward the inflated balloon, creating the fenestration. *C*, Fluoroscopic image shows dilation of the fenestration with the balloon catheter. *D*, Angiogram with injection of the false lumen shows flow to both lower extremities after fenestration.

were considered *static*, caused by the dissecting hematoma extending into a branch vessel and producing narrowing, or *dynamic*, caused by a dissection flap prolapsing into the origin of the branch vessel or narrowing the true lumen above it. Twelve patients were treated with endovascular stents combined with fenestration, eight with fenestration alone, and four with stents alone. Endovascular therapy did not lower false lumen pressure; however, the treatments eliminated the pressure gradients between the true and false lumens. Flow was restored in 71 (92%) of 77 arteries. The 30-day mortality rate was 25%. Two patients died during follow-up of complications of an expanding false lumen. Overall, prognosis appeared to be related to the ischemic injury sustained before the percutaneous intervention.

Inoue and coworkers[18] reported successful endovascular stent grafting of the descending thoracic aorta and the left subclavian artery in a patient with type B dissection originating just beyond the left subclavian artery. The stent graft, constructed of a Dacron graft supported by multiple rings of flexible nickel titanium wire, had a tapered configuration measuring 34 mm in diameter at the proximal end and 28 mm in diameter at the distal end; it was 21 cm long. The stent graft incorporated several thorns to ensure fixation to the aortic wall. A side branch graft, measuring 8 mm in diameter and 3 cm long, was placed into the left subclavian artery. After intraoperative aortography, the right femoral artery was surgically isolated under local anesthesia, and a transverse arteriotomy was performed. A 22-Fr sheath was introduced into the descending thoracic aorta over a 0.038-inch guide wire placed through the femoral arteriotomy under fluoroscopic guidance. The branch stent graft and its carrying system were introduced within the sheath and advanced to the descending thoracic aorta using fluoroscopic guidance. After the graft was positioned at the predetermined target point, the free end of a detachable wire attached to the side branch graft was caught and pulled back by a gooseneck snare wire, which was inserted percutaneously through the left brachial artery. After the side branch graft had been placed in the left subclavian artery, the compactly folded prosthesis was deployed by removal of a nickel titanium wire, allowing rapid self-expansion of the branched graft. The branched graft was released from the carrying system and pressed against the aortic wall by balloon inflation. One month after the successful deployment of the stent graft, aortography and CT demonstrated that the false lumen had completely thrombosed.

Conclusions

Endovascular stent grafting of descending thoracic aortic aneurysms is an alternative to open surgical repair for high-risk patients. Patients who are likely to benefit include the very elderly; those with markedly compromised cardiac, pulmonary, or renal status; and individuals who have undergone previous complex operations on the descending thoracic aorta. Endovascular stent grafting is a useful adjunct for patients with abdominal and descending thoracic aortic aneurysms that need to be treated concomitantly. Results suggest that a less invasive approach may be associated with less early morbidity compared with open thoracotomy and repair. Endovascular techniques for aortic dissection have been successfully employed for the treatment of associated peripheral vascular complications. Assessment of the efficacy of these endovascular techniques, particularly stent grafting for aortic aneurysmal disease, awaits 5- to 10-year follow-up investigations.

References

1. Bickerstaff LK, Pairolero PC, Hollier LH, et al. Thoracic aortic aneurysms: a population-based study. Surgery 1982;92:1103–1108.
2. Borst HG, Jurmann M, Buhner B, et al. Risk of replacement of descending aorta with a standardized left heart bypass technique. J Thorac Cardiovasc Surg 1994;107:126–133.
3. Borst HG, Laas J. Surgical treatment of thoracic aortic aneurysms. *In* Karp RB, Laks H, Wechsler AS (eds). Advances in Cardiac Surgery, vol 4. St. Louis: Mosby–Year Book, 1993:47–87.
4. Cartier R, Orszulak TA, Pairolero PC, et al. Circulatory support during crossclamping of the descending thoracic aorta. J Thorac Cardiovasc Surg 1990;99:1038–1047.
5. Crawford ES, Walker HSJ, Saleh SA, et al. Graft replacement of aneurysm in descending thoracic aorta: results without bypass or shunting. Surgery 1981;89:73–85.
6. Dake MD, Miller DC, Semba CP, et al. Transluminal placement of endovascular stent-grafts for the treatment of descending thoracic aortic aneurysms. N Engl J Med 1994;331:1729–1734.
7. DeBakey ME, McCollum CH, Graham JM. Surgical treatment of aneurysms of the descending thoracic aorta. J Cardiovasc Surg 1978;19:571–576.
8. DeSanctis RW, Eagle KA. Aortic dissection. Curr Probl Cardiol 1989;14:227–278.

9. Fann JI, Dake MD, Semba CP, et al. Endovascular stent-grafting after arch aneurysm repair using the "elephant trunk." Ann Thorac Surg 1995;60:1102–1105.
10. Fann JI, Miller DC. Aortic dissection. Ann Vasc Surg 1995;9:311–323.
11. Fann JI, Miller DC. Descending thoracic aortic aneurysms. In Baue AE, Geha AS, Hammond GL, Laks H, Naunheim KS (eds). Glenn's Thoracic and Cardiovascular Surgery, ed 6. Stamford: Appleton & Lange, 1995:2255–2272.
12. Fann JI, Mitchell RS, Dake MD, et al. The results of endovascular grafting of descending thoracic aortic aneurysms. In Yao JST (ed). Vascular Surgery: Twenty Years of Progress. Stamford: Appleton & Lange, 1996:241–254.
13. Fann JI, Sarris GE, Mitchell RS, et al. Treatment of patients with acute aortic dissection presenting with peripheral vascular complications. Ann Surg 1990;212:705–713.
14. Fann JI, Smith JA, Miller DC, et al. Surgical management of aortic dissection over a 30-year period. Circulation 1995;92(suppl II):113–121.
15. Glower DD, Fann JI, Speier RH, et al. Comparison of medical and surgical therapy for uncomplicated descending aortic dissection. Circulation 1990;82(suppl IV):39–46.
16. Hamerlijnck RP, Rutsaert RR, DeGeest R, et al. Surgical correction of descending thoracic aortic aneurysms under simple aortic cross-clamping. J Vasc Surg 1989;9:568–573.
17. Hata M, Zuguchi M, Saito H, et al. Stent angioplasty for renovascular disease associated with acute aortic dissection. Ann Thorac Surg 1997;63:244–246.
18. Inoue K, Sato M, Iwase T, et al. Clinical endovascular placement of branched graft for type B aortic dissection. J Thorac Cardiovasc Surg 1996;112:1111–1113.
19. Laschinger JC, Izumoto H, Kouchoukos NT. Evolving concepts in prevention of spinal cord injury during operations on the descending thoracic and thoracoabdominal aorta. Ann Thorac Surg 1987;44:667–674.
20. Livesay JJ, Cooley DA, Ventemiglia RA, et al. Surgical experience in descending thoracic aneurysmectomy with and without adjuncts to avoid ischemia. Ann Thorac Surg 1985;39:37–46.
21. Marty-Ane G, Serres-Cousine O, Laborde JC, et al. Use of endovascular stents for acute aortic dissection: an experimental study. Ann Vasc Surg 1994;8:434–442.
22. McNamara JJ, Pressler VM. Natural history of arteriosclerotic thoracic aortic aneurysms. Ann Thorac Surg 1978;26:468–473.
23. Miller DC. Acute dissection of the descending thoracic aorta. Chest Surg Clin North Am 1992;2:347–378.
24. Miller DC. Surgical management of aortic dissections: indications, perioperative management, and long-term results. In Doroghazi RM, Slater EE (eds): Aortic Dissection. New York: McGraw-Hill, 1983:193–243.
25. Mitchell RS, Dake MD, Semba CP, et al. Endovascular stent-graft repair of thoracic aortic aneurysms. J Thorac Cardiovasc Surg 1996;111:1054–1062.
26. Moon MR, Dake MD, Pelc LR, et al. Intravascular stenting of acute experimental type B dissections. J Surg Res 1993;54:381–388.
27. Moon MR, Mitchell RS, Dake MD, et al. Simultaneous abdominal aortic replacement and thoracic aortic stent-graft placement for multilevel aortic disease. J Vasc Surg 1997;25:332–340.
28. Moreno-Cabral CE, Miller DC, Mitchell RS, et al. Degenerative and atherosclerotic aneurysms of the thoracic aorta. J Thorac Cardiovasc Surg 1984;88:1020–1032.
29. Najafi H, Javid H, Hunter J, et al. Descending aortic aneurysmectomy without adjuncts to avoid ischemia. Ann Thorac Surg 1980;30:326–335.
30. Pressler V, McNamara JJ. Aneurysm of the thoracic aorta. J Thorac Cardiovasc Surg 1985;89:50–54.
31. Pressler V, McNamara JJ. Thoracic aortic aneurysm: natural history and treatment. J Thorac Cardiovasc Surg 1980;79:489–498.
32. Rubin GD, Walker PJ, Dake MD, et al. Three-dimensional spiral computed tomographic angiography: an alternative imaging modality for the abdominal aorta and its branches. J Vasc Surg 1993;18:656–665.
33. Schepens MA, Defauw JJ, Hamerlijnck RP, et al. Risk assessment of acute renal failure after thoracoabdominal aortic aneurysm surgery. Ann Surg 1994;219:400–407.
34. Slonim SM, Nyman Y, Semba CP, et al. Aortic dissection: percutaneous management of ischemic complications with endovascular stents and balloon fenestration. J Vasc Surg 1996;23:241–253.
35. Slonim SM, Nyman UR, Semba CP, et al. True lumen obliteration in complicated aortic dissection: endovascular treatment. Radiology 1996;201:161–166.
36. Svensson LG, Patel V, Robinson MF, et al. Influence of preservation or perfusion of intraoperatively identified spinal cord blood supply on spinal motor evoked potentials and paraplegia after aortic surgery. J Vasc Surg 1991;13:355–365.
37. Trent MS, Parsonnet V, Shoenfeld R, et al. A balloon-expandable intravascular stent for obliterating aortic dissection. J Vasc Surg 1990;11:707–717.
38. von Segesser LK, Killer I, Jenni R, et al. Improved distal circulatory support for repair of descending thoracic aortic aneurysms. Ann Thorac Surg 1993;56:1373–1380.
39. Walker PJ, Dake MD, Mitchell RS, et al. The use of endovascular techniques for the treatment of complications of aortic dissection. J Vasc Surg 1993;18:1042–1051.

40. Williams DM, Brothers TE, Messina LM. Relief of mesenteric ischemia in type III aortic dissection with percutaneous fenestration of the aortic septum. Radiology 1990;174:450–452.
41. Williams DM, Lee DY, Hamilton BH, et al. The dissected aorta: percutaneous treatment of ischemic complications—principles and results. J Vasc Interv Radiol 1997;8:605–625.
42. Yoshida H, Yasuda K, Tanabe T. New approach to aortic dissection: development of an insertable aortic prosthesis. Ann Thorac Surg 1994;58:806–810.

CHAPTER 10

Transluminally Placed Endovascular Grafts for the Treatment of Aortoiliac Aneurysms

Takao Ohki, M.D., Frank J. Veith, M.D.,
Michael L. Marin, M.D., Luis A. Sanchez, M.D.,
William D. Suggs, M.D., Jacob Cynamon, M.D.,
and Reese A. Wain, M.D.

The outcome of standard surgical abdominal aortic aneurysm (AAA) repair has proven to be excellent, with mortality rates in the range of 3% to 5%.[1] However, standard AAA repair is not perfect, and the quality of life after this repair is impaired by postoperative pain, sexual dysfunction, and a lengthy hospital stay resulting in high health care costs. All these negative effects are related to the large incision and extensive tissue dissection. Mortality and morbidity increase with the presence of associated diseases, and a mortality rate of 60% has been reported for high-risk patients.[2] The standard repair is also extremely difficult in patients with multiple abdominal operations with extensive scarring and infection.

Endovascular grafting is an alternative treatment to standard open aneurysm repair. Endovascular grafts (EVGs) can be inserted through remote arterial access sites to treat aortoiliac aneurysms, thereby avoiding the need to directly expose the diseased artery through a large incision or an extensive dissection.

This chapter describes some of the fundamental issues of endovascular AAA repair and reviews our experience with the use of EVGs for the treatment of AAAs at the Montefiore Medical Center in New York.

Selection Criteria for Endovascular Repair

Certain anatomic features and conditions must exist before attempting EVG placement for AAAs:

1. A segment of normal aorta at least 1.5 to 2 cm long (proximal neck) distal to the renal ostia and proximal to the aneurysm must be present.
2. A distal aortic neck at least 1.5 to 2 cm long proximal to the aortic bifurcation must be present if a tube graft is to be employed.
3. If the site selected for distal implantation is the iliac artery, its morphology must be adequate for seating an attachment system.
4. The common and external iliac and the femoral arteries must be of sufficient caliber to allow passage of the introducer sheath or must be amenable to balloon dilatation to facilitate passage.

5. The iliac vessels cannot be excessively tortuous.

6. Aberrant vessels, such as an indispensable accessory renal artery, must not be present in the excluded segment of aorta.

7. The patient cannot depend on the inferior mesenteric artery for intestinal perfusion, because this vessel will be excluded from the circulation.

8. Some investigators require that there be no angle greater than 60 to 75 degrees between the suprarenal aorta and the aneurysm's proximal neck.[3, 4]

If these conditions are not met, the procedure usually is contraindicated.

Choice of Endovascular Grafts Based on Anatomic Classification and Patient Health Status

AAAs have been classified into five distinct groups according to the morphology and the extent of the aneurysm (Fig. 10–1).[5, 6] The appropriate EVG for the treatment of a given aneurysm is chosen on the basis of this classification. Because these procedures are still under investigation, each operation is performed under a Food and Drug Administration Investigational Device Exemption that allows the use of the device in low-risk or high-risk patients. The choice of device can be further specified according to the health status of the patient along with the anatomic classification.

The Parodi graft, the Montefiore graft, the Talent graft, and the Nottingham graft are predominantly used for high-risk surgical patients (ie, compassionate use). The Chuter bifurcated graft, the Endovascular Technologies (EVT) graft, the Vanguard graft, the White-Yu Endovascular Graft Attachment Devices (GAD) graft,[7, 8] and the Corvita graft are being evaluated in good surgical risk patients.

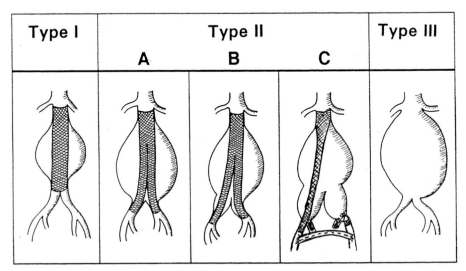

Figure 10–1. Morphometric classification of abdominal aortic aneurysms and possible endovascular graft configurations. Type I: Abdominal aortic aneurysm with sufficient proximal (≥15 mm) and distal (≥10 mm) aortic neck (tube graft). Type IIA: Proximal neck (≥15 mm) and absence of distal aortic involvement (bifurcated graft). Type IIB: Proximal neck (≥15 mm) with proximal common iliac artery involvement (bifurcated graft). Type IIC: Proximal neck (≥15 mm) with iliac artery involvement to the iliac bifurcation (aortouniiiliac graft with contralateral iliac occlusion, femorofemoral bypass, and coil embolization of hypogastric arteries). Type III: Proximal neck (<15 mm) grafts that permit suprarenal stent placement.

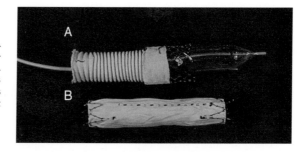

Figure 10–2. *A,* Parodi graft. A modified Palmaz stent (p) is sutured to a crimped Dacron graft. *B,* Endovascular Technologies (EVT) graft. Self-expanding stents with metallic hooks ensure graft fixation.

Devices Designed for Type I Abdominal Aortic Aneurysms

First-generation EVGs were tube grafts that could treat only aneurysms categorized as type I (Fig. 10–2).[9, 10] This type of stented graft was limited by the fact that patients with type I comprised only 10% to 11% of all AAAs.[6, 11] The high incidence of incomplete aneurysm exclusion (ie, endoleaks) originating from the distal fixation site also hampered the value of this type of graft (Fig. 10–3). The Parodi tube graft (see Fig. 10–2*A*), the EVT tube graft (Fig. 10–4*A* and see Fig. 10–2*B*), the Vanguard tube graft, the Talent tube graft, the White-Yu Endovascular GAD graft (Fig. 10–5),[7, 8] and the Corvita tube graft (Fig. 10–6) are of this design.

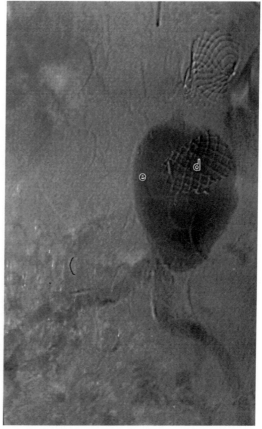

Figure 10–3. Angiogram taken 1 year after endovascular aortic aneurysm repair with a Parodi tube graft. The distal fixation stent (d) has been dislodged into the aneurysm, and a large endoleak (e) is apparent. This patient subsequently underwent surgical repair of the aneurysm.

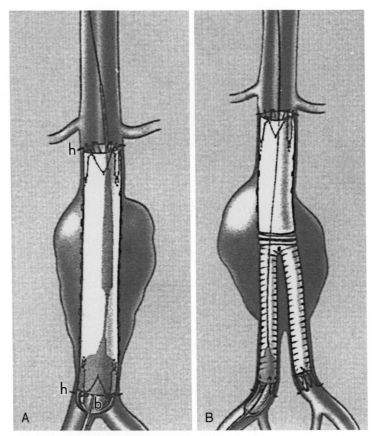

Figure 10-4. Schematic of EVT tube graft and bifurcated graft. *A*, Tube graft. A balloon (b) is inflated at either end of the graft to ensure penetration of the metallic hooks (h) into the aorta wall after graft deployment. *B*, Bifurcated graft.

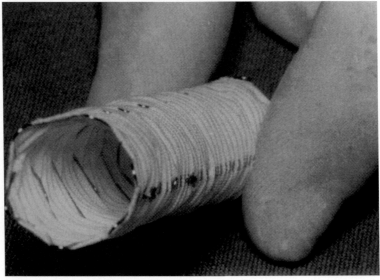

Figure 10-5. The White-Yu endovascular GAD graft, demonstrating the integrated wire forms along the length of the polyester graft body. (From White GH, Yu W, May J, et al. Three year experience with the White-Yu endovascular GAD graft for transluminal repair of aortic and iliac aneurysms. J Endovasc Surg 1997;4:124–136.)

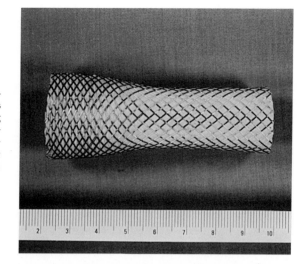

Figure 10–6. The Corvita endoluminal vascular graft (tube) is fabricated from a self-expanding stent of braided wire. The polycarbonate elastomer lines the luminal surface of the stent, and the graft has a flare at the proximal end to ensure fixation.

Devices Designed for Type IIA and IIB Abdominal Aortic Aneurysms

Developmental efforts in stent graft design have focused on devices that can treat types IIA and IIB AAAs (see Fig. 10–1). These grafts are bifurcated, and the distal fixation sites are in the common iliac arteries. The Chuter graft (Fig. 10–7)[12–14] was the first graft that had a bifurcated design. The EVT bifurcated graft (Fig. 10–4B), the Vanguard graft (Fig. 10–8A),[15] the Talent graft (Fig. 10–8B), the White-Yu Endovascular GAD bifurcated graft,[8] the Corvita bifurcated graft, and the AneuRx graft[16] fall into this category.

Figure 10–7. The Chuter bifurcated graft. The delivery system is inserted over the wire through a right femoral arteriotomy into the proximal aorta. The proximal stent is deployed immediately below the renal arteries. The cross-femoral catheter is used to pull the left limb catheter from the right femoral to the left. (From Chuter TAM, Wendt G, Hopkinson BR, et al. European experience with a system for bifurcated stent-graft insertion. J Endovasc Surg 1997;4:13–22.)

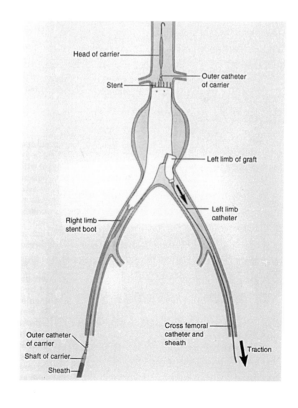

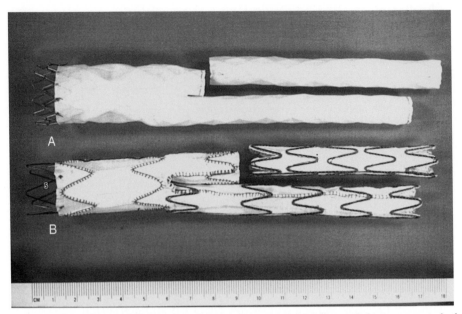

Figure 10–8. *A*, The Vanguard endovascular graft is a modular bifurcated device composed of a main graft and a separate contralateral limb component. The distal landing zone of the contralateral limb can be adjusted by changing the amount of graft overlap between the two grafts. The nitinol frame is located on the luminal surface of the graft. *B*, Talent endovascular bifurcated spring graft is also a modular bifurcated graft. The nitinol framework of the main body is located on the luminal surface, and the framework of the iliac component (i) is on the outer surface of the graft to decrease metal exposure to circulating blood. The uncovered proximal portion of the stent (s) has wide openings that permit suprarenal placement of the graft.

Devices Designed for Type IIC Abdominal Aortic Aneurysms

AAAs with extensive iliac artery involvement can be treated only with aorto-uniiliac grafts in combination with a standard femorofemoral bypass, placement of a contralateral iliac artery occluder device, and embolization of the ipsilateral hypogastric artery. The Parodi graft (Fig. 10–9*A*), the Montefiore graft (Figs. 10–9*B* and 10–10),[17] the Nottingham graft,[17] the Leicester graft,[18, 19] and the EVT aortoiliac graft were designed to treat this type of AAA.

Devices Designed for Type III Abdominal Aortic Aneurysms

Although type III AAAs are generally thought to be unsuitable for endovascular repair, certain EVGs with bare proximal stents that have wide interstices permit the proximal-fixation stent to be placed above the lowest renal artery. Such devices include the Montefiore graft,[20] the Chuter bifurcated graft,[4, 14] the Leicester device,[7, 19] and the Talent graft.

Montefiore Experience With Endovascular Grafts
Parodi Graft Versus the Montefiore Graft

The endovascular graft program at Montefiore Medical Center in New York began in November 1992, when the first stent graft repair of an AAA in North America was performed.[21] Since then, we have treated more than 40

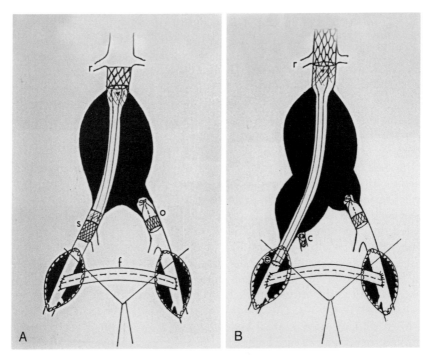

Figure 10–9. *A,* Parodi-type graft. The proximal stent is placed below the renal arteries (r), and the distal end of the graft is fixed with a second stent (s) in the iliac artery. A standard femorofemoral bypass (f) and placement of an occluder device (o) in the contralateral iliac artery completes the procedure. *B,* Montefiore "one-size-fits-all" graft. The bare portion of the proximal stent is placed above the renal arteries (r), and the distal end of the graft is brought out of the insertion arteriotomy site, where it is cut to the appropriate length. A hand-sewn endoluminal anastomosis (e) is then performed below the embolization coils (c).

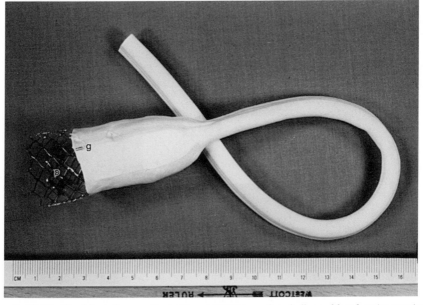

Figure 10–10. The Montefiore graft. A 10-mm IMPRA graft is balloon dilated at its proximal end prior to construction of the device. A large Palmaz stent (P-5014) (p) is then sutured to the proximal end of the graft using four U stitches. A gold marker (g) placed at the proximal end of the graft allows visualization of the proximal end of the graft with the fluoroscope, which is used to place it just below the lowest renal artery.

AAAs using EVGs. We have experience with the EVT tube and bifurcated grafts (Fig. 10–11), the Talent bifurcated graft (Fig. 10–12), and several types of home-made grafts. Most cases were performed using one of the home-made grafts, including the Parodi graft (ie, aorto-aortic and aortoiliac straight grafts) and the Montefiore graft (ie, aortofemoral graft). Initially, we used the Parodi aortoiliac grafts for AAAs that were not suited for tube grafts (Fig. 10–13 and see Fig. 10–9*A*). However, as we gained experience, we modified it into a Montefiore aortofemoral graft (see Fig. 10–9*B*) because of some difficulties we encountered with the Parodi graft. The first difficulty was calculating the exact measurement of the length of the graft. Because the Parodi device required placement of a second stent to fix the distal end of the graft, it was crucial to obtain an accurate measurement of the graft. In complex AAAs, we found this difficult to carry out despite the use of all the recommended imaging methods.

The Montefiore "one-size-fits-all" device employs a graft that is long enough so that the distal end of the graft emerges from the arteriotomy site used for insertion. The surgeon can tailor the length of the graft by cutting the excess graft at the arteriotomy site, followed by a hand-sewn endoluminal anastomosis (Fig. 10–14). This modification obviated the need for the precise and often difficult preoperative assessment of graft length. This feature also permitted treatment of an aneurysm with extensive external iliac artery involvement.

Other limitations of the Parodi graft were its inability to treat AAAs with short, proximal necks (<1.5 cm) and the frequent occurrence of proximal endoleaks. To overcome these problems, we began to deploy the bare portion

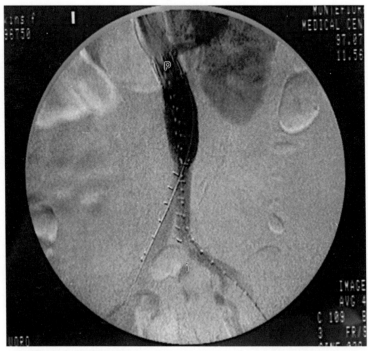

Figure 10–11. Angiogram of a completed endovascular repair of an aortic aneurysm using the bifurcated EVT graft. A proximal attachment device (p) is placed immediately below the renal artery, and the limbs of the graft are fixed in both common iliac arteries, thereby preserving internal iliac artery flow (i). Metallic markers placed on the surface of the graft show the absence of a twist in the graft.

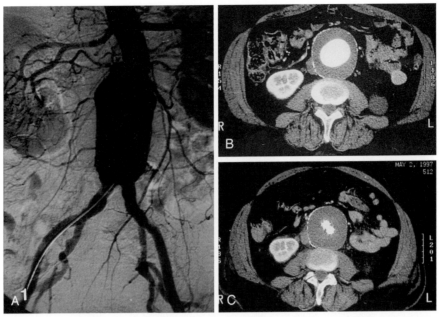

Figure 10–12. Endovascular repair of an abdominal aortic aneurysm using a Talent endovascular bifurcated spring graft. *A,* Preoperative angiogram reveals a large aortic aneurysm with a long proximal neck. The lack of a distal aortic cuff requires a bifurcated graft. *B,* Preoperative enhanced computed tomographic (CT) scan reveals a 7.8-cm aneurysm with mural thrombus. *C,* Postoperative enhanced CT scan. The contrast is confined to the limbs of the Talent graft, and the aneurysm is completely excluded from the circulation.

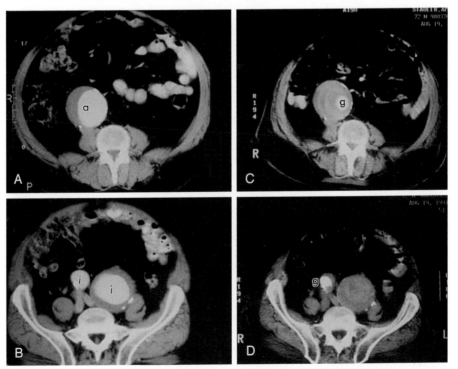

Figure 10–13. *A* and *B,* Endovascular repair of an abdominal aortic aneurysm (a) and bilateral common iliac artery aneurysms (i). *C* and *D,* After insertion of an endovascular graft (g), the aortic aneurysm and the bilateral common iliac artery aneurysms have thrombosed.

Illustration continued on following page

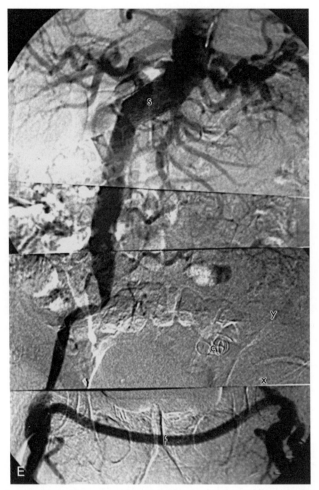

Figure 10–13 *Continued.* *E,* Postoperative angiogram demonstrates the completed reconstruction. Embolization coils within the origin of the left internal iliac artery (c) prevent backflow from this vessel into the left common iliac artery aneurysm. Ligation of the proximal left common femoral artery at point x, followed by the creation of a femorofemoral bypass (f), restores circulation to the lower extremities; s, proximal stent fixation site.

of the proximal stent across the orifice of the renal artery to obtain maximum contact between the proximal attachment device and the proximal aortic neck.

Construction of the Montefiore Device

Our EVG was constructed from 8- or 10-mm polytetrafluoroethylene (PTFE) grafts (ie, Gore-Tex thin-walled grafts, W. L. Gore and Associates, Flagstaff, AZ; Impra Company, Tempe, AZ). The proximal 4-cm portion of each graft was expanded to 30 mm to accommodate the diameter of the proximal aortic neck (Fig. 10–15A). Expansion was accomplished by means of gradual dilation using 10 atm of pressure with an esophageal dilatation balloon (Medi-tech Inc., Watertown, MA). The graft was then sutured to a Palmaz stent (P-5014, Johnson and Johnson Interventional Systems, Warren, NJ) with four U-shaped stitches placed to overlap one half the length of the stent.

The stent graft was then crimped onto a 35-mm balloon and front loaded into a 23-Fr sheath (Fig. 10–15B). The 35-mm balloon catheter had a second balloon at the tip of the catheter. This balloon functioned to create a smooth

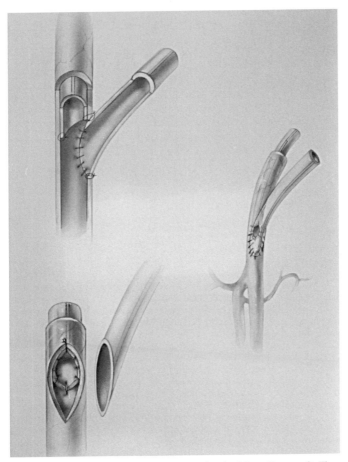

Figure 10–14. Management of the distal anastomosis for the Montefiore graft. The endovascular graft is long enough to emerge from the arteriotomy site at the femoral artery. The graft is then cut to an appropriate length, and a hand-sewn endoluminal anastomosis is carried out. The femorofemoral graft anastomosis was performed over the arteriotomy. (From Ohki T, Marin ML, Veith FJ, et al. Endovascular aorto-uni-iliac grafts and femoro-femoral bypass for bilateral limb-threatening ischemia. J Vasc Surg 1996;24:984–997.)

transition zone at the distal end of the delivery sheath and to occlude the sheath, which permitted pressurization of the sheath when saline was injected from the flush port. The pressurization provided variable pushability and flexibility of the sheath, depending on the amount of pressure applied. This feature facilitates insertion of the delivery sheath through diseased and tortuous iliac arteries.

The occluder device, which is placed in the contralateral iliac artery to prevent retrograde filling of the aneurysm, was also made from PTFE and a Palmaz stent (Fig. 10–15C). PTFE suture material was used as two ligatures to occlude one end of the expanded PTFE graft. A Palmaz 4014 stent was attached to the other end of the expanded PTFE graft by means of four U-shaped stitches. The occluder device was loaded onto an angioplasty balloon and then inserted into an 18-Fr sheath. A separate balloon catheter was used to create a smooth transition zone at the distal end of the sheath.

Coil Embolization of the Hypogastric Artery

Coil embolization of the hypogastric artery ipsilateral to the graft insertion site was carried out for Parodi type aortoiliac grafts if the graft crossed the

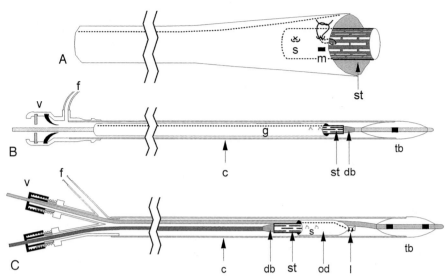

Figure 10–15. *A,* Montefiore "one-size-fits-all" graft. The proximal end of the graft is predilated with an esophageal balloon. A Palmaz 5014 stent (st) is sutured to the graft using four diametrically opposed U sutures (s) so that one half of the stent protrudes from the graft. A radiopaque gold marker (m) is sutured to the graft to denote the proximal end of the graft under the fluoroscope. In all cases, the length of the graft is 40 cm so that the distal end of the graft always emerges from the arteriotomy site. *B,* The delivery system consists of a single balloon catheter that has two balloons on a single shaft. The tip balloon (tb) functions as a tapered tip to the catheter system and allows pressurization of the flexible sheath (c) after saline is injected from the flush port (f). The stent graft is mounted onto the independent deploying balloon (db). st, stent; g, graft; v, hemostatic valve mechanism. *C,* Occluder device and delivery system. The occluder device (od) is constructed from a PTFE graft (s) sutured to a Palmaz stent (st). One end of the graft is ligated with two sutures (l) to prevent flow. The occluder device is mounted onto a deployment balloon (db). A separate balloon catheter serves as the tip balloon (tb). c, sheath; f, flush port; v, hemostatic valve mechanism.

hypogastric orifice. Coil embolization was performed at the time of the preoperative angiogram. Coil embolization was routinely performed for all Montefiore aortofemoral grafts.

Operative and Adjunct Techniques

Each procedure was performed in an operating room with the patient prepared for conversion to a standard open vascular surgical procedure if required. Bilateral surgical exposure of the common femoral arteries was followed by insertion of a diagnostic catheter into the aorta through one of these vessels. The location of the renal artery, aortoiliac bifurcation, and hypogastric arteries and the site for proximal graft implantation were identified.

A delivery catheter containing the EVG was then advanced over a wire. If difficulty was encountered advancing the device through a diseased, tortuous iliac artery, one of the following techniques was used. First, pressurization of the delivery catheter was performed, which in many cases is sufficient to insert the device. If this failed, additional proximal dissection of the external iliac artery from the surrounding tissue through a groin incision was carried out. This maneuver usually straightens any tortuosity in the external iliac artery. A snare wire was introduced from a left brachial artery puncture site to capture the guide wire introduced from the groin. By applying tension on both ends of the through-and-through guide wire, most of the tortuosity of the aortoiliac system was significantly reduced, and the introduction of the delivery system was always successful (Fig. 10–16). Our current threshold for this technique is very low, and we apply it as soon as we encounter any difficulties with device introduction. If stenosis in the iliac system was encountered, balloon dilatation before insertion of the device was undertaken.

After confirmation of the location of the lowest renal artery, the proximal stent was deployed in this proximal attachment site by inflating the deployment balloon under fluoroscopic guidance. During balloon inflation, the patient's blood pressure is lowered to a mean of 60 to 70 mm Hg, or asystole was temporarily induced by means of an intravenous bolus injection of adenosine (12 to 30 mg). The cephalad end of the graft material in the Montefiore graft was marked with a gold marker for fluoroscopic visualization. The graft was deployed so that this marker was placed just below the lowest renal artery. The bare stent above the gold marker covered the orifice of the renal artery.

After the EVG is deployed, an occluder device is placed in the contralateral common or external iliac artery, depending on the presence or absence of a common iliac artery aneurysm. A standard femorofemoral crossover graft was constructed.

Completion arteriograms and intravascular ultrasonography (IVUS) were performed to ensure technical satisfaction and the absence of an endoleak. IVUS can identify many lesions such as compression of the EVG or dissection of the iliac artery caused by the insertion of the graft, both of which are not always apparent on angiograms (Fig. 10–17).[22] Graft compressions and arterial dissections were treated by additional balloon dilatation or by the placement of a Palmaz stent or a Wallstent. If an endoleak resulted from low deployment of the proximal stent, a PTFE-covered Palmaz stent was deployed proximal to the previously deployed graft to seal the leakage. If it resulted from

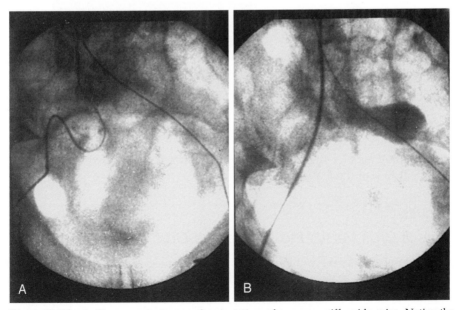

Figure 10–16. *A,* Fluoroscopic image after insertion of a super stiff guide wire. Notice the marked tortuosity of the iliac vessels. *B,* The tortuosity of the iliac vessels can be reduced by capturing the guide wire with a snare introduced from a brachial artery puncture and by applying tension on both ends of the wire.

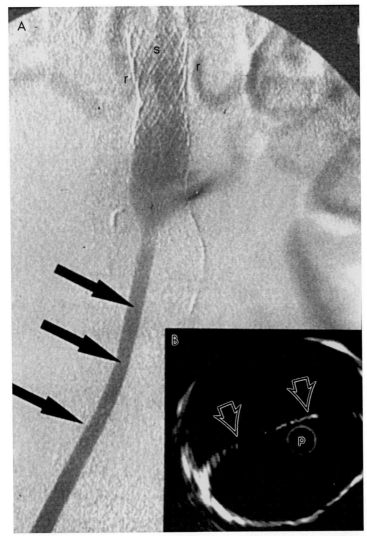

Figure 10–17. *A,* Angiogram after completion of an endovascular repair of an abdominal aortic aneurysm. The aneurysm has been excluded, and good flow is preserved through the endovascular graft. s, proximal fixation stent; r, renal artery. *B,* However, intravascular ultrasonography (IVUS) reveals compression of the endovascular graft at the sites denoted by the *arrows* in *A.* *Open arrows,* endovascular grafts; p, IVUS probe.

underdeployment of the stent, further dilatation of the proximal stent was sufficient to seal the leakage.

Results

Parodi Graft Versus the Montefiore Graft

Forty-one AAAs were treated endovascularly; eight were treated with the Parodi aortoiliac graft and 13 with the Montefiore aortofemoral graft. The remaining cases were treated with the EVT graft (eg, tube, bifurcated, aortoiliac), the bifurcated Talent graft, or the Parodi tube graft. There was no difference in the mean size of the AAAs or length of the proximal neck between the groups treated with the Parodi aortoiliac graft and the Montefiore aortofemoral graft (Table 10–1). However, when using the Montefiore graft,

Table 10–1.
Endovascular Repair with the Parodi Graft and Montefiore Graft

Graft	Cases	Mean Age	Mean Size of AAA	Mean Length of Proximal Neck	Range of Proximal Neck Length	Endoleaks
Parodi AI	8	76 y	6.8 cm	18 mm	10–30 mm	4 (50%)
Montefiore AF	13	78 y	6.8 cm	21 mm	6–35 mm	4 (31%)

AAA, abdominal aortic aneurysm; AI, aortoiliac; AF, aortofemoral.

we were able to treat aneurysms with a proximal neck length of 6 mm. The rate of endoleaks seemed to be lower with the Montefiore graft (50% versus 31%). There was one death in each group.

Endovascular Repair of Iliac Aneurysm

From 1993 through 1997, we treated 22 iliac artery aneurysms using EVGs. There were 18 men and 1 woman with a mean age of 72 years (range, 51 to 88 years). Nineteen common iliac (11 right, 8 left) and three internal iliac (two right, one left) artery aneurysms received EVGs. Eight patients (42%) had previous aortic surgery, and 16 (84%) had significant comorbid medical illnesses. Seventeen patients received epidural anesthesia, one patient was treated under general anesthesia, and one patient was treated under local anesthesia. One patient presented preoperatively with embolization from the aneurysm, and the remaining patients were asymptomatic. All of the EVGs were constructed from Palmaz stents and PTFE grafts in a manner similar to that described previously. All procedures were performed in the operating room under fluoroscopic guidance and arterial access was obtained by surgical exposure. The repairs were performed with one of the various techniques shown in Figure 10–18.

Procedure-related complications were limited to three cases (16%) (ie, one case each of embolization, hematoma, and colonic mucosal ischemia). A small reduction in the aneurysmal diameter was seen in 90% of the iliac artery aneurysms treated (Table 10–2). The remainder of the lesions were unchanged, with no aneurysm showing an increase in cross-sectional diameter on computed tomography images with follow-up to 3 years (mean, 16 months).

Table 10–2.
Endovascular Repair of Isolated Iliac Artery Aneurysms:
Outcome According to Type of Repair

Factor	Type of Repair*				
	A	B	C	D	E
Number of EVG procedures†	3	8	2	3	3
Endoleaks	0	0	1	0	0
Thromboses	0	0	0	1	0
Extrinsic graft compression (supplemental stent required)	0	1	0	1	0
Percent reduction in aneurysm diameter (mean + SD)	1.30 ± 1.83	5.30 ± 3.30	3.33 ± 1.44	11.10 ± 9.71	5.52 ± 5.25

*According to the type of repair shown in Figure 10–18.
†In some instances, the distal stent was eliminated, and the graft was anastomosed directly to the common femoral artery. EVG = endovascular grafts.

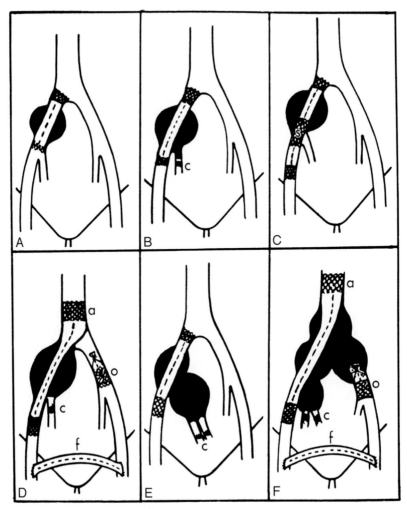

Figure 10–18. Techniques for the endoluminal repair of aortoiliac aneurysms: *A,* A localized common iliac artery aneurysm is treated with stents anchoring the endovascular graft proximal and distal to the aneurysm. *B* and *C,* If the aneurysm of the common iliac artery extends to the hypogastric vessel, placement of occlusion coils in the internal iliac artery (c) or deployment of an additional stent within the endovascular graft is performed to prevent retrograde flow from the hypogastric artery into the common iliac artery aneurysm. *D* and *E,* If there is no proximal neck of the iliac aneurysm (d) or for common iliac artery aneurysms with aortic aneurysms (f), a large aortic stent (a) is placed in the distal aorta. Before graft insertion, an occlusion coil is placed in the hypogastric artery or its branches (c). To perfuse the contralateral limb, a standard femorofemoral bypass (f) is performed. An occluder device (o) is inserted in the contralateral common iliac artery to prevent backflow perfusion of the aneurysms. *F,* For a wide mouth opening to an internal iliac artery aneurysm, the anterior and posterior divisions of the hypogastric artery are individually coil embolized (c), and the endovascular graft is secured with a stent above and below the origin of the aneurysmal artery, functionally excluding it from the circulation. In any of these four reconstruction techniques, the second (distal) stent, which is responsible for fixing the distal portion of the graft to the arterial wall, may be eliminated by extending the endovascular graft to the common femoral artery (ie, site of device insertion) and performing an endoluminal anastomosis as described in Figure 10–13. (From Marin ML, Veith FJ, Lyon RT, et al. Transfemoral endovascular repair of iliac artery aneurysms. Am J Surg 1995;170:179–182.)

Conclusions

EVG repair has been investigated in clinical trials since 1991. During this period, a variety of devices were developed, and guidelines[23] for their use and reporting standards [24] have been established. Several questions regarding the use of EVGs were raised, most of which still remain unanswered. These questions include the ethical and legal aspects[25] of EVG use, who should perform these procedures, and, most importantly, its efficacy and effectiveness.

After the first successful report of endovascular grafting for the treatment of AAAs by Parodi,[9] the indications for endovascular grafting were expanded to include arterial occlusive disease,[26, 27] occluded grafts,[28] peripheral aneurysms,[29, 30] and traumatic arterial lesions.[31, 32] Based on reported results, some of these indications, such as endovascular grafting for traumatic central arterial lesions and isolated iliac aneurysmal disease in high-risk surgical patients, seem to be justified. Although the treatment of AAAs with EVGs appears to interest physicians and manufacturers, the safety and long-term efficacy of this treatment remain to be proven. Data are needed because of the rate of mortality and the significant rate of complications, including endoleaks and distal embolization, and because of the availability of standard aneurysm repair techniques that have been proven safe and durable. Further investigation is required before endovascular repair of AAAs is widely used.

Several additional issues are of concern regarding the endovascular repair of aortic aneurysms, including occlusion of the hypogastric artery using a coil. It has been thought that occlusion of the hypogastric artery might be harmful or lethal. Iliopoulos and coworkers[33] described their experience with this occlusion, which led to lethal complications such as lower extremity paralysis, buttock necrosis, anal and bladder sphincteric dysfunction, and colorectal ischemia. However, our experience failed to confirm their findings.[34] We have intentionally occluded 48 hypogastric arteries to facilitate the endovascular repair of abdominal aortic and iliac artery aneurysms, and only 9% resulted in nonlethal consequences. These complications included three buttock claudications and one colonic mucosal ischemia. None required additional intervention, and all resolved with conservative therapy. We therefore believe unilateral coil embolization of hypogastric artery occlusion can be safely performed. Bilateral hypogastric artery occlusion may be required in cases in which bilateral common iliac arteries are aneurysmal. The safety of this procedure has yet to be proven.

Another issue is the management of endoleaks. There seems to be uniform agreement that large endoleaks should be aggressively treated. Rupture of AAAs after endovascular repair with large endoleaks has been reported.[9, 35] However, the appropriate treatment of endoleaks that have spontaneously sealed remains a matter of considerable debate. To address this issue, experimental aneurysms were created in canines and repaired with EVGs with small endoleaks.[36] These endoleaks were 4 mm in diameter, were spontaneously sealed, and could not be detected on postoperative angiograms. The aneurysmal pressure was chronically measured with a pressure transducer implanted in the aneurysmal wall. This study revealed that aneurysmal pressure in the control groups that had complete endovascular repair without endoleaks decreased significantly, whereas the pressure in the animals with endoleaks remained elevated at 80% of systemic pressure. On the basis of these results, we believe that angiographic closure of an endoleak does not provide protection from rupture and that all detected endoleaks, regardless of closure, should be treated if possible.

Although placement of the bare portion of the stent above the renal artery reduced the endoleak incidence, the consequence of this action on the renal artery remains a concern. Nasim and associates[19] reported that in five patients in whom the renal arteries were covered by stents only one patient's renal artery became occluded. This study also showed no changes in serum creatinine levels before and after stent placement. We placed the bare portion of the stent across the renal artery in 15 patients and did not encounter any renal artery occlusions or renal dysfunction as measured by serum creatinine levels.

Although several issues still must be answered, the procedure provides a means of treating patients whose comorbid illnesses make conventional repair dangerous or impossible. Shrinkage of the AAA has been observed when these grafts were successfully deployed.[37–40] Long-term follow-up of patients treated with EVGs is not yet available, but the initial early and midterm results are promising.

References

1. Ernst CB: Abdominal aortic aneurysm. N Engl J Med 1993;328:1167–1172.
2. McCombs RP, Roberts B. Acute renal failure after resection of abdominal aortic aneurysm. Surg Gynecol Obstet 1970;148:175–179.
3. Moore WS. The EVT tube and bifurcated endograft systems: technical considerations and clinical summary. J Endovasc Surg 1997;4:182–194.
4. Chuter TAM, Risberg BO, Hopkinson BR. Clinical experience with a bifurcated endovascular graft for abdominal aortic aneurysm repair. J Vasc Surg 1996;24:655–666.
5. Schumacher H, Allenberg JR, Eckstein HH. Morphological classification of abdominal aortic aneurysm in selection of patients for endovascular grafting. Br J Surg 1996;83:949–950.
6. Schumacher H, Eckstein HH, Kallinowski F, et al. Morphometry and classification in abdominal aortic aneurysms: patient selection for endovascular and open surgery. J Endovasc Surg 1997;4:39–44.
7. May J, White G, Waugh R, et al. Treatment of complex abdominal aortic aneurysms by a combination of endoluminal and extraluminal aortofemoral grafts. J Vasc Surg 1994;19:824–833.
8. White GH, Yu W, May J. Three year experience with the White-Yu endovascular GAD graft for transluminal repair of aortic and iliac aneurysms. J Endovasc Surg 1997;4:124–136.
9. Parodi JC, Palmaz JC, Barone HD. Transfemoral intraluminal graft implantation for abdominal aortic aneurysms. Ann Vasc Surg 1991;5:491–499.
10. Moore WS, Vescera CL. Repair of abdominal aortic aneurysm by transfemoral endovascular graft placement. Ann Surg 1994;220:331–341.
11. Chuter RAM, Green RM, Ouriel K, et al. Infrarenal aortic aneurysm morphology: implications for transfemoral repair. J Vasc Surg 1994;20:44–50.
12. Chuter TAM, Donayre C, Wendt G. Bifurcated stent-grafts for endovascular repair of abdominal aortic aneurysm: preliminary case reports. Surg Endosc 1994;8:800–802.
13. Chuter TAM, Green RM, Ouriel K, et al. Transfemoral endovascular aortic graft placement. J Vasc Surg 1993;18:185–197.
14. Chuter TAM, Wendt G, Hopkinson BR. European experience with a system for bifurcated stent-graft insertion. J Endovasc Surg 1997;4:13–22.
15. Blum U, Voshage G, Lammer J, et al. Endoluminal stent-grafts for infrarenal abdominal aortic aneurysms. N Engl J Med 1997;336:13–20.
16. Allen RC, White RA, Zarins CK, et al. What are the characteristics of the ideal endovascular graft for abdominal aortic aneurysm exclusion? J Endovasc Surg 1997;4:195–202.
17. Yusef SW, Whitaker SC, Chuter TAM. Early results of endovascular aortic aneurysm surgery with aortouniiiliac graft, contralateral iliac occlusion, and femorofemoral bypass. J Vasc Surg 1997;25:165–172.
18. Thompson MM, Sayers RD, Nasim A. Aortomonoiliac endovascular grafting: difficult solutions to difficult aneurysms. J Endovasc Surg 1997;4:174–181.
19. Nasim A, Thompson MM, Sayers RD, et al. Investigation of the relationship between aortic stent position and renal function. J Endovasc Surg 1995;2:90–91.
20. Wain RA, Marin ML, Veith FJ, et al. Endoleaks after endovascular graft treatment of aortic aneurysms: classification, risk factors, and outcome. J Vasc Surg 1998;27:69–80.
21. Parodi JC, Marin ML, Veith FJ. Transfemoral, endovascular stented graft repair of an abdominal aortic aneurysm. Arch Surg 1995;130:549–552.
22. Lyon RT, Marin ML, Veith FJ, et al. Intravascular ultrasound for intraoperative assessment of endovascular graft procedures. Proceedings of the 11th Annual Meeting of the Eastern Vascular Society; Atlantic City, NJ, 1997.
23. Veith FJ, Abbott WM, Yao JST, et al. Guidelines for development and use of transluminally placed endovascular prosthetic grafts in the arterial system. J Vasc Surg 1995;21:670–685.
24. Ahn SS, Rutherford RB, Johnston KW, et al. Ad Hoc Committee for standardized reporting practices in vascular surgery for the Society for Vascular Surgery/International Society for Cardiovascular Surgery: reporting standards for infrarenal endovascular abdominal aortic aneurysm repair. J Vasc Surg 1997;25:405–410.
25. Veith FJ, Marin ML. Ethical and legal issues related to endovascular graft investigation and early usage. J Endovasc Surg 1997;4:66–71.

26. Marin ML, Veith FJ, Cynamon J, et al. Transfemoral endovascular stented graft treatment of aorto-iliac and femoropopliteal occlusive disease for limb salvage. Am J Surg 1994;168:154–162.
27. Ohki T, Marin ML, Veith FJ, et al. Endovascular aorto-uni-iliac grafts and femorofemoral bypass for bilateral limb-threatening ischemia. J Vasc Surg 1996;245:984–997.
28. Sanchez LA, Marin ML, Veith FJ, et al. Placement of endovascular stented grafts via remote access sites: a new approach to the treatment of failed aortoiliofemoral reconstructions. Ann Vasc Surg 1995;9:1–8.
29. Marin ML, Veith FJ, Lyon RT, et al. Transfemoral endovascular repair of iliac artery aneurysms. Am J Surg 1995;170:179–182.
30. Tazavi MK, Dake MD, Semba CP, et al. Percutaneous endoluminal placement of stent-graft for the treatment of isolated iliac artery aneurysms. Radiology 1995;197:801–804.
31. Marin ML, Veith FJ, Panetta TF, et al. Percutaneous transfemoral stented graft repair of a traumatic femoral arteriovenous fistula. J Vasc Surg 1993;18:299–302.
32. Ohki T, Veith FJ, Marin ML, et al. Endovascular approaches for traumatic arterial lesions. Semin Vasc Surg, 1997;10:242–256.
33. Iliopoulos JI, Horanitz PE, Pierce GE, et al. The critical hypogastric circulation. Am J Surg 1987;154:671–675.
34. Marin ML, Veith FJ, Ohki T, et al. Intentional internal iliac artery occlusion to facilitate endovascular repair of aortoiliac aneurysms and occlusions. Proceedings of the 21st Annual Meeting of the Society of Southern Vascular Surgeons; Coronado, CA, 1997.
35. Lumsden AB, Allen RC, Chaikof EL, et al. Delayed rupture of aortic aneurysms following endovascular stent grafting. Am J Surg 1995;170:174–178.
36. Bettina M, Sanchez LA, Ohki T, et al. Endoleak after endovascular graft repair of experimental aortic aneurysms: Does coil embolization with angiographic "seal" lower intraaneurysmal pressure? J Vasc Surg 1998;27:454–462.
37. May J, White GH, Yu W, et al. A prospective study of changes in morphology and dimensions of abdominal aortic aneurysms following endoluminal repair: a preliminary report. J Endovasc Surg 1995;2:343–347.
38. Matsumura JS, Pearce WH, McCarthy JW, et al. Reduction in aortic aneurysm size: early results after endovascular graft placement. J Vasc Surg 1997;25:113–123.
39. Malina M, Ivancev K, Chuter TMA, et al. Changing aneurysmal morphology after endovascular grafting: relation to leakage or persistent perfusion. J Endovasc Surg 1997;4:23–30.
40. Balm R, Katee R, Blankensteijn JD, et al. CT-angiography of abdominal aortic aneurysms after transfemoral endovascular aneurysm management. Eur J Endovasc Surg 1996;12:182–188.

Surgical Approaches and Techniques for Treating Challenging Abdominal Aortic Aneurysms

Midline Versus Retroperitoneal Approach for Abdominal Aortic Aneurysm Surgery

Gregorio A. Sicard, M.D., and
Boulos Toursarkissian, M.D.

The transperitoneal approach is the most frequently used surgical access by surgeons operating on the infrarenal abdominal aorta. During the past decade, the retroperitoneal approach has experienced a resurgence of popularity based on the results of several retrospective and a few prospective studies demonstrating the many advantages of this approach over the more traditional transabdominal exposure.[4–9, 11–15]

The retroperitoneal approach was first used by John Abernathy in 1796 to ligate an aneurysm of the external iliac artery.[1] It was also the approach used by DuBost in 1951 in his landmark operation on an abdominal aortic aneurysm.[5] In 1980, Williams and collaborators expanded its use for surgery on the juxtarenal and suprarenal aorta.[4–9, 11–15] Since then, multiple studies have demonstrated the benefits and versatility of this approach.[6–9, 11–15] Despite these reports, its routine use in aortic reconstruction remains controversial.[2, 3]

In addition to its benefits, the retroperitoneal approach has many indications for its use (Table 11–1). Originally, the primary recommended use was for the so-called hostile abdomen, a term that encompassed multiple abdominal operations, previous pelvic or abdominal irradiation, prior transabdominal aortic surgery, and the presence of enteric or urinary stoma. During the past decade, other indications have been added for this versatile exposure, including morbid obesity, patients with ascites or peritoneal dialysis, inflammatory

Table 11–1.
Indications for and Relative Contraindications to the Retroperitoneal Approach for Aortic Revascularization in Aneurysmal Disease

Indications
- Hostile abdomen (eg, multiple abdominal procedures, urinary or enteric stomas, previous transabdominal aortic surgery, and prior pelvic or abdominal irradiation)
- Obesity
- Ascites or peritoneal dialysis
- Inflammatory aneurysm
- Aneurysm associated with horseshoe kidney or renal ectopia
- Juxtarenal or suprarenal aortic aneurysm

Relative Contraindications
- Previous left retroperitoneal operation
- Ruptured infrarenal aortic aneurysm
- Associated long or distal right renal artery stenosis

aortic aneurysms, juxtarenal aortic aneurysms, anastomotic aortic aneurysms, and aortic abnormalities associated with a horseshoe kidney or renal ectopia. Even though most surgeons with experience agree with the indications, the most debatable issue remains its use in routine aortic reconstruction.[2, 3]

The few relative contraindications to a retroperitoneal approach to the aorta include prior left retroperitoneal surgery; a free, noncontained aortic or left iliac aneurysm rupture; and a long, right renal artery stenosis extending well beyond its origin. Although not frequently found, a duplicated left-sided vena cava has been reported as another relative contraindication for the left retroperitoneal approach, although a right retroperitoneal aortic exposure is feasible in those cases. Moreover, an anticipated need for an anastomosis to the right external iliac artery is a relative contraindication, unless an additional right-sided kidney transplantation–like counterincision is carried out. In this situation, we prefer to carry the right limb to the right femoral position, unless contraindicated by local factors in the femoral area.

Multiple retrospective studies in the 1980s suggested that patients undergoing surgery using a retroperitoneal approach had more benign postoperative courses (Table 11–2).[6, 8, 9, 11, 12, 14] Collectively, these studies reported a lower incidence of postoperative paralytic ileus and shorter hospital stays. Other advantages included less intraoperative hypothermia, lower third-spacing fluid losses, and a lower incidence of respiratory problems. Hudson and colleagues[7] reported a lower production of prostaglandin metabolites in patients undergoing retroperitoneal compared with transabdominal vascular operations, metabolites that can cause adverse cardiac and hemodynamic changes.

These studies led to extensive debate and a call for prospective randomized studies. Three such studies have been published (Table 11–3).[3, 4, 13] The first randomized study report by Cambria and associates[3] randomized 54 patients to a retroperitoneal approach and 59 to a transabdominal approach. Although the incidence of paralytic ileus was lower in the retroperitoneal group, there were no differences in overall complications or in length of hospital stay. In the second study by Darling and collaborators,[4] a total of 27 patients were randomized. In that study, patients undergoing the retroperitoneal approach had a quicker return to a normal diet and a shorter hospital stay. In the third study, published by our group,[13] a total of 145 patients undergoing infrarenal aortic reconstruction (81 for aneurysms and 64 for occlusive disease) were randomized. The retroperitoneal group (70 patients) had significantly fewer postoperative complications compared with the transabdominal group (75 patients). This difference primarily reflected a decrease in paralytic ileus. Although hospital stay was decreased for the retroperitoneal group (9.9 versus 12.9 days), the difference did not reach statistical significance. Nevertheless, the length of intensive care unit stay and the overall cost of hospitalization were reduced for patients undergoing the retroperitoneal approach.

The in-hospital mortality rate was 0% for the retroperitoneal group and 1.4% for the transabdominal group, a difference that was not statistically significant. The incidence of incisional hernia was 10% for the retroperitoneal group, which was not significantly different from that for the transabdominal group. Neither our study nor the one by Cambria and colleagues demonstrated any significant differences in pulmonary complications between the two approaches. This can be attributed to the widespread use of postoperative epidural analgesia in patients undergoing major abdominal operations, a practice that was not as common in the previous decade, during which most of the retrospective studies were carried out.[6, 8, 9, 11, 12, 14]

Table 11–2.
Retrospective Studies of Transabdominal and Retroperitoneal Approaches in Aortic Surgery

Author (year)	No. of Patients		Paralytic Ileus*			Hospital Length of Stay (Days)			Mortality		
	Retro	*Trans*	*Retro*	*Trans*	*P Value*	*Retro*	*Trans*	*P Value*	*Retro*	*Trans*	*P Value*
Wilkens (1985)[14]	84	49	0.5%	50%		15	19	<0.05	5%	9%	NS
Johnson (1986)[8]	298	161	1%	6%	<0.001	12	17	<0.05	4%	3.7%	NS
Peck (1986)[11]	200	70	18%	19%	<0.001	7	10	NS	1.5%	2.8%	NS
Sicard (1987)[12]	54	50	0%	6%	<0.001	10	14	<0.02	1.9%	1.9%	NS
Leather (1989)[9]	193	106	0.5%	10.4%	<0.02	7	12	<0.02	3.6%	3.8%	NS
Gregory (1989)[6]	53	119	3.3%	4.9%	<0.01	9	13	<0.01	0%	4.2%	NS

Retro, retroperitoneal approach; Trans, transabdominal approach; NS, not significant.
*Based on individual study definitions of paralytic ileus.

Table 11-3.
Randomized, Prospective Trials of Transabdominal and Retroperitoneal Approaches in Aortic Surgery

Author (year)	No. of Patients		Paralytic Ileus*			Hospital Length of Stay (Days)			Mortality		
	Retro	Trans	Retro	Trans	P Value	Retro	Trans	P Value	Retro	Trans	P Value
Cambria (1990)[3]	54	59	3.5 d	4.0 d	<0.02	10.3	12.5	NS	0%	1.7%	NS
Darling (1992)[4]	15	12	2.1 d	4.0 d	<0.03	6.7	9.0	0.16	0%	0%	NS
Sicard (1995)[13]	70	75	0 d	11%	0.005	9.9	12.9	0.10	0%	3.0%	NS

Retro, retroperitoneal approach; Trans, transabdominal approach; NS, not significant.
*Based on individual study definitions of paralytic ileus.

Retroperitoneal Approach

The patient is positioned on a self-molding, vacuum-operated beanbag, with the left shoulder elevated 60 degrees off the table and the hips allowed to fall back as parallel to the table as possible. The left arm is rested on a Mayo stand with appropriate cushioning. The patient is positioned such that the kidney rest is halfway between the iliac crest and the costal margin. The kidney rest is maximally elevated, and the table is flexed into a jackknife position to allow a maximum opening of the space between the ribs and the iliac crest (Fig. 11–1). The legs may need to be supported on pillows. The beanbag is then suctioned to stabilize the positioning. If the surgeon antici-pates the need for suprarenal clamping, the left shoulder should be elevated closer to 90 degrees to allow the incision to be extended higher and more posteriorly. Positioning should also anticipate the possible need for right groin access if an aortofemoral bypass is contemplated; this can often be helped by rotating the table to the patient's left in due time.

The type of incision is dictated to some degree by the anticipated level of aortic disease. For a standard infrarenal exposure, the incision is started about 2 inches (5 cm) below the umbilicus at the lateral border of the left rectus and curved posteriorly and gently to the tip or superior border of the 12th rib; this incision can subsequently be extended posteriorly or the 12th rib resected. If the aneurysm is inflammatory, juxtarenal, or involves a chronic contained rupture, the incision should be carried into the inferior border of the 11th rib or into the 10th intercostal space (see Fig. 11–1).

The external oblique, internal oblique, and transversus abdominis muscles

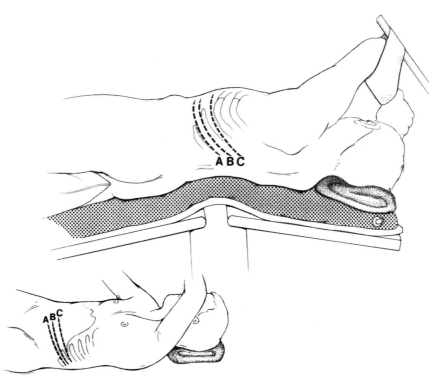

Figure 11–1. Patient positioning for a retroperitoneal approach to the infrarenal aorta and the location of incisions. Incision A is used for routine infrarenal exposure. Incision B is used for more complicated cases (ie, juxtarenal or inflammatory aneurysms), and incision C is used for suprarenal exposure of the aorta.

are divided with electrocautery. The lateral edge of the left rectus muscle may be partially divided for more medial exposure. The retroperitoneal space is best entered at the junction of the lateral border of the rectus to the lateral abdominal wall muscles by dividing the transversalis fascia and mobilizing the peritoneum medially and cephalad until the left ureter and left gonadal vein, adherent to the peritoneal envelope, are identified. The ureter is mobilized laterally along with periureteral fat with the use of a vessel loop to avoid later traction injury; this maneuver also helps in the posterior descent of the kidney. The gonadal vein is traced up to its junction with the left renal vein, where the gonadal vessel is ligated and divided. The kidney and its surrounding envelope are mobilized off the peritoneal sac and allowed to fall back against the posterior abdominal wall (Fig. 11–2). These latter two maneuvers help open the area of the juxtarenal aorta for dissection of the aortic neck. Depending on the level needed for aortic clamping, the left kidney can be mobilized anteriorly (Fig. 11–3). Several lumbar veins draining into the left renal vein should be ligated if additional juxtarenal or suprarenal exposure is required.

A Finochietto-type thoracic retractor is sutured to the abdominal wall with 2-0 silk to open the space between the costal margin and the iliac crest and to help maintain a static exposure (see Fig. 11–2). An Omni-type, self-retaining retractor is used as well for exposure, avoiding unnecessary motion of the intraabdominal contents and possible accidental injury to the spleen. The left common iliac artery is identified low in the wound and can be dissected for clamping; the proximal right common iliac artery can be similarly exposed;

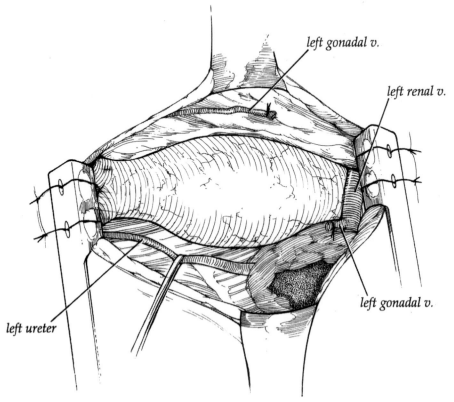

left gonadal v.

left renal v.

left gonadal v.

left ureter

Figure 11–2. Exposure achieved after the left ureter and kidney have been mobilized and the gonadal vein ligated.

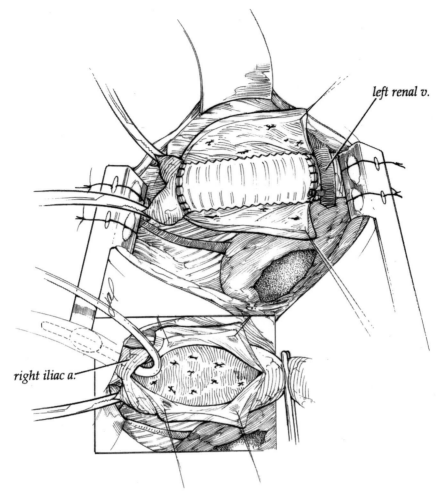

left renal v.

right iliac a:

Figure 11–3. Tube graft repair of aortic aneurysm using the retroperitoneal approach. If the proximal right iliac artery is difficult to clamp, endoluminal control with a balloon catheter is advisable *(inset).*

however, if more distal exposure is required or if the view is obscured by a large aneurysm, it is best to control backbleeding from the right iliac endoluminally after the aorta has been opened using a 6- or 9-Fr, Pruitt-type balloon occlusion-irrigation catheter (see Fig. 11–3, *inset*). Injury to the iliac veins is thereby avoided. It is often helpful to place a splanchnic-type retractor on the Omni inside the aneurysmal sac after it has been opened to retract its right wall and the peritoneal sac laterally, thereby enhancing exposure of the proximal and distal aortic neck and the proximal right iliac artery. The inferior mesenteric artery is best sutured endoluminally after the aorta has been opened. If the inferior mesenteric artery must be reimplanted, backbleeding can be controlled with a small balloon-occlusion catheter and reimplanted into the aortic graft in a Carrel patch fashion. The exposure achieved through this approach allows a tube graft repair of an aortic aneurysm, with or without external clamping of the right common iliac artery (see Fig. 11–3).

For juxtarenal aneurysms, it is usually possible to crossclamp the aorta between the renal arteries and the superior mesenteric artery (Fig. 11–4). Alternatively, the supraceliac aorta can be clamped after dividing the left crus

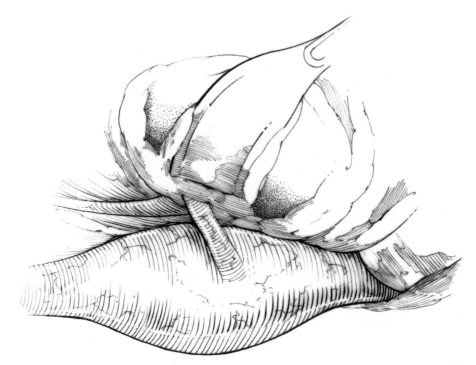

Figure 11–4. Retroperitoneal exposure of a juxtarenal abdominal aortic aneurysm. The left kidney has been mobilized anteromedially.

of the diaphragm for additional exposure of the suprarenal aorta up to the distal thoracic aorta. This approach frequently necessitates extending the incision back into the 10th or 11th interspace, depending on the desired level of proximal control. The superior margin of the diaphragm should be radially incised for 2 to 4 cm to allow for adequate retraction of the suprarenal aorta (Fig. 11–5). If the left renal artery is involved, a beveled graft to include the right renal artery is sutured, and the left renal artery is reimplanted in the lateral face of the graft to avoid kinking of the renal artery when the left kidney falls back into its fossa (Fig. 11–6).

   If an aortobifemoral bypass is deemed necessary, after completion of the proximal aortic anastomosis, blunt finger dissection is started immediately atop the right common iliac and femoral artery until the fingers meet and create a *tissue-free tunnel* (Fig. 11–7). The table is rotated to the left to allow better exposure of the right femoral area. A blunt-tipped clamp (eg, Crafoord aortic clamp) can then be passed from the groin into the left retroperitoneum and used to pass the graft limb down (Fig. 11–8). Passage of the left limb is easier because the iliac artery space was previously dissected. Staying on top of the vessels maintains the graft limbs behind the ureters (Fig. 11–9).

   In cases of inflammatory aneurysms, we prefer to have ureteral stents placed retrograde before the start of the aortic procedure to facilitate identification of the ureters. In these cases, the incision is placed in the 11th or 10th intercostal space, depending on the body habitus of the patient, and retroperitoneal dissection is carried out posterior to Gerota's fascia, allowing mobilization of the left kidney superiorly and medially (Fig. 11–10). Because the inflammatory process frequently stops at the inferior border of the left renal vein, this approach allows dissection of the juxtarenal aorta and frequently allows placement of an infrarenal aortic clamp (Fig. 11–11). Because

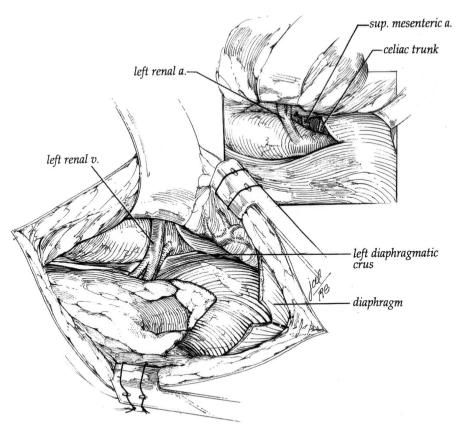

Figure 11–5. Suprarenal exposure of aorta with the kidney up or down. Notice the division of the left diaphragmatic crura and exposure of the superior mesenteric arteries and celiac axis *(inset).*

the inflammatory process usually involves the region of the iliac arteries, no attempt should be made to dissect these vessels free.

After the left ureter (with the stent in place) is identified, it is mobilized to identify its course in relation to the aneurysmal sac and to avoid injury when the aorta is opened. After the proximal aortic clamp is applied, the aneurysm is opened posterior and lateral to the left ureter, and the iliac arteries are controlled endoluminally (Fig. 11–12).

The retroperitoneal approach has been extremely useful in the surgical management of aortic aneurysms associated with a horseshoe kidney and renal ectopia. This approach completely avoids the need for extensive mobilization or division of the renal isthmus and its associated complications. Moreover, any reimplantation of accessory renal arteries can be incorporated into the anastomotic suture line or reimplanted onto the graft. O'Hara and coworkers[10] reported a decrease in intraoperative and postoperative complications when the retroperitoneal approach was used for this condition.

Closure of the incision may be carried out in one layer of interrupted figure-of-eight sutures or two layers of running suture, with the inner layer comprising the transversus abdominis and internal oblique muscles. Closure is facilitated by lowering the kidney rest and unflexing the operating table. Any opening in the diaphragm is closed with interrupted, nonabsorbable sutures. It is not always necessary to place a chest tube; if the defect is small, air may be aspirated out of the chest through a small red rubber catheter as

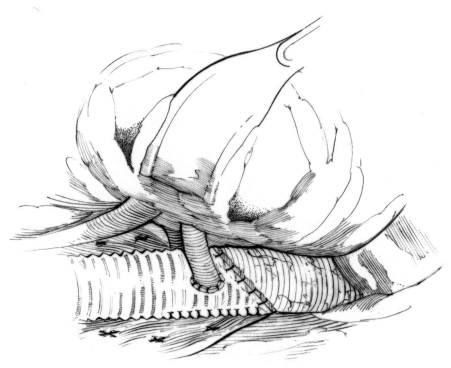

Figure 11–6. Repair of a juxatrenal aortic aneurysm with reimplantation of the left renal artery.

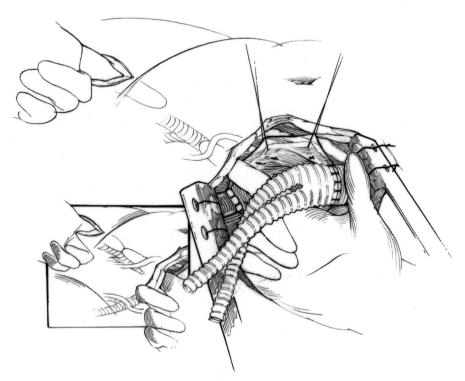

Figure 11–7. Aortobifemoral graft through the retroperitoneal approach, with creation of a right limb tunnel.

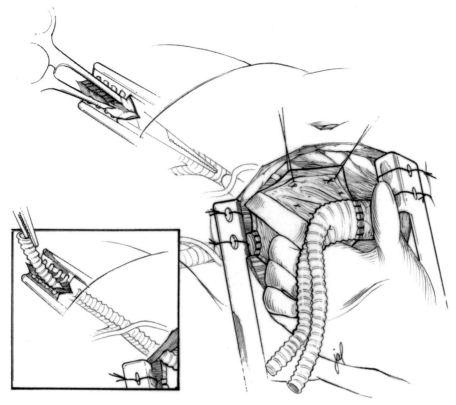

Figure 11-8. Aortobifemoral graft, with passage of a blunt tip clamp and pulling of right limb into femoral region *(inset).*

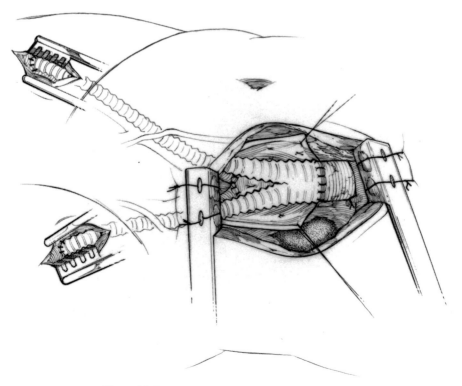

Figure 11-9. Completed aortobifemoral bypass graft.

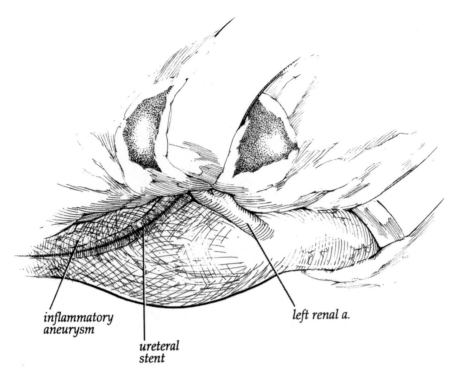

inflammatory aneurysm

ureteral stent

left renal a.

Figure 11–10. Retroperitoneal exposure of an inflammatory abdominal aortic aneurysm. Notice the ureteral stent and anteromedial rotation of the left kidney.

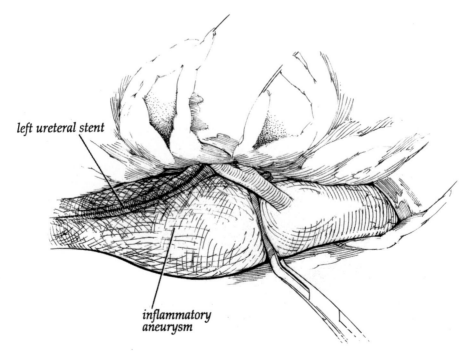

left ureteral stent

inflammatory aneurysm

Figure 11–11. Aortic crossclamping in an inflammatory abdominal aortic aneurysm.

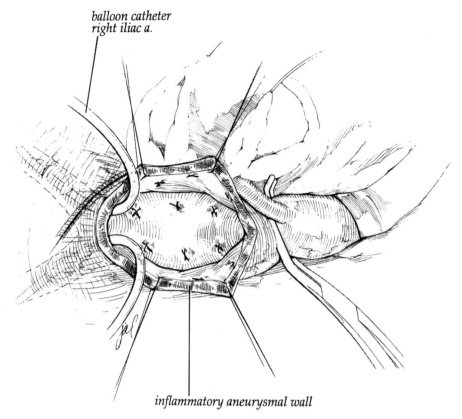

balloon catheter
right iliac a.

inflammatory aneurysmal wall

Figure 11–12. Control of inflammatory aortic aneurysm using intraluminal balloon catheters in the iliac arteries.

the sutures are tightened. In selected cases, we leave a closed-suction drain of the Jackson-Pratt variety in the retroperitoneal space behind the left kidney for 24 hours postoperatively.

Conclusions

The retroperitoneal approach to the aorta is a useful and versatile approach for the treatment of aortic aneurysms and should be part of the armamentarium of every vascular surgeon. It has many advantages over the transabdominal route in a large number of cases.

References

1. Abernathy J. Surgical Observations. London: Longman & O'Rees, 1804:209–231.
2. Brewster D. Transabdominal versus retroperitoneal approach for abdominal aortic aneurysm repair: current status of controversy. Semin Vasc Surg 1995;8:144–154.
3. Cambria RP, Brewster DC, Abbott WM, et al. Transperitoneal versus retroperitoneal approach for aortic reconstruction: a randomized prospective study. J Vasc Surg 1990;11:314–325.
4. Darling RC III, Shah DM, McClellan WR, et al. Decreased morbidity associated with retroperitoneal exclusion treatment for abdominal aortic aneurysm. J Cardiovasc Surg 1992;33:65–69.
5. DuBost G, Allary M, Oeconomos N. Resection of an aneurysm of the abdominal aorta: reestablishment of the continuity by a preserved human arterial graft with results after five months. Arch Surg 1952;64:405–408.
6. Gregory RT, Wheeler JR, Snyder SO, et al. Retroperitoneal approach to aortic surgery. J Cardiovasc Surg 1989;30:185–189.
7. Hudson JC, Wurm WH, O'Donnell TF Jr. Hemodynamic and prostacyclin release in the early

phases of aortic surgery: comparison of transabdominal and retroperitoneal approaches. J Vasc Surg 1988;7:190–198.

8. Johnson JN, McLoughlin GA, Wake PN, Helsby CR. Comparison of extraperitoneal and transperitoneal methods of aortoiliac reconstruction. J Cardiovasc Surg 1986;27:561–564.

9. Leather RP, Shah DM, Kaufman JL, et al. Comparative analysis of retroperitoneal and transperitoneal aortic replacement of aneurysms. Surg Gynecol Obstet 1989;168:387–393.

10. O'Hara PG, Hakaim AG, Hertzer NR, et al. Surgical management of aortic aneurysm and coexistent horseshoe kidney: review of a 31-year experience. J Vasc Surg 1993;17:940–947.

11. Peck IJ, McReynolds DG, Baker DH, Eastman AB. Extraperitoneal approach for aortoiliac reconstruction of the abdominal aorta. Am J Surg 1986;151:620–623.

12. Sicard GA, Freeman MC, Vander Woude JC, et al. Comparison between the transabdominal and retroperitoneal approach for reconstruction of the infrarenal abdominal aorta. J Vasc Surg 1987;5:19–27.

13. Sicard GA, Reilly JM, Rubin BG, et al. Transabdominal versus retroperitoneal incision for abdominal aortic surgery: report of a prospective randomized trial. J Vasc Surg 1995;21:174–183.

14. Wilkens FGJ, Widdershoven GMJ, Kirks RS. The retroperitoneal approach to aortoiliac vessels. Angiology 1985;7:31–37.

15. Williams GM, Ricotta J, Zinner M, Burdick J. The extended retroperitoneal approach for treatment of extensive atherosclerosis of the aorta and renal vessels. Surgery 1980;88:846–855.

Concomitant Aortic Aneurysm Repair and Other Abdominal Surgery

John W. Hallett, Jr., M.D.

The coincidental presence of an abdominal aortic aneurysm (AAA) and other intraabdominal disease can challenge a surgeon's judgment.[1–6] In some cases, the technical problems associated with the concurrent diseases become problematic, prompting several questions. Do both conditions require surgical intervention? If so, which should receive priority? What are the risks of a one-stage or two-stage approach to the concurrent conditions? The answers to these questions remain debatable, and this chapter focuses on principles of judgment and technique that result in the best short- and long-term outcomes.

Principles of Treating Aneurysms and Coexisting Disease

Most experienced surgeons follow the dictum that AAA repair should not be combined with other intraabdominal procedures that may result in bacterial contamination from the gastrointestinal or genitourinary systems. Concern about perioperative graft contamination, gastrointestinal or urinary anastomotic leaks, and subsequent abscess formation is justifiable. However, certain circumstances may motivate the surgeon to combine aneurysm repair with other procedures. Other factors favor staging the operations.

Gallbladder Disease

Cholelithiasis is the most common concurrent abdominal disease found in AAA patients (Fig. 12–1). Estimates of prevalence range from 5% to 20%. Most patients with gallstones are asymptomatic. Asymptomatic cholelithiasis rarely causes acute symptoms after AAA repair. In a review of 703 AAA patients by Ouriel and colleagues,[5] only 1.1% had acute postoperative cholecystitis, and the underlying cause was calculus cholecystitis in 75% of these patients. In a literature review of 131 patients who underwent aortic surgery without concomitant cholecystectomy for cholelithiasis, the prevalence of acute postoperative cholecystitis was 3.8%.[5, 7–10] In contrast, infectious or other biliary tract complications occurred in 2.4% of 287 patients who underwent concurrent AAA repair and cholecystectomy; the mortality rate was 14.3% for the patients with complications.

These pooled data indicate that the following approach is rational. Most gallstones that produce no symptoms can be left alone. Cholecystectomy

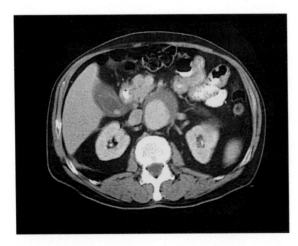

Figure 12–1. This 68-year-old patient presented with acute cholecystitis. A large, juxtarenal abdominal aortic aneurysm was discovered on abdominal computed tomography.

should be considered with AAA repair when gallbladder disease is apparent: the patient has had recent symptoms of cholecystitis, the gallbladder appears chronically inflamed, multiple stones are present, or common duct stones are palpable. Although laparoscopic cholecystectomy can be performed preoperatively in patients with symptoms of gallstone disease and can be followed at a later date with AAA repair, my colleagues and I have observed several patients in whom bile and gallstone spillage was evident 4 to 6 weeks after laparoscopic cholecystectomy and at the time of AAA repair.

Colorectal, Prostate, and Kidney Tumors

The dilemma in treating colorectal tumors is whether they should be resected before or after aneurysm repair (Fig. 12–2).[4, 6, 11] If a tumor is found incidentally during elective aneurysm repair, my colleagues and I repair the

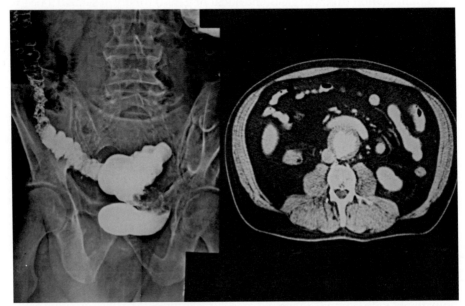

Figure 12–2. This 72-year-old patient presented with obstipation due to a rectosigmoid colonic carcinoma. An incidental abdominal aortic aneurysm was suspected on abdominal palpation and confirmed by computed tomography.

aneurysm first and return 3 to 6 weeks later to resect the tumor. If the tumor and the aneurysm are recognized preoperatively, we address the more pressing problem first. For example, an obstructing colonic tumor is relieved before repair of a smaller (4 to 6 cm) aneurysm. Occasionally, we encounter the combination of a tender or large aneurysm and an almost totally obstructive colonic tumor. When both diseases require correction during the same operation, the aneurysm is repaired first, and the retroperitoneum is completely closed before the bowel resection. Bowel resection is followed by creation of a colostomy and a Hartmann pouch. At a later date, the colostomy can be closed.

The literature contains few cases of combined aneurysm and colon cancer. Each review gives essentially the same recommendations that are outlined in this chapter. More than 30 years ago, Szilagyi and colleagues[6] concluded that the symptomatic lesion should be treated first. If neither is symptomatic, they recommend treating the AAA if it is larger than 6 cm and treating the cancer first if the AAA is less than 6 cm in diameter. If the cancer is metastatic, the AAA repair should be considered only if the aneurysm is causing symptoms (Fig. 12–3).

Prostatic cancer is another common malignancy that may be found when an AAA is recognized. Occasionally, the patient is a candidate for a radical prostatectomy, which includes iliac node dissection. When prostatectomy is indicated, my colleagues and I tend to repair the aortoiliac aneurysms first if they are 5 cm or larger and sample the iliac nodes simultaneously. The radical prostatectomy is delayed until the patient has recovered from the AAA repair (usually 6 to 8 weeks). In the case of smaller (<5 cm) AAAs, radical prostatectomy is performed first, and the AAA is monitored for expansion.

Renal cell carcinomas occasionally coexist with a large (>5 cm) AAA. In

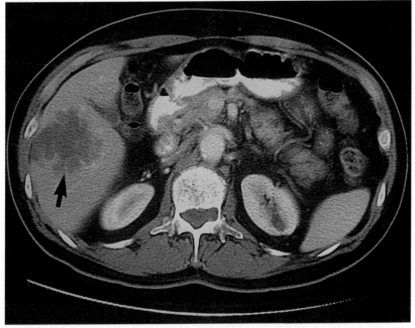

Figure 12–3. This patient was referred for an abdominal aortic aneurysm (not seen on this computed tomography [CT] cut) and vague right upper quadrant pain. Five years earlier, he had a left colectomy for carcinoma. This CT cut shows hepatic metastasis.

such cases, my coworkers and I have not been hesitant to combine a radical nephrectomy with an AAA repair.

Hernias

Inguinal hernias are common abdominal conditions in AAA patients. Inguinal hernias and recurrent incisional hernias may be related to the same systemic connective tissue disorder that results in the aneurysm. My colleagues and I usually repair symptomatic inguinal hernias first. The elective AAA repair follows after the patient has recovered from the herniorrhaphy. Although hernia repair can be combined successfully in many patients with AAA repair, systemic anticoagulation may predispose the patient to inguinal hematoma. Postoperative coughing and abdominal distention may also increase the risk of perioperative weakening or disruption of a hernia repair. We seldom combine these two procedures.

Mayo Clinic Experience

To ascertain the results of treating gastrointestinal disease concurrent with an AAA, I reviewed the records for 479 consecutive patients treated at the Mayo Clinic. Forty-seven patients (9.8%) were identified with 53 gastrointestinal disorders (Table 12–1). The most common conditions were cholelithiasis (4.8%), colonic diverticular disease (3.3%), colorectal neoplasm (1.5%), pancreatic disease (1%), and portal hypertension due to liver cirrhosis (0.5%). In this group of 47 patients, the 36 men and 11 women had a mean age of 71.9 years (range, 57 to 84 years). Mean follow-up was 29.3 months (range, 1 to 96 months).

The patients were treated following the principles previously outlined. The 30-day mortality rate was 0%, and the long-term mortality rate was 17% (8 of 47). No late graft infections have been discovered in these patients.

Conclusions

Although the appropriate surgical management of patients with other abdominal disease or conditions concomitant with AAA depends on the type and clinical activity of the associated condition, certain guidelines are available. The symptomatic condition takes priority. In the long run, however, both conditions require surgical attention if the quality and length of life are to be maximized. If operations are staged, most patients require at least 4 to 6 weeks for recovery before the second operation, and some patients need longer periods. If both conditions are asymptomatic, a larger AAA (>6 cm)

Table 12–1.
Concomitant Gastrointestinal Diseases in 479 Consecutive Patients Undergoing Elective Abdominal Aortic Aneurysm Repair at the Mayo Clinic

Condition	Patients
Cholelithiasis	23
Diverticular disease	16
Colorectal neoplasm	7
Pancreatic disease	5
Portal hypertension	2

is managed first. If the AAA is smaller, the other condition takes priority, and the AAA is rechecked in 6 to 8 weeks for expansion.

When the AAA and the other intraabdominal disease are both symptomatic, it is reasonable to repair the aneurysm first, achieve complete retroperitoneal coverage, and then finish with the operation for the concomitant disease. Such combinations are rare but can be accomplished successfully with precise surgical technique. As endovascular grafting for AAAs finds its place, the management of concomitant intraabdominal disease and aneurysms may require innovative tactics.

References

1. Hallett JW Jr, Bower TC, Cherry KJ, et al. Selection and preparation of high-risk patients for repair of abdominal aortic aneurysms. Mayo Clin Proc 1994;69:763–768.
2. Nevitt MP, Ballard DJ, Hallett JW Jr. Prognosis of abdominal aortic aneurysms: a population-based study. N Engl J Med 1989;321:1009–1014.
3. Lierz MF, Davis BE, Noble MJ, et al. Management of abdominal aortic aneurysm and invasive transitional cell carcinoma of bladder. J Urol 1993;149:476–479.
4. Nora JD, Pairolero PC, Nivatvongs S, et al. Concomitant abdominal aortic aneurysm and colorectal carcinoma: priority of resection. J Vasc Surg 1989;9:630–636.
5. Ouriel K, Green RM, Ricotta JJ, et al. Acute acalculous cholecystitis complicating abdominal aortic aneurysm resection. J Vasc Surg 1984;1:646–648.
6. Szilagyi DE, Elliot JP, Berguer R. Coincidental malignancy and abdominal aortic aneurysm. Arch Surg 1967;95:402–411.
7. String ST. Cholelithiasis and aortic reconstruction. J Vasc Surg 1984;1:664–667.
8. Thomas JH, McCroskey BL, Iliopoulos JI, et al. Aortoiliac reconstruction combined with nonvascular operations. Am J Surg 1983;146:784–787.
9. Ameli FM, Weiss M, Provan JL, Johnston KW. Safety of cholecystectomy with abdominal aortic surgery. Can J Surg 1987;30:170–173.
10. Bickerstaff LK, Hollier KH, Van Peenen HJ, et al. Abdominal aortic aneurysm repair combined with a second surgical procedure—morbidity and mortality. Surgery 1984;95:487–491.
11. Lobatto VJ, Rothenberg RE, LaRaja RD, Georgiou J. Coexistence of abdominal aortic aneurysm and carcinoma of the colon: a dilemma. J Vasc Surg 1985;2:724–726.

Concomitant Aortic Aneurysm Repair and Coronary Artery Bypass

Douglas J. Wirthlin, M.D., and
Jonathan P. Gertler, M.D.

Concomitant abdominal aortic aneurysm (AAA) repair and coronary artery bypass (CAB) is a surgical strategy used at some centers to treat high-risk cardiac patients with AAA. The incidence of coronary artery disease (CAD) among patients with AAA is high, and most short- and long-term mortality after AAA repair correlates with extent of CAD. Hertzer and colleagues[1] observed a 40% to 60% incidence of CAD among patients with AAA and found that up to one third of patients scheduled for AAA repair had CAD severe enough to warrant coronary artery bypass (CAB).[2] More than 25% of patients with three-vessel CAD develop myocardial ischemia after AAA repair,[3] and CAD is responsible for approximately 50% of postoperative mortality.[4, 5] Moreover, reports of long-term survival showed that CAD was responsible for 38%[6] to 65%[7] of late deaths after AAA repair.

These observations have prompted strategies to diagnose and treat CAD before AAA repair, and these approaches have significantly reduced the morbidity and mortality after AAA resection. Roger and coworkers[8] demonstrated that uncorrected CAD increased the risk of death nearly twofold after AAA reconstruction, and Toal and colleagues[9] observed significantly decreased mortality (2.3% from 8%) with selective evaluation of CAD and CAB before AAA repair. In the Coronary Artery Surgery Study (CASS), perioperative mortality was significantly increased for patients with CAD without prior CAB compared with similar patients who had previous CAB.[10] Thus, detection and treatment of CAD improves short- and long-term outcomes after AAA repair.

The mainstay of treatment for patients with both severe CAD and AAA is CAB or angioplasty, followed by AAA resection after a short recovery period (ie, staged approach). Concomitant AAA repair and CAB have been introduced for specific high-risk patients or because of potential medical and economic advantages. This chapter reviews the indications and results of combined CAB and AAA repair.

Combined Coronary Artery Bypass and Abdominal Aortic Aneurysm Repair

Overview

Reis and associates[11] were the first to publish results of combined CAB and AAA. Their report was published at the time when combining carotid endarterectomy (CEA) with CAB was becoming widely accepted. During this period, there were two premises for combining CAB with other noncardiac surgery. First, additional cardiac procedures performed simultaneously with CAB do not significantly increase morbidity and mortality. Second, each comorbidity, such as carotid artery disease and CAD, independently worsen the surgical outcome of treating either disease separately. Reis reported three cases of combined CAB and AAA repair, and all patients survived without cardiac morbidity. However, unlike combined CAB and CEA, simultaneous CAB and AAA has not achieved wide acceptance, and the literature is limited. Table 13–1 gives an overview of published reports.

One reason for the limited acceptance of combined CAB and AAA is the increased magnitude of surgery created by combining two major operations. When the early results of CAB combined with noncardiac surgery were presented in 1978, a surgeon commented, "These case reports only prove that some people are tough enough to survive an insult of this magnitude."[12] This concern may explain why a smaller operation, CEA combined with CAB, has been accepted while concomitant CAB and AAA has not. However, Korompai and colleagues,[13] proponents of combined procedures, suggest that, in selected patients, lesser procedures fail to correct the entire problem and are poorly tolerated.

Another reason for limited acceptance is that outcomes after a staged approach are excellent. Most patients with severe CAD and AAA are effectively treated with AAA repair staged after CAB, yielding low perioperative mortality (1.2% to 2.3%) and morbidity (2.4%).[4, 9, 14] Likewise, using a staged approach at our institution, Cambria and associates[15] observed a 2% mortality rate for 202 aortic reconstructions. Similarly, in a series of 106 AAA repairs in high-risk patients in which CAB was used selectively and staged before AAA, Hollier and coworkers[16] observed a 5.6% perioperative mortality rate. Staged CAB and AAA has become the standard of treatment for patients with both severe CAD and AAA.

Staged CAB and AAA resection is possible when the AAA can be repaired electively. However, a subset of patients present with severe CAD and symptomatic AAA, and the urgency of the AAA does not allow a staged approach. Dalton and associates[17] were the first to report this scenario as a rationale for combining AAA repair with CAB and reported no deaths in three cases. Whittemore and colleagues used the combined procedure successfully in 2 of 110 AAA repairs. In their 11-year experience, simultaneous CAB and AAA was used in 6 of 227 AAA repairs, and they observed no perioperative mortality and no cardiac morbidity.[19] Others have accepted this rationale and have reported their experience using combined CAB and AAA in this subset of patients.[20–27] Overall, the results of simultaneous procedures in this subset of patients have been good (see Table 13–1), and building on this experience, selected centers have expanded the indications for concomitant CAB and AAA to include CAD and asymptomatic AAA both to avoid the risk of AAA rupture after CAB,[28] and to reduce medical cost and patient convalescence time.[29, 30]

Despite the enthusiasm in some centers for concomitant CAB and AAA, the literature is limited by the small number of reports and number of patients. Patient numbers range from 1 to 21, with only four studies reporting more than 10 patients (see Table 13–1) suggesting that even among proponents of combined procedures, the use of simultaneous CAB and AAA is very selective. Another limitation of the literature is the variability of indications, patient selection, and surgical technique, which must be considered when interpreting the reported results of concomitant CAB and AAA. Accordingly,

Table 13–1.
Overview of Reports of Concomitant Abdominal Aortic Aneurysm Repair and Coronary Artery Bypass

Author	Year	Length of Study	Number of Patients (AAA/other)	Indications	CPB and CPB Time	30-day Mortality (%)	Morbidity (%)
Autschbach[20]	1995	4 yr 3 mo	21/4	Symptomatic AAA	On (?)	10.5	52
Black[46]	1995	Case reports	3	Asymptomatic AAA	On 149 min	0	0
Mohr[22]	1995	3 yr 4 mo	21/4	Impaired LVF & symptomatic AAA	On 131 min	12	40
Vicaretti[21]	1994	4 yr	15	Symptomatic AAA	Off 74 min	6.7	20
Blackbourne[28]	1994	5 yr 7 mo	6	Asymptomatic AAA, risk of AAA rupture	5 on, 1 off (?)	0	0
Taylor[23]	1993	Case report	1	Symptomatic AAA	Off (?)	0	0
Westaby[24]	1992	Case series	8	Impaired LVF & symptomatic AAA	On	25	?
Hinkamp[29]	1991	4 yr	17	Good LVF & asymptomatic AAA	Off (?)	5.9	18
Grebenik[26]	1989	Case report	1	Symptomatic AAA	On 174 min	0	100
Hoy[61]	1989	Case report	1	Asymptomatic AAA	Off (?)	0	0
Emery[25]	1988	Case series	2	Symptomatic AAA	Off, cannulas in place (?)	0	?
Reul[27]	1986	8 yr	11	Symptomatic AAA	On/off (?)	4	6
Ruby[19]	1985	11 yr	6	Symptomatic AAA	Off (?)	0	0
David[30]	1985	4 yr	4/10	Asymptomatic AAA	Off (?)	0	0
Korompai[13]	1982	?	5/58	Asymptomatic AAA	On/off (?)	4.7	?
Dalton[17]	1978	6.5 yr	3/68	Symptomatic AAA	?	2.9	0
Reis[11]	1977	Case series	3/7	Asymptomatic AAA	Off (?)	0	33

AAA, abdominal aortic aneurysm; CPB, cardiopulmonary bypass; LVF, left ventricular function.

this review discusses the results of combined CAB and AAA in the context of indications, patient selection, and surgical technique.

Indications

Concomitant CAB and AAA has been recommended for the following reasons: symptomatic AAA concurrent with severe CAD, AAA and severe CAD to avoid the risk of AAA rupture with the staged approach, and AAA and severe CAD to reduce medical costs and patient convalescence. Of these indications, concomitant CAB and AAA for symptomatic or leaking AAA in the presence of severe CAD is the most accepted and appears the most clinically sound. In situations of severe CAD concurrent with symptomatic AAA, AAA rupture poses the most immediate risk,[31–33] but AAA repair in the setting of severe CAD is associated with significant perioperative mortality (3% to 19%).[3, 5, 7, 34] Simultaneous CAB and AAA repair is a potential solution to this clinical dilemma.

Severe Coronary Artery Disease and Symptomatic Abdominal Aortic Aneurysm

The reported incidence of severe CAD concurrent with a symptomatic AAA ranges from 3%[19] to 11%[22] of all treated AAAs. The incidence of this subset of patients depends on the definition of symptomatic aneurysm and determination of the severity of CAD. In our series of 202 aortic reconstructions, CAB was deemed necessary in only 9% of patients,[15] and in a series of 422 AAA resections reported by Brown and colleagues,[4] only six patients required CAB. The need for CAB prior to AAA repair ranges from 1% to 30% and may depend on the treatment center.[2, 4, 15]

The urgency of AAA repair also varies. In one report that recommended combined procedures for symptomatic or "significant" AAAs, only three of 15 patients presented with a symptomatic AAA.[21] In another report, only patients with acutely expanding AAAs and symptoms, large AAAs and symptoms, or leaking AAAs underwent combined procedures.[20] Autschbach and coworkers provided the most specific indications for this approach: the extent of aortic disease must justify immediate intervention (ie, leaking AAA, prone to rupture, symptomatic patient, or enlarging aneurysm) and the severity of CAD must justify CAB (ie, unstable angina, left main disease, triple-vessel disease, or stable angina with poor left ventricular function).[20] Using these criteria, 21 of 259 patients with AAA (8%) underwent CAB simultaneous with AAA repair during a 4-year period.

The perioperative mortality after concomitant CAB and AAA for severe CAD and symptomatic AAA ranges from 0% to 25%[17, 19–24, 27] and from 0% to 12%[20–22, 27] when only series with more than 10 patients are considered. There was only one cardiac-related death[22] in a total of 98 patients. The cardiac morbidity and mortality after combined procedures are similar to results after elective AAA repair, and the perioperative mortality (in reports of more than 10 patients) is slightly higher than reported mortality for elective AAA repair (0% to 7%). The increased early mortality for combined procedures may reflect a population of higher-risk patients. For example, presentation with a symptomatic AAA correlates with increased perioperative morbidity and mortality compared with presentation with an asymptomatic AAA.[31] All of the patients treated with combined procedures had severe CAD, and 66 of the 98 patients had impaired left ventricular ejection fraction (LVEF). The highest perioperative mortality (12% to 25%) was reported for patients with CAD and low LVEF.[22, 24] Severe CAD, impaired LVEF, and symptomatic AAA significantly increased the perioperative risks, and most of these patients were refused AAA resection by other centers and referred specifically for concomitant CAB and AAA.[24] The long-term survival after combined AAA and CAB was favorable (81% at 2 years).[22]

Similar to early mortality, the perioperative morbidity was higher compared with that for elective AAA and ranged from 0% to 52% (see Table 13–1) with the highest morbidity (20% to 52%) observed in patients with low LVEF.[20–22] Only 1 of 98 patients had a myocardial infarction, and 17 of 98 complications were pulmonary (Table 13–2). Seven patients developed renal complications, and three had bleeding complications. There were no sternal or abdominal wound complications.

These results suggest that concomitant AAA and CAB is a feasible treatment option for patients with severe CAD and symptomatic AAA. Supporting this conclusion, Reul and colleagues[27] retrospectively compared the timing of CAB before vascular procedures in 1093 patients and observed no difference in perioperative mortality (4%), cardiac mortality (3%), and morbidity (6%) between combined procedures and AAA repair staged after CAB during the same admission. Mortality (0.1%) and cardiac morbidity (3%) were significantly lower in the third group, patients who underwent staged procedures during separate admissions (average of 24 months apart).[27] These data suggest that vascular procedures staged shortly after CAB offer no cardiac advantage compared with combined procedures and that urgent vascular procedures are higher risk than nonurgent procedures. Combining CAB with AAA appears to be appropriate for this subset of high-risk patients.

Risk of Aneurysm Rupture With the Staged Approach

The risk and mortality of AAA rupture has been well described, but until recently, there have been only anecdotal reports of AAA rupture after CAB.[14, 35, 36] Blackbourne and coworkers[28] reviewed 23 patients who underwent CAB and AAA to determine the optimal timing of AAA repair after CAB. Patients were divided into two groups: patients who had AAA repair 2 weeks or less after CAB (six combined procedures were included in this group) and patients who had AAA repair between 2 weeks and 6 months after CAB. Average AAA size in the group treated between 2 weeks and 6 months was 5.7 cm, compared with 7.3 cm in the group treated within 2 weeks ($P < 0.05$). They observed a 33% AAA rupture rate when AAA repair was performed longer than 2 weeks after CAB. They also observed no perioperative deaths or cardiac morbidity in the six combined procedures. From their experience, they

Table 13–2.
Morbidity Related to Cardiopulmonary Bypass

			Complications					
CPB	Patients	Early Mortality	MI	Bleeding	Pulmonary	Renal	Neurologic	Wound
On	67	8 (12%)	1 (1.5%)	4 (6%)	15 (22%)	9 (13%)	7 (10%)	0
Off	76	3 (3%)	2 (2.6%)	3 (4%)	2 (2.6%)	3 (4%)	0	1 (1%)

CPB, cardiopulmonary bypass; MI, myocardial infarction.

made two recommendations: AAA should be repaired within 2 weeks of CAB, and combined AAA repair and CAB is a safe option for treating patients with severe CAD and AAA.[28] This was the first report to consider risk of rupture a rationale for concomittant CAB and AAA, but the study was criticized for small patient numbers and potentially overrepresenting the AAA rupture rate after CAB.[37]

Risk of AAA rupture after CAB remains a concern. In an attempt to explain the pathophysiology, Dobrin[38] has suggested that elastase causes aneurysmal dilation and that collagenase causes aneurysm rupture.[38] Both proteases are elevated perioperatively, and collagenase activity is greatest at 7 days.[39–41] It is possible that increased collagenase activity perioperatively may weaken the aneurysm wall, making it more susceptible to rupture. Clinically, the reported AAA rupture rate after an unrelated operative procedure ranges from 3%[42] to 25%,[43] and as observed by Swanson and colleagues,[44] it occurs within 36 days (mean, 10 days) after laparotomy. These reports included a total of 13 patients with AAA sizes ranging from 5.0 to 13 cm, and most presented with AAAs larger than 8 cm, suggesting that aneurysm size may have been more of a factor than laparotomy. AAA rupture after CAB ranges from 2.9%[35] to 10%.[36] In a series of 246 patients treated at the Cleveland Clinic for AAA repair, 70 patients underwent CAB before AAA resection. Of these 70, two patients (2.9%) experienced AAA rupture after CAB.[35] During this series, a high rupture rate (42%) was observed for untreated AAA, suggesting that the two ruptures after CAB may have reflected the natural history of AAA rather than increased rate after CAB.[35] Findings at a molecular level support the hypothesis of increased AAA rupture after CAB. However, clinical observations vary and do not clearly suggest an increased rupture rate after CAB. Performing concomitant procedures for this rationale is unfounded.

Economic Rationale for Concomitant Operations

Another proposed rationale for combined AAA and CAB in patients with nonurgent AAAs is the potential cost benefit and shortened convalescence. Korompai and associates[13] first suggested a cost savings for concomitant AAA repair and CAB and reported costs of approximately $28,500 for staged procedures and $20,000 for combined procedures. Later, David[30] reviewed 26 consecutive patients during a 4-year period who required both CAB and AAA repair and compared medical costs of the staged approach to the combined approach. Most combined procedures were performed during the second half of the study, after espousing the concept of simultaneous procedures. There were four AAA resections and eight operations for aortoiliac disease in the combined group and five AAA resections and nine operations for aortoiliac disease in the staged group. The perioperative mortality (0%) and morbidity (40%) were the same for both groups, but the costs of care in terms of blood transfusions (4.2 versus 7.5 units), operating room time (231 versus 290 minutes), time in the intensive care unit (2.6 versus 3.7 days), and length of hospitalization (14 versus 29 days) were significantly less ($P < 0.05$) for combined procedures compared with staged procedures. David[30] also observed that patients undergoing combined procedures returned to work earlier (2.9 versus 6.4 months) and mentioned that the delay in the staged group resulted mostly from the recovery period between operations.

The cost savings and shortened patient convalescence shown by David[30] has not been replicated. Autschbach and coworkers[20] reviewed economic factors in their series of 25 high-risk patients with symptomatic AAAs and observed only decreased operating time (230 versus 318 minutes) when comparing combined with staged procedures. However, treatment of symptomatic AAAs in high-risk patients costs significantly more than elective treatment of AAAs,[45] which may partially explain why Autschbach did not observe a cost advantage.

Overall, it is unclear whether concomitant AAA repair and CAB provides any economic advantage over staged operations and, more importantly, whether combining procedures is safe when treating asymptomatic AAAs. Reul and associates[27] suggested that with increasing economic pressure on medical care, there may be increased demand for combined procedures.[27] However, less aggressive approaches to cost containment exist, such as care pathways and endovascular therapies, and the economic rationale for combined AAA and CAB should be entertained only when the safety is verified.

Surgical Technique

Simultaneous CAB and AAA repair introduces new variables (eg, urgency of each procedure, number of surgical teams, use of cardiopulmonary bypass [CPB], and dose and timing of heparin administration) that may alter established surgical technique. The following discussion addresses each step in concomitant AAA repair and CAB and the impact of each variable on outcome.

Surgical Teams and Timing

In most reported series, a team of cardiovascular surgeons performed the simultaneous procedure. In one report, a single cardiovascular surgeon performed the entire procedure and remarked that the CPB time could be reduced by using a team approach.[46] In two other reports, a team of cardiovascular surgeons performed the CAB, and a team of vascular surgeons resected the AAA after completion of the CAB.[19, 23] It is difficult to determine which approach is best because of limited data on operative time and CPB time. It seems logical that a team approach would shorten operative time and potentially affect outcome. Korompai and colleagues[13] give the most detailed discussion of timing and coordination of steps, and Figure 13–1 gives an example of their operative approach to concomitant CAB and AAA resection.

Anesthesia and Coronary Artery Bypass

In all reports, CAB was performed before AAA resection, and the specifics of anesthesia and CAB varied little compared with CAB alone. The patient is draped for sternotomy, laparotomy, and saphenous vein harvesting. Standard intraoperative monitoring is used for CAB.[20, 21] After completion of CAB, AAA resection can be started, and decisions regarding use of continued CPB, heparinization, and rewarming must be made.

Cardiopulmonary Bypass

Of all of the technical aspects of concomitant CAB and AAA, use of CPB has generated the most discussion. In the 19 reports reviewed in this chapter, six used CPB in all cases, two used CPB selectively, one discontinued CPB but left the canulas in place, seven discontinued CPB, and one did not state

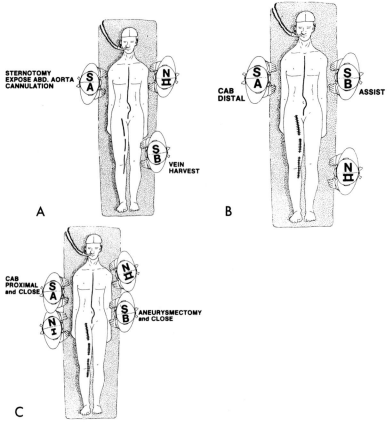

Figure 13–1. Coordinated steps of concomitant coronary artery bypass and abdominal aortic aneurysm repair. (From Korompai FL, Hayward MB, Knight WL. Noncardiac operations combined with coronary artery bypass. Surg Clin North Am 1982;62:221.)

whether CPB was used. Most of the larger and later reports used CPB during AAA repair (see Table 13–1).

Proponents of CPB during AAA argue that it reduces the hemodynamic consequences of aortic clamping and provides added myocardial protection during AAA resection (ie, the same rationale for recommending combined procedures for patients with low LVEF).[22, 24, 26] The adverse hemodynamic and cardiac consequences of aortic surgery have been described in several investigations.[47–54] Aortic crossclamping causes an acute rise in afterload and systemic vascular resistance and a decrease in the cardiac index.[47] After aortic crossclamping, the cardiac index decreases more for patients with AAA than patients with aortoiliac disease[48] and more for patients with CAD than those without.[49] Gooding and colleagues[49] also observed that, unlike patients without CAD, pulmonary capillary wedge pressure (PCWP) increased in patients with CAD after aortic clamping, and Attia and coworkers[50] reported that rises in PCWP during aortic clamping could lead to myocardial ischemia.[50] Harpole and associates[51] observed increased wall stress after aortic clamping in patients with and without CAD and suggested that increased wall stress could lead to global ventricular dysfunction and myocardial ischemia. The pathophysiologic consequences of aortic crossclamping are more severe in patients with CAD and are more likely to lead to myocardial ischemia, suggesting a beneficial role of CPB during AAA repair. Moreover, Westaby and coworkers[24] observed no hemodynamic changes during aortic crossclamping while on CPB.

Although coronary revascularization before AAA may also provide cardiac protection against the adverse effects of aortic crossclamping, a recovery period may be necessary for the heart to overcome the effects of cardioplegic arrest.[22] Right and left ventricular functions significantly decrease after CAB and do not return to baseline levels 24 to 48 hours postoperatively.[52, 53] Mangano and colleagues[54] observed a reduction in ventricular function after bypass and found that the reduction in function was greatest in patients with a LVEF of less than 45% preoperatively. These results support the continued use of CPB during AAA repair, especially in patients with impaired LVEF.

In addition to cardiac protection during aortic crossclamping, continued CPB has several other advantages. CPB gives more control over temperature regulation, and controlled hypothermia can be used to protect the spinal cord, kidneys, and visceral organs, especially in the setting of temporary supraceliac crossclamping.[24, 46] Black and associates[46] also suggested that there is minimal pressure in the aorta while on bypass, which may decrease clamp injury to the aorta and embolization. While on CPB, use of cardiotomy suctioning and rapid autotransfusion of intraabdominal blood loss is possible.[20, 24, 46] Emery and colleagues[25] recommend leaving the CPB cannulas in place and continuing full heparinization to permit immediate access to CPB in case a cardiovascular event or technical problem occurs during AAA repair. They presented a case of combined CAB and AAA in which an intraoperative aortic dissection occurred at the proximal anastomosis of the coronary grafts. The CPB cannulas had been left in place, and the patient was fully heparinized, allowing them to rapidly put the patient on CPB and repair the dissection.[25]

The advantages of CPB must be weighed against the potential complications of prolonged CPB. In studies that reported CPB times, the average time ranged from 122 to 174 minutes[22, 24, 26, 46] when CPB was continued during AAA resection, compared with 74 minutes[21] when CPB was discontinued before AAA resection. Prolonged CPB can cause activation of acute inflammatory components,[55] platelet activation and dysfunctional aggregation,[56] and consumption of coagulation components.[56] These changes may increase the risk of bleeding and acute lung injury after CPB.

Perioperative mortality was higher when CPB was continued during AAA repair (0% to 25%), compared with mortality for AAA repair off CPB (0% to 6.7%). This finding may be partially explained by the differences in patient population. For example, AAA repair off CPB was performed on patients with asymptomatic AAA and normal LVEF, whereas CPB during AAA repair was used primarily in higher risk patients.

Table 13–2 summarizes the morbidity after combined CAB and AAA, separating outcomes by use of CPB. Postoperative myocardial infarction, bleeding, and wound complications were not influenced by CPB use. However, pulmonary, renal, and neurologic complications were increased when CPB was continued during AAA resection. These differences may be attributed to a higher-risk patient population, but pulmonary, renal, and neurologic complications could also be related to prolonged CPB times.

The exact indications for CPB are unclear. CPB does appear to provide cardiac protection, especially in patients with low LVEF, and may be necessary in treating these high-risk patients. However, perioperative morbidity may be increased with prolonged CPB times, suggesting that CPB should be used selectively. Alternatively, steps of the combined procedure should be coordinated between two teams to shorten CPB times when CPB is deemed necessary during AAA repair.

Heparinization

Heparinization is determined in large part by the use of CPB, and several strategies are presented in the literature. David[30] reversed heparin after CAB and used local heparin during AAA resection. Reul and colleagues[27] did not reverse heparin and used the same heparinization during AAA repair. In another report, heparin was reversed with one half of the calculated dose of protamine, followed by AAA repair without further heparinization.[29] Several surgeons reverse heparin after CAB and reheparinize only as needed during AAA repair.[20–22]

Abdominal Aortic Aneurysm Repair

AAA repair in combined procedures varies little from AAA resection performed alone. In most cases, the sternotomy is left open, which provides excellent exposure of the abdominal aorta and easy access to the supraceliac aorta.[24] Bleeding complications are a major concern with combined procedures, and several surgeons stress the importance of meticulous hemostasis and minimal dissection.[23, 46] As recommended by Autschbach and coworkers,[20] a shielded prosthesis is mandatory. Mohr[22] was the only investigator to report intraoperative blood loss, which ranged from 1500 to 2700 mL in 25 combined procedures.[22] Average use of blood products per report ranged from 4 to 8 units of packed red blood cells, 0 to 12 units of fresh-frozen plasma, and 0 to 12 units of platelets.[22, 26, 29, 30] The operative time ranged from 3.83 to 6.6 hours.[20–22, 30]

Alternative Approaches

Alternative approaches for treating patients with severe CAD and AAA exist and should be considered when determining the need for combined CAB and AAA. Nonresectional treatment has been recommended for selected high-risk patients,[57] and perioperative mortality of 7% has been reported using this approach.[58] Partial (femoral-femoral) CPB during AAA repair was used successfully in two patients with severely impaired LVEF.[59]

Endovascular therapies provide the most promising potential treatment alternative. Several groups have observed high technical success rates, low perioperative mortality rates, and low morbidity rates with endovascular repair of AAA.[62–64] In their initial experience of endovascular treatment of 30 AAAs, Brewster and colleagues[60] had a 93% technical success rate and observed decreased systemic complications, blood loss, intensive care unit stay, and hospitalization compared with 28 similar patients who underwent traditional AAA repair. The long-term outcomes after endovascular AAA repairs must be evaluated before catheter-based interventions replace traditional AAA repairs.

Conclusions

The data on concomitant AAA repair and CAB are sparse, but several investigators have reported reasonable results with combined procedures. Combined procedures should be performed only in selected patients at centers where there is ample experience with concomitant AAA repair and CAB. In our view, the only strong indication for this procedure is severe CAD with a symptomatic or ruptured AAA requiring urgent treatment. The optimal coordination of specific steps and surgical teams should be determined at each center, adhering to the principles that CPB time should be minimized and CPB should be used selectively for patients with severe LVEF. Further development of endovascular treatment of AAA may obviate the need for concomitant AAA repair and CAB.

References

1. Hertzer NR. Basic data concerning associated coronary artery disease in peripheral vascular patients. Anna Vasc Surg 1987;1:616–620.
2. Hertzer NR, Beren EG, Young JR, et al. Coronary artery disease in peripheral vascular patients: a classification of 100 coronary angiograms and results of surgical management. Ann Surg 1984;199:223–233.
3. Blombery PA, Ferguson IA, Rosengarten DS, et al. The role of coronary artery disease in complications of abdominal aortic aneurysm surgery. Surgery 1985;101:150–155.
4. Brown OW, Hollier LH, Pairolero PC, et al. Abdominal aortic aneurysm and coronary artery disease. Arch Surg 1981;116:1484–1488.
5. Hertzer NR. Fatal myocardial infarction following abdominal aortic aneurysm resection: three hundred forty-three patients followed 6–11 years prospectively. Ann Surg 1980;192:667–673.
6. Hollier LH, Plate G, O'Brien PC, et al. Late survival after abdominal aortic aneurysm repair: influence of coronary artery disease. J Vasc Surg 1984;1:290–299.
7. Jamieson WRE, Janusz MT, Miyagishima RT, et al. Influence of ischemic heart disease on early and late mortality after surgery for peripheral occlusive vascular disease. Circulation 1982;66:192–197.
8. Roger VL, Ballard DJ, Hallett JW et al. Influence of coronary artery disease on morbidity and mortality after abdominal aortic aneurysmectomy: a population-based study, 1971–1987. J Am Coll Cardiol 1989;14:1245–1252.
9. Toal KW, Jaccocks MA, Elkins RC. Preoperative coronary artery bypass grafting in patients undergoing abdominal aortic reconstruction. Am J Surg 1984;148:825–829.
10. Foster ED, Davis KB, Carpenter JA, et al. Risk of noncardiac operation in patients with defined coronary disease: the Coronary Artery Surgery Study (CASS) registry experience. Ann Thorac Surg 1986;41:42–50.
11. Reis RL, Hannah H. Management of patients with severe, coexistent coronary artery and peripheral vascular disease. J Thorac Cardiovasc Surg 1977;73:909–918.
12. American College of Chest Physicians annual meeting. Report presented to the Committee for Cardiovascular Surgery; Washington, DC, 1978.
13. Korompai FL, Hayward RH, Knight WL. Noncardiac operations combined with coronary artery bypass. Surg Clin North Am 1982;62:215–224.
14. Suggs WD, Smith III RB, Wintraub WS, et al. Selective screening for coronary artery disease in patients undergoing elective repair of abdominal aortic aneurysms. J Vasc Surg 1993;18:349–357.
15. Cambria RP, Brewster DC, Abbott WA, et al. The impact of selective use of dipyridamole-thallium scans and surgical factors on the current morbidity of aortic surgery. J Vasc Surg 1992;15:43–50.
16. Hollier LH, Reigel MM, Kazmier FJ, et al. Conventional repair of abdominal aortic aneurysm in the high-risk patient: a plea for abandonment of nonresective treatment. J Vasc Surg 1986;3:712–717.
17. Dalton ML, Parker TM, Mistrot JJ, et al. Concomitant coronary artery bypass and major noncardiac surgery. J Thorac Cardiovasc Surg 1978;75:621–624.
18. Whittemore AD, Clowes AW, Hechtman HB, et al. Aortic aneurysm repair: reduced operative mortality associated with maintenance of optimal cardiac performance. Ann Surg 1980;192:414–421.
19. Ruby ST, Whittemore AD, Couch NP, et al. Coronary artery disease in patients requiring abdominal aortic aneurysm repair. Ann Surg 1985;201:758–764.
20. Autschbach R, Falk V, Walther T, et al. Simultaneous coronary bypass and abdominal aortic surgery in patients with severe coronary disease—indications and results. Eur J Cardiothorac Surg 1995;9:678–684.
21. Vicaretti M, Fletcher JP, Richardson A, et al. Combined coronary artery bypass grafting and abdominal aortic aneurysm repair. Cardiovasc Surg 1994;2:340–343.
22. Mohr FW, Falk V, Autschbach R, et al. One-stage surgery of coronary arteries and abdominal aorta in patients with impaired left ventricular function. Circulation 1995;91:379–385.
23. Taylor SM, Fujitani RM, Myers JC, et al. Combined coronary artery bypass and abdominal

aortic aneurysmectomy: appropriate management in selected cases. South Med J 1993;86:974–976.

24. Westaby S, Parry A, Grebenik CR, et al. Combined cardiac and abdominal aortic aneurysm operations: the dual operation on cardiopulmonary bypass. J Thorac Cardiovasc Surg 1992;104:990–995.
25. Emery RW, Ott RA, Bernhard V, et al. Surgical approach to combined coronary revascularization and abdominal aortic aneurysmectomy. J Cardiovasc Surg 1988;29:143–145.
26. Grebenik CR, Trinca JJ. Abdominal aortic aneurysm repair and coronary artery grafting as a combined procedure on coardiopulmonary bypass. J Cardiothorac Anesth 1989;3:473–476.
27. Reul CJ, Cooley DA, Duncan JM, et al. The effect of coronary bypass on the outcome of peripheral vascular operations in 1093 patients. J Vasc Surg 1986;3:788–798.
28. Blackbourne LH, Tribble CG, Langenburg SE, et al. Optimal timing of abdominal aortic aneurysm repair after coronary artery revascularization. Ann Surg 1994;219:693–698.
29. Hinkamp TJ, Pifarre R, Bakhos M, et al. Combined myocardial revascularization and abdominal aortic aneurysm repair. Ann Thorac Surg 1991;51:470–472.
30. David TE. Combined cardiac and abdominal aortic surgery. Circulation 1985;72(suppl II):18–21.
31. Sullivan CA, Rohrer MJ, Cutler BS. Clinical management of the symptomatic but unruptured abdominal aortic aneurysm. J Vasc Surg 1990;11:799–803.
32. Jensen BS, Vestersgaard-Andersen T. The natural history of abdominal aortic aneurysm [see comments]. Eur J Vasc Surg 1989;3:135–139.
33. Satta J, Laara E, Reinila A, et al. The rupture type determines the outcome for ruptured abdominal aortic aneurysm patients. Ann Chir Gynaecol 1997;86:24–29.
34. Crawford ES, Saleh SA, Babb III JW, et al. Infrarenal abdominal aortic aneurysm factors influencing survival after operations performed over a 25-year period. Ann Surg 1981;193:699–709.
35. Hertzer NR, Young JR, Beren EG, et al. Late results of coronary bypass in patients with infrarenal aortic aneurysms. Ann Surg 1987;205:360–367.
36. Smith RB III. *In* discussion of Ruby ST. Coronary artery disease in patients requiring abdominal aortic aneurysm repair. Ann Surg 1985;201:763.
37. Dean RH. *In* discussion of Blackbourne LH et al. Ann Surg 1994;219:696–697.
38. Dobrin PB. Pathophysiology and pathogenesis of aortic aneurysms: current concepts. Surg Clin North Am 1989;69:687–703.
39. Hunt TK, Winkle WV. Fundamentals of wound management in surgery. *In* Wound Healing: Normal Repair. South Plainfield, NJ: Chirurgecom, 1976.
40. Busuttil RW, Abou-Zamzam AM, Machleder HI. Collagenase activity of the human aorta. Arch Surg 1980;115:1373–1378.
41. Cohen J. *In* discussion of Durham SJ, Steed DL, Moosa HH, et al. Probability of rupture of an abdominal aortic aneurysm after an unrelated operative procedure: a prospective study. J Vasc Surg 1991;13:248–252.
42. Durham SJ, Steed DL, Moosa HH, et al. Probability of rupture of an abdominal aortic aneurysm after an unrelated operative procedure: a prospective study. J Vasc Surg 1991;13:248–252.
43. Nora JD, Pairolero PC, Niratuongs S, et al. Concomitant abdominal aortic aneurysm and colorectal carcinoma: priority of resection. J Vasc Surg 1989;9:630–636.
44. Swanson RJ, Littooy FN, Hunt TK, et al. Laparotomy as a precipitating factor in the rupture of intraabdominal aneurysms. Arch Surg 1980;115:299–304.
45. Breckwoldt WL, Mackey WC, Donnell Jr TF. The economic implications of high-risk abdominal aortic aneurysms. J Vasc Surg 1991;13:798–803; discussion 803–804.
46. Black JJM, Desai JB. Combined coronary artery bypass surgery and abdominal aneurysm repair. J R Soc Med 1995;88:350–352.
47. Fiser WP, Thompson BW, Thompson AR, et al. Nuclear cardiac ejection fraction and cardiac index in abdominal aortic surgery. Surgery 1983;94:736–739.
48. Dunn E, Prager RL, Fry W, et al. The effect of abdominal aortic cross-clamping on myocardial function. J Surg Res 1977;22:463–468.
49. Gooding JM, Archie JP, McDowell H. Hemodynamic response to infrarenal aortic cross-clamping in patients with and without coronary artery disease. Criti Care Med 1980;8:382–385.
50. Attia R, Murphy JD, Snider M, et al. Myocardial ischemia due to infrarenal aortic cross-clamping during aortic surgery in patients with severe coronary artery disease. Circulation 1976;53:961–964.
51. Harpole DH, Clements FM, Quill T, et al. Right and left ventricular performance during and after abdominal aortic aneurysm repair. Ann Surg 1989;209:356–362.
52. Breisblatt WB, Stein KL, Wolfe CJ, et al. Acute myocardial dysfunction and recovery: a common occurrence after coronary bypass surgery. J Am Coll Cardiol 1990;15:1261–1269.
53. Roberts AJ, Spies SM, Sanders JH, et al. Serial assessment of left ventricular performance following coronary artery bypass grafting: early postoperative results with myocardial protection afforded by multidose hypothermic potassium crystalloid cardioplegia. J Thorac Cardiovasc Surg 1981;81:69–84.
54. Mangano DT. Biventricular function after myocardial revascularization in humans: deterioration and recovery patterns during the first 24 hours. Anesthesiology 1985;62:571–577.

55. Colman RW. Platelet and neutrophil activation in cardiopulmonary bypass. Ann Thorac Surg 1990;49:32–34.
56. Rinder CS, Bohnert J, Rinder HM, et al. Platelet activation and aggregation during cardiopulmonary bypass. Anesthesiology 1991;75:388–393.
57. Pevec WC, Holcroft JW, Blaisdell FW. Ligation and extraanatomic arterial reconstruction for the treatment of aneurysms of the abdominal aorta [review]. J Vasc Surg 1994;20:629–636.
58. Karmody AM, Leather RP, Goldman M, et al. The current position of nonresective treatment for abdominal aortic aneurysm. Surgery 1983;94:591–597.
59. Fiore WM, Ouriel K, Green R, et al. High-risk aortic aneurysm repair with partial cardiopulmonary bypass. J Vasc Surg 1987;6:563–565.
60. Brewster DC, Geller SC, Kaufman JA, et al. Initial experience with endovascular aneurysm repair: comparison of early results with conventional open repair. J Vasc Surg (In press).
61. Hoy FBY, Brody N, Gomez RC. Concomitant vascular procedures in conjunction with myocardial revascularization: all or none? A report of a case. Can J Surg 1989;32:442–444.
62. Chuter TA, Risberg B, Hopkinson BR, et al. Clinical experience with a bifurcated endovascular graft for abdominal aortic aneurysm repair. J Vasc Surg 1996;24:655–666.
63. Blum V, Langer M, Spillner G, et al. Abdominal aortic aneurysms: preliminary technical and clinical results with transfemoral placement of endovascular self-expanding stent-grafts. Radiology 1996;198:25–31.
64. Moore WS, Rutherford RB. Transfemoral endovascular repair of abdominal aortic aneurysm: results of the North American EVT Phase I trial. J Vasc Surg 1996;23:543–53.

Complicated Abdominal Aortic Aneurysm Repair

Roy Greenberg, M.D., and Richard Green, M.D.

The treatment of abdominal aortic aneurysms has evolved significantly over the years. Unfortunately, surgery for even the simplest aneurysm carries significant morbidity and mortality in the range of 3% to 5%. Most aneurysms are infrarenal, but 2% to 20% extend to a pararenal or suprarenal location.[1, 2] Some aneurysms are inflammatory, and a number of patients have aberrant anatomy. Concomitant visceral or renal artery disease is also prevalent in this patient population. These complicating factors increase the complexity of aneurysm repair and the potential for morbidity and mortality. An understanding of aneurysm pathophysiology, use of preoperative imaging techniques, and a surgeon well versed in the various exposures and methods of repair allow for optimal results.

Molecular Aspects of Aneurysmal Disease

The search is underway for a molecular mechanism that can predict the formation of an infrarenal aneurysm, the rate of expansion, risk of rupture, cause of a severe inflammatory reaction, or extension into the more proximal aortic branches. The fundamental characteristics of the aortic wall are important. The resistance of an artery to aneurysmal dilation is thought to be related to the lamellar structure of the arterial wall. The lamellar arrangement of the infrarenal abdominal aorta differs from the more proximal aorta and is often cited as an explanation for the high frequency of infrarenal aortic dilation in preference to other locations. The relative abundance of smooth muscle cells, collagen, and elastin differ markedly in aneurysms, atherosclerotic disease, and normal aortas. Apoptosis of smooth muscle cells has been associated with wall degeneration and pathologic dilation.[3] Pathologic examination of aortic aneurysms has demonstrated globally abnormal cellular populations with undefined origins.

The relative concentrations of collagen and elastin appear to be closely linked to aneurysm formation. Elastin is primarily responsible for wall recoil, and the collagen is associated with wall strength. Genetic mutations involving type III collagen or elastic fibers have been detected in patients with inherited aneurysm syndromes.[4] The status of elastic matrices, increased concentrations of elastin-degrading proteinases, and diminished amounts of their associated inhibitors[3, 4] have been correlated with aneurysm formation. Paradoxically, the total content of aortic elastin is not significantly altered in infrarenal or suprarenal aneurysms.[4] However, the surface area of an aneurysmal aorta is much greater than that of a normal aorta, and the total amount of elastin may be more dispersed in these pathologic cases. In contrast to nonspecific aneurysms, inflammatory aneurysms have a markedly decreased total elastin content, which may reflect the increased concentration of macrophages and neutrophils and their associated release of elastin degradation proteins. Despite the prevalence of some degree of inflammation in nonspecific aneurysms, the cause and effect relationship of this phenomenon has not been established.[4]

The spectrum of inflammation in aneurysmal disease ranges from the development of lymphoid follicles seen in severe forms of inflammatory aneurysms to mild changes detectable only on microscopic investigation. The process is pathologically identical to idiopathic retroperitoneal fibrosis, which is seen more commonly in the setting of a nondilated aorta.[5] The aortic wall histology differs markedly between inflammatory and nonspecific aneurysms. The surrounding chronic periaortitis is predominately B cells enveloped by T lymphocytes, representing follicle formation. Adhesion molecules (primarily ICAM-1 and VCAM-1) are abundant and probably dominate the formation of new lymphoid follicles by perpetuation of the inflammatory response.[5] Quantitative levels of adhesion molecules appear to correlate strongly with the degree of inflammation. A variety of matrix metalloproteinases, interleukins, and other chemoattractants participate in the formation of all types of aneurysms to some extent but are often exaggerated in inflammatory aneurysms.[6, 7] The thrombus itself, present in most aneurysms, is biologically active and may be integrally involved with further expansion, extension, or inflammation of the aneurysm.[8]

Infections may be causative factors. *Chlamydia pneumoniae* and cytomegalovirus infections have been implicated in the formation of inflammatory and noninflammatory aneurysms.[9, 10]

The demonstration of pathologic differences between inflammatory and nonspecific aneurysms predicts different causes and clinical sequelae. No such differences have been found in patients with different degrees of aneurysmal disease (suprarenal versus infrarenal). Undetected intrinsic structural defects, hemodynamic properties, or other extrinsic factors may explain the extension or formation of aneurysms in the pararenal or suprarenal location.

Preoperative Patient Evaluation

Imaging

The preoperative evaluation of aneurysmal dilation of the abdominal aorta is essential. Accurate knowledge of the relevant anatomy enables the ideal surgical management of these complex patients. Pararenal aneurysms have no infrarenal segment of nondilated aorta. Suprarenal aneurysms must involve at least one of the renal artery orifices. Inflammatory aneurysms typically have a thick rind of surrounding adherent tissue in conjunction with a pathologic inflammatory response not seen with nonspecific aneurysms. Preoperative discrimination between infrarenal aortic aneurysms and more complex conditions is imperative. Attention must be directed to determination of an acceptable sewing neck, the extent of aneurysmal disease, and the presence of occlusive disease in the renal, superior mesenteric, inferior mesenteric, or celiac arteries. Without this information, preoperative patient preparation and the most appropriate operative approach cannot occur.

B-mode ultrasonography is an effective tool for screening patients for aneurysmal disease. The ease of use, noninvasive nature, and low cost make this an ideal initial evaluation. Many studies have confirmed the accuracy of

B-mode ultrasonography to detect changes in aneurysmal diameter over time.[11] However, details regarding the aneurysm neck, aortic bifurcation, or involvement of renal and visceral vessels cannot be accurately performed with ultrasonography.[12] Consequently, physicians rely on various alternative imaging modalities, including computed tomography (CT) scans, magnetic resonance (MR) imaging techniques, and angiography to help delineate the anatomy. Controversy over the ideal imaging technique is expressed in the radiology and surgical literature.[11–21] The advent of endovascular aneurysm repair has placed emphasis on the detailed assessment of aneurysm morphology.

Historically, conventional aortography has been viewed as the gold standard of aortic aneurysm imaging. This method allows a detailed look at the vascular anatomy and intraluminal architecture. Precise delineation of anomalous renal vasculature, stenoses of the renal or mesenteric vessels, and the amount of iliac arteriosclerosis is possible. The intraluminal nature of this study precludes data regarding the overall size of the aneurysm or extent of intramural calcification, and it conveys no information about the surrounding organs. The length of the neck, extent of thrombus, and dilation of iliac vessels are not well established with angiography alone and can occasionally be misleading. The invasive nature of the study portends potential complications, including hematoma of the puncture site, embolism, allergic reactions to dye, and contrast-induced renal failure. Surgeons differ about the necessity of preoperative angiography in the setting of infrarenal aneurysms. Johnston and Scobie's[22] series from 1988 demonstrated that preoperative angiography did not significantly affect operative decision making about routine infrarenal aortic aneurysms. A meta-analysis of 680 patients with aortic aneurysms had concomitant occlusive lesions that were angiographically detected.[23] The clinical significance of these lesions is unknown. It is our practice to perform aortography on patients with complex aneurysms, those with simultaneous symptoms attributable to occlusive disease, and candidates for endovascular aneurysm repair.

Conventional CT has been used for more than 20 years to evelute aneurysms. However, calculations regarding the aneurysm neck or size made from conventional axial images assumes that the axis of the aneurysm is perpendicular to the image slice. This was found by Ouriel and colleagues[24] to be an inaccurate method of measurement. Modifications in scanning techniques have allowed clinicians to more accurately evaluate aneurysm morphology.

Improved resolution, alternative methods of data acquisition, and more sophisticated computer software have resulted from the development of spiral CT scanning. Patients are placed on a table moving at a designated speed through a rotating scanner that continuously acquires data. The data is stored in a three-dimensional format, denoted as voxels. Excellent spatial resolution is obtained by the use of special protocols involving timed contrast administration and specific scanning parameters that enable detailed assessment of aneurysm morphology and associated visceral vessel pathology. Scanning protocols have been designed to provide directed assessment of the pararenal aorta, depicting accurate information regarding the status of renal and visceral vessels. The accuracy of this morphologic data has been confirmed by numerous investigators.[14, 15]

Data can be displayed with conventional axial images or in a three-dimensional format. The technique can be further modified by using large amounts of contrast and timed imaging to selectively evaluate the arterial tree. This process is called *CT angiography*. This provides excellent information regarding the relationships of visceral vessels to the aneurysm.[12, 17] CT angiographic evaluation of concurrent disease in branch vessels and demonstration of small or anomalous vessels may still be inferior to conventional angiography. Rubin and associates[17] correlated CT angiographic interpretations with surgical findings. The sensitivity and specificity of CT angiography for the detection of renal arterial stenoses was 92% and 83%, respectively.[17] However, accurate arterial data is often obtained at the expense of information about the surrounding organs.

Intravascular ultrasonography (IVUS) is frequently used for the assessment of aneurysms. IVUS technology is extremely accurate in locating the aneurysm neck, involvement of visceral vessels, and distal cuff evaluation. Substantial information regarding the morphology of the aneurysm, thrombus, and surrounding plaque can be obtained.[21] The accuracy of the IVUS images has created doubt about detailed measurements obtained from other imaging techniques.[21] IVUS imaging is best performed in conjunction with fluoroscopic guidance. It is particularly useful for sizing and the placement of endovascular devices. It has additional applications in the evaluation of stent placement and incomplete expansion.

MR angiography has received much attention. The renal artery ostia were located in 90% of cases, but the presence of anomalous vasculature decreases the sensitivity to 50%.[14] Like spiral CT scanning, a high spatial resolution is obtained by the use of specific image processing programs and experienced technologists. Current MR techniques may be suboptimal for the detection of stenoses in renal and visceral vessels, but future advances prompt optimism among radiologists. A distinct advantage of MR over CT scanning is the ability to interrogate the aneurysm wall. Inflammatory aneurysms are accurately differentiated from those without inflammatory components using specially designed protocols. Tennant and colleagues[20] noticed a characteristic onion-skin appearance of the wall of inflammatory aneurysms on the T1-weighted images and STIR sequences (Fig. 14–1).

Careful evaluation of the ureters in patients with suspected inflammatory aneurysms can be helpful. The normal lateral displacement of ureters by noninflammatory aneurysms is reversed in the setting of severe inflammation. As the ureters become encased in fibrotic material, they deviate medially. This

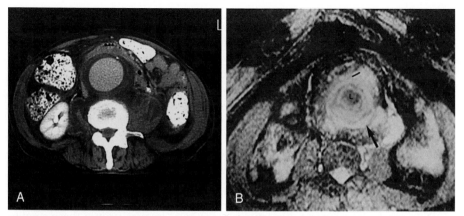

Figure 14–1. *A,* The computed tomographic characteristics of an inflammatory aneurysm include a rind of 1 cm or larger. *B,* The magnetic resonance image demonstrates the onion-skin appearance created by the inflammatory component of the aneurysm.

can be seen by using CT or MR imaging in addition to intravenous pyelography studies.[25]

Medical Workup

Cardiopulmonary Assessment

The morbidity and mortality of patients with complex aortic aneurysms are higher than for those requiring standard infrarenal repair. Nearly 60% of perioperative and late deaths of aneurysm patients result from coronary arterial disease.[26] The need for objective preoperative cardiac testing is best determined by the presence of symptoms attributable to coronary vascular disease, evidence of ischemia or previous myocardial infarction confirmed by electrocardiography, or a history of congestive heart failure. Patients with these risk factors must undergo a functional assessment of the coronary circulation. The ejection fraction, although commonly used in preoperative decision making, is not a good predictor of postoperative myocardial events.[27] Dipyridamole-thallium and dobutamine echocargiography have largely replaced exercise stress tests in determination of stress-induced ischemia in the patient with peripheral vascular disease.[28] The routine use of coronary angiography is not recommended in the absence of a positive functional test result.[29] Evaluation of myocardial function and treatment decisions should be made in the context of the overall patient situation. Careful consideration of the risk-benefit ratio of aneurysm repair and coronary revascularization must be emphasized in the preoperative period. Intraoperative monitoring devices are frequently necessary for optimal intraoperative management of complex aortic cases.

Pulmonary function is also critical. Prolonged postoperative intubation, although not desired, often is necessary. Pulmonary function tests are helpful in predicting postoperative difficulties or in establishing the surgical risks and potential benefits of preoperative or postoperative bronchodilators.

Renal Assessment

Baseline renal function is the most reliable predictor of postoperative renal complications.[1] Intrinsic or parenchymal renal disease must be differentiated from renovascular disease to determine the potential benefits of revascularization. The presence of hypertension, uremia, or an elevated serum creatinine level indicates the need for detailed renal evaluation. In the setting of renal insufficiency, the size of both kidneys should be measured using ultrasonography or CT. Careful use of contrast agents in this setting is advisable. The functional status of the kidneys must be assessed with serum and urine evaluations. Warm ischemia time, the use of suprarenal clamping techniques, and atheroemboli all contribute to postoperative renal deterioration. Meticulous monitoring and rapid treatment of intraoperative and postoperative hypotension can deter further renal dysfunction. Uremic patients should be dialyzed preoperatively to provide an optimal fluid balance and platelet function.

Risk of Rupture

The decision to operate on any abdominal aneurysm portrays the surgeon's belief that the risk of aneurysm rupture is greater than the morbidity and mortality associated with operative repair. Numerous individuals have attempted to quantify factors predicting aneurysm rupture. The maximal diameter of the aneurysm is the single most important factor. Extrapolation of data pertaining to infrarenal aortic aneurysms is the only means of assessing the risk of rupture of more complex aneurysms. The Society for Vascular Surgery and the International Society for Cardiovascular Surgery guidelines for aneurysm repair indicate that the rupture risk rises significantly with a maximal diameter greater than 5.0 cm.[30] Additional criteria include an expansion rate greater than 0.5 cm/year. Chronic obstructive pulmonary disease and systemic hypertension also are associated with a higher rate of rupture.[31, 32] Imaging limitations must be considered when measurements are taken from CT scans. There are no special data for patients with pararenal or inflammatory aneurysms; consequently, the risk of rupture is extrapolated from information regarding infrarenal aneurysms.

Operative Techniques for the Complicated Aortic Aneurysm

Exposure of Pararenal Aneurysms

Successful complex aneurysm repair requires a knowledgeable surgeon, meticulous and expeditious technique, and proper patient selection. Exposure can be obtained using one of three methods. The operative approach depends on the surgeon's expertise, the preoperative determination of proximal clamp location, and associated problems, such as iliac artery aneurysms, renal artery stenoses, and the patient's body habitus. Proper patient positioning is imperative for any of the operative approaches.

In the first method, a left flank retroperitoneal approach provides unimpeded exposure and continuous control of the subdiaphragmatic aorta. The incision is from the 11th interspace to the border of the rectus muscle. Care is taken to enter the retroperitoneal space laterally and to avoid violating the peritoneal cavity. The left ureter must be identified and carefully retracted for aortic exposure. This approach is useful in short, obese patients or in those with hostile abdomens. In the setting of severe right iliac or renal artery disease, this dissection may prove difficult in terms of distal exposure.

In the second method, a midline, transperitoneal approach with transcrural exposure of the supraceliac aorta provides discontinuous aortic control, allowing repair of juxtarenal aneurysms and some suprarenal aneurysms. This approach involves the least amount of dissection and allows exposure of both renal arteries in addition to the entire iliac system. If the aorta is normal at the level of the superior mesenteric artery, the aneurysm can usually be repaired with this approach. If more exposure is required, conversion to the third option is easily accomplished.

In the third method, a midline, transperitoneal approach with medial visceral rotation provides the most flexibility of the three methods. It allows complete and continuous exposure of the subdiaphragmatic aorta, its branches, and iliac systems.

Regardless of the preferred exposure method, the surgeon should be familiar with the different approaches. They provide the necessary flexibility to care for any complex aneurysm in the presence or absence of concomitant disease.

Aortic Clamping and Grafting

Systemic vascular resistance increases as a result of aortic clamping, causing myocardial strain and higher oxygen consumption. The more proximal the clamp, the more significant is the rise in afterload, and the more severe is the myocardial stress. Modulation of intraoperative preload and afterload help to diminish the effects of increased afterload on myocardial oxygen demand. Preoperative knowledge of the desired clamp location helps anesthesia personnel to optimize monitoring and pharmacotherapy. Frequent communication between the anesthesiologist and surgeon is imperative for optimizing patient care.

Dissection around the aorta in the presence of a complex aneurysm is dangerous. Adherence of the aorta to surrounding tissues in the region of the left renal vein should deter the surgeon from further exploration of the juxtarenal segment. We favor supraceliac clamping in any patient if the ability to clamp the infrarenal cuff is questionable. This method does not increase the morbidity or mortality and probably provides for a safer operation than the alternatives.[33] The proximal anastomosis of a juxtarenal aneurysm repair often includes the lower margins of the renal arteries. Suprarenal aneurysms can be repaired using a beveled anastomosis, incorporating the renals in a patch-like fashion. Occasionally, a separate graft limb is required. The choice of graft material, although often controversial, has little bearing in long-term outcome.[34]

Concomitant Renal Artery Issues

Involvement of the renal artery in the operative care of aneurysm patients can take three forms. Anomalous renal arteries, renal artery stenosis, and renal arterial aneurysms are all potential difficulties. Anomalous renal vasculature is present in approximately 23% of patients. Most often, this takes the form of an additional renal artery on one side.[2] Reimplantation of all renal arteries should be attempted, especially if the diameter is greater than 2 mm.

Concomitant renal artery stenosis and aortic pathology is frequently found. The natural history of untreated disease in this situation is one of slow progression, worsening hypertension, and deterioration of renal function.[35] Aggressive treatment is therefore indicated. Severe renal arterial occlusive disease occurred in 15.3% of 65 patients with juxtarenal and suprarenal aneurysms evaluated by Allen and colleagues.[36] In Qvarfordt's[2] series of 77 patients with pararenal aneurysms, 49% of the renal arteries had evidence of atherosclerotic disease. The disease usually is unilateral.[37] The patients benefiting most from renal arterial reconstruction were those demonstrating evidence of baseline renal dysfunction with an elevated serum creatinine level.[2] In this series, hypertensive patients without elevated creatinine levels often improved after renal artery reconstruction, but nearly one fourth of the group suffered a deterioration in renal function after aneurysm repair. Numerous surgeons report increased mortality in the setting of a combined renal artery and aortic aneurysm procedure.[38–40] It is unclear whether this finding represents a specific patient population or the addition of another procedure with aneurysm repair. Most vascular surgeons favor an aggressive approach to the simultaneous presentation of this disease.

There are various methods of renal arterial repair. The use of a transaortic renal endarterectomy is advocated by some surgeons,[2] and direct or indirect reimplantation is favored by others.[1] Autotransplantation can be performed in situations requiring significant distal vessel reconstruction. No single technique of renal artery reconstruction has proven superior to others; surgical ingenuity is often required in these situations (Fig. 14–2).

One of the critical predictors of postoperative renal dysfunction is warm

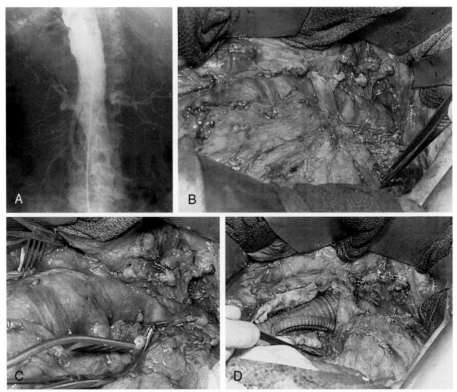

Figure 14–2. *A*, The angiogram demonstrates an infrarenal aneurysm with a left renal artery stenosis. *B*, The medial visceral rotation technique leaves the left kidney down. Notice the left renal vein over the neck of the aneurysm. *C*, Transection of the left renal vein was necessary to obtain adequate exposure of the left renal artery, which was repaired with a graft off the aortic graft. *D*, The left renal vein was then reconstructed.

ischemic time. In a review of several studies, Allen found that decreased total ischemic time and perfusion of the kidney with a hypothermic solution improved renal preservation.[1] This observation was supported by Svensson and Crawford.[41] The use of hypothermic perfusion systems can be somewhat cumbersome. Simpler methods involve the application of ice over the kidney or injection of the renal orifice with cooled Ringer's lactate. Aneurysms of the renal arteries are uncommonly seen in conjunction with aortic aneurysms. They should be resected in conjunction with the aortic aneurysm and an autogenous or artificial graft used as a conduit.

Inflammatory Aneurysms

Most surgeons recognize the shiny, pale fibrosis in the retroperitoneum of patients with inflammatory aneurysms (Fig. 14–3). These patients often have more symptoms than their counterparts with atherosclerosis.[42] This condition often clouds the presentation and results in emergent surgery for potential rupture. Improved imaging techniques discussed in the previous sections may eliminate this problem for the hemodynamically stable patient. Unfortunately, the presence of retroperitoneal fibrosis predicts a challenging operation, difficult postoperative management, and increased morbidity and mortality. The duodenum is nearly always adherent to the anterior aortic wall. Efforts at separation of these two structures should not be attempted. The risk of enterotomy is exceptionally high, and contamination of the field results in

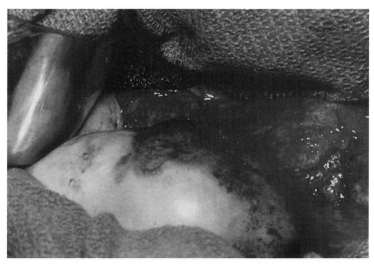

Figure 14–3. The classic, shiny white appearance of an inflammatory aneurysm is demonstrated in this photograph.

disaster. The vena cava, left renal vein, sigmoid colon, and small bowel are also frequently adherent.[43] In these situations, it is advisable to minimize dissection in the region of inflammation.

Supraceliac clamping has been shown to be safe and effective.[16, 33, 42] If the supraceliac aorta is involved, an alternative is to obtain proximal controls with an intraaortic balloon.[44, 45] We have found that placement through an axillary artery is superior to more caudal access techniques. Although controversial, some surgeons advocate a retroperitoneal approach because of adherent viscera.[46] The paucity of posterior aortic inflammatory involvement, even in the setting of severe fibrosis, is another benefit of retorperitoneal repair. However, distal control of the right iliac or right renal artery is challenging with this approach. Extreme fibrosis pulls the ureters in a medial fashion. Without ureteral stents, their exact location is difficult to ascertain, and dissection around the common iliacs is treacherous. An ideal method of establishing proximal and distal control is the placement of a supraceliac clamp, followed by an aortotomy with rapid placement of balloon-occluding catheters in both common iliacs. This method minimizes dissection in an inflammatory field.

The proximal anastomosis is best performed from within the aorta. Placement of sutures in the posterior wall is not difficult. The anterior and lateral walls are best anastomosed using a horizontal mattress suture technique. The use of a V-7 or MH needle allows full-thickness purchase of the aortic wall. The distal anastomosis can be constructed in the usual fashion.

Ureterolysis is often considered at the conclusion of the aneurysm repair. Obstruction of the urogenital system manifests in 10% to 20% of patients.[43] Urine leaks are sometimes difficult to isolate and indicate a high risk of graft infection.[47] For this reason, we are reluctant to proceed with any complex ureteral dissection, even in the setting of impending obstruction. If ureteral involvement is anticipated preoperatively, stents should be placed before exploration. In the setting of unknown ureteral involvement, we recommend a minimal dissection technique and the use of postoperative stents or nephrostomy tubes to temporize drainage. Spontaneous resolution of ureteral obstruction is common.[42]

Many surgeons have noticed a clinical regression of the retroperitoneal fibrosis after aneurysm resection.[42, 48] The clinical improvements after aneurysmectomy have been correlated with histologic or radiographic resolution of disease. Stella and colleagues[49] reported complete postoperative regression of fibrosis in 47% of patients, partial resolution in 21%, and no change in the remaining 32%. The extent of postoperative improvement appeared to correlate with the cellular density of the periaortic inflammatory tissue.

Horseshoe Kidney

The horseshoe kidney is the most common anomaly of renal fusion. The incidence is approximately 0.25% of the general population.[50] Stones and urinary tract infections are more common in these patients. Two renal masses are typically connected by an isthmus, most commonly located between the lower poles, but the position is variable (Fig. 14–4).

The isthmus often has a separate blood supply arising from the aorta or either renal artery. Ureteral abnormalities, including multiplicity and aberrant locations, are also prevalent. Preoperative evaluation requires CT scanning, evaluation of the arterial system with angiography, and assessment of the ureteral system with an intravenous pyelogram. More than one half of the patients with horseshoe kidneys have three to five arteries arising from the aorta. Another 14% have a blood supply derived from other vessels. In these situations, only 20% of patients have single renal arteries bilaterally.[45]

The location of the anomalous blood supply, ureteral evaluation, and size of the isthmus help determine the most feasible method of repair. A transperitoneal approach provides ideal exposure to anomalous arteries and ureters. However, some surgeons express concern regarding division of the isthmus to obtain aortic exposure.[50] If the isthmus is bulky and divided, renal ischemia and urine leakage can follow.[51] However, in our series of eight patients,[52] the results of which were confirmed by two other evaluations,[53, 54] there was no loss of renal function or urinary leaks as a result of isthmus division. The alternative approach is through the left retroperitoneum. This method elevates the left kidney to expose the aorta without requiring division of any renal tissue.[45, 55] Exposure of anomalous arteries, ureters, and the right renal and iliac system are potentially compromised in this situation.

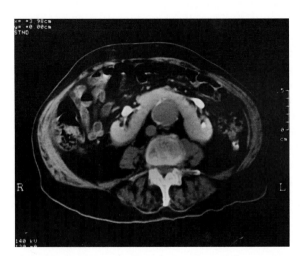

Figure 14–4. A computed tomography scan demonstrates the typical appearance of a fused horseshoe kidney.

Conclusions

Patients with complex aortic issues are best served by a physician familiar with the associated pathophysiology, imaging modalities, preoperative evaluation, and a variety of operative approaches. Therapeutic decisions must be made in the context of the risks and benefits for the patient. Technologic advances have improved renal preservation, provided more accurate imaging modalities, and helped the management of the physiologic effects of aortic clamping. The use of endovascular stent grafts in the setting of an inflammatory aneurysm has been reported,[56] but this technology is not capable of handling the complex morpholgy of pararenal aneurysms. Continued advances in patient care and meticulous technique with complete preoperative patient preparation should provide excellent surgical results for this complex problem.

References

1. Allen B, Anderson C, Rubin B, et al. Preservation of renal function in juxtarenal and suprarenal abdominal aortic aneurysm repair. J Vasc Surg 1993;17:948–958.
2. Qvarfordt P, Stoney R, Reilly L, et al. Management of pararenal aneurysm of the abdominal aorta. J Vasc Surg 1986;3:84–93.
3. Lopez-Candales A, Holmes D, Liao S, et al. Decreased vascular smooth muscle cell density in medial degeneration of human abdominal aortic aneurysms. Am J Pathol 1997;150:993–1007.
4. Cenacchi G, Guiducci F, Pasquinelli G, et al. The morphology of elastin in nonspecific and inflammatory abdominal aortic aneurysms. J Submicrosc Cytol Pathol 1995;27:75–81.
5. Ramshaw A, Parums D. The distribution of adhesion molecules in chronic periaortitis. Histopathology 1994;24:23–32.
6. Koch A, Kunkel S, Pearce W, et al. Enhanced production of the chemotactic cytokines interleukin-8 and monocyte chemoattractant protein-1 in human abdominal aortic aneurysms. Am J Pathol 1993;142:1423–1431.
7. Holmes D, Wester W, Thompson R, Reilly J. Prostaglandin E_2 synthesis and cyclooxygenase expression in abdominal aortic aneurysms. J Vasc Surg 1997;25:810–815.
8. Adolph R, Vorp D, Steed D, et al. Cellular content and permeability of intraluminal thrombus in abdominal aortic aneurysm. J Vasc Surg 1997;25:916–926.
9. Juvonen J, Juvonen T, Laurila A, et al. Demonstration of *Chlamydia pneumoniae* in the walls of abdominal aortic aneurysms. J Vasc Surg 1997;25:499–505.
10. Yonemitsu Y, Nakagawa K, Tanaka R, et al. In situ detection of frequent and active infection of human cytomegalovirus in inflammatory abdominal aortic aneurysms: possible pathogenic role in sustained chronic inflammatory reaction. Lab Invest 1996;74:723–736.
11. Gomes M, Choyke P. Pre-operative evaluation of abdominal aortic aneurysms: ultrasound or computed tomography? J Cardiovasc Surg 1987;28:159–165.
12. Balm R, Eikelboom B, van Leeuwen M, Noordzij J. Spiral CT-angiography of the aorta. Eur J Vasc Surg 1994;8:544–551.
13. Cohen R, Siegel C, Korobkin M, et al. Abdominal aortic aneurysms: CT evaluation of renal artery involvement. Radiology 1995;194:751–756.
14. Costello P, Gaa J. Spiral CT angiography of abdominal aortic aneurysms. Radiographics 1995;15:397–406.
15. Gomes M, Davros W, Zeman R. Preoperative assessment of abdominal aortic aneurysm: the value of helical and three-dimensional computed tomography. J Vasc Surg 1994;20:367–376.
16. Kneimeyer H, Kolvenbach R, Rhode E, et al. Inflammatory aneurysm of the aorta: diagnosis, therapy and results. Chirurg 1990;61:27–31.
17. Rubin G, Walker P, Dake M, et al. Three-dimensional spiral computed tomographic angiography: an alternative imaging modality for the abdominal aorta and its branches. J Vasc Surg 1993;18:656–664.
18. Salaman R, Shandall A, Morgan R, et al. Intravenous digital subtraction angiography versus computed tomography in the assessment of abdominal aortic aneurysm. Br J Surg 1994;81:661–663.
19. Stanley R. Which techniques should I use for the evaluation of abdominal aortic aneurysm—sonography, CT, MR imaging, or angiography—and when should I use each? Am J Roentgenol 1994;163:1262–1263.
20. Tennant W, Hartnell G, Baird R, Horrocks M. Radiologic investigation of abdominal aortic aneurysm disease: comparison of three modalities in staging and the detection of inflammatory changes. J Vasc Surg 1993;17:703–709.
21. White R, Scoccianti M, Back M, et al. Innovations in vascular imaging: arteriography, three-

dimensional CT scans, and two- and three dimensional intravascular ultrasound evaluation of an abdominal aortic aneurysm. Ann Vasc Surg 1994;8:285–289.

22. Johnston K, Scobie T. Multicenter prospective study of nonruptured abdominal aortic aneurysms, I. Population and operative management. J Vasc Surg 1988;7:69–81.
23. Goldstone J. Aneurysms of the aorta and iliac arteries. *In* Moore W (ed). Vascular Surgery: a Comprehensive Review. Philadelphia: WB Saunders, 1998.
24. Ouriel K, Green R, Donayer C, et al. An evaluation of new methods of expressing aortic aneurysm size: relationship to rupture. J Vasc Surg 1992;15:12–20.
25. Curci J. Modes of presentation and management of inflammatory aneurysms of the abdominal aorta. J Am Coll Surg 1994;178:573–580.
26. Yeager R, Moneta G. Assessing cardiac risk in vascular surgical patients: current status. Perspect Vasc Surg 1989;2:18–39.
27. Halm E, Browner W, Tubau J, et al. Echocardiography for assessing cardiac risk in patients having noncardiac surgery. Ann Intern Med 1996;125:433–441.
28. Eichelberger J, Schwartz K, Black E, et al. Predictive value of dobutamine echocardiography just before noncardiac vascular surgery. Am J Cardiol 1993;72:602–607.
29. Report of the American College of Cardiology/American Heart Association Task Force on Practice Guidelines. Executive summary of the ACC/AHA Task Force Report: guidelines for perioperative cardiovascular evaluation for noncardiac surgery. Anesth Analg 1996;82:854–860.
30. Johnstone K, Rutherford R, Tilson D, et al. Suggested standards for reporting on arterial aneurysms. J Vasc Surg 1991;13:452–458.
31. Cronenwett J, Murphy T, Zelenock G, et al. Actuarial analysis of variables associated with rupture of small aortic aneurysms. Surgery 1985;98:472–483.
32. Cronenwett J. Variables that affect the expansion rate and rupture of abdominal aortic aneurysms. Ann N Y Acad Sci 1996;800:56–67.
33. Green R, Ricotta J, Ouriel K, et al. Results of supraceliac aortic clamping in the difficult elective resection of infrarenal aortic aneurysms. J Vasc Surg 1989;9:124–134.
34. Erdoes L, Bernhard V. Prosthetic vascular grafts: materials and their properties. *In* Ouriel K (ed). Lower Extremity Vascular Disease. Philadelphia: WB Saunders, 1995.
35. Tollefson D, Ernst C. Natural history of atherosclerotic renal artery stenosis associated with aortic disease. J Vasc Surg 1991;14:327–331.
36. Allen B, Anderson C, Rubin B, et al. Preservation of renal function in juxtarenal and suprarenal abdominal aortic aneurysm repair. J Vasc Surg 1993;17:948–958.
37. Chaikof E, Smith R, Salam A, et al. Ischemic nephropathy and concomitant aortic disease: a ten year experience. J Vasc Surg 1994;19:135–148.
38. Diehl J, Cali R, Herzer N, Beven E. Complications of abdominal aortic reconstruction. Ann Surg 1983;197:49–56.
39. Ernst C, Stanley J, Marshall F, Fry W. Renal revascularization for arteriosclerotic renovascular hypertension. Surgery 1973;73:859–867.
40. Dean R, Keyser J, Dupont W, et al. Aortic and renal vascular disease: factors affecting the value of combined procedures. Ann Surg 1984;197:49–56.
41. Svensson L, Crawford E, Hess K, et al. Thoracoabdominal aortic aneurysms associated with celiac, superior mesenteric, and renal artery occlusive disease: methods and analysis of results in 271 patients. J Vasc Surg 1992;16:378–390.
42. Crawford J, Stowe C, Safi H, et al. Inflammatory aneurysms of the aorta. J Vasc Surg 1985;2:113–124.
43. Pietre P, Gabrielli F, Prati P, Baldette G. Clinical aspects and treatment of inflammatory abdominal aortic aneurysms. Int J Angiol 1995;14:368–374.
44. Fiorani P, Faraglia V, Speciale F, et al. Extraperitoneal approach for repair of inflammatory abdominal aortic aneurysm. J Vasc Surg 1991;13:692–697.
45. Green R. Management of complicated abdominal aortic aneurysms: juxtarenal aneurysms, horseshoe kidney, inflammatory aneurysms. *In* Calligaro K, Dougherty M (eds). Current Diagnosis and Treatment of Aortic and Peripheral Arterial Aneurysms. Philadelphia: Access Medical Group, 1997.
46. Sterpetti A, Hunter W, Feldhaus R, et al. Inflammatory aneurysms of the abdominal aorta: incidence, pathologic, and etiologic considerations. J Vasc Surg 1989;9:633–650.
47. Loughlin K, Kearney G, Helfrich W, Carey R. Ureteral obstruction secondary to perianeurysmal fibrosis. Urology 1984;24:332–336.
48. Gans R, Hoorntje S, Rauwerds J, et al. The inflammatory abdominal aortic aneurysm: prevalence, clinical features and diagnostic evaluation. Neth J Med 1993;43:105–115.
49. Stella A, Gargiulo M, Faggioli G, et al. Postoperative course of inflammatory abdominal aortic aneurysms. Ann Vasc Surg 1993;7:229–238.
50. O'Hara P, Hakaim A, Hertzer N, et al. Surgical management of aortic aneurysms and horseshoe kidney: review of 31 years' experience. J Vasc Surg 1993;18:586.
51. Glenn J. Analysis of 51 patients with horseshoe kidney. N Engl J Med 1959;261:684–687.
52. Shortell C, Welch E, Ouriel K, et al. Operative management of coexistent aortic disease and horseshoe kidney. Ann Vasc Surg 1995;9:123–128.
53. Crawford E, Coselli J, Hazim J, et al. The impact of renal fusion and extopia on aortic surgery. J Vasc Surg 1988;8:375–383.

54. Sidell P, Pairolero P, Payne W, et al. Horseshoe kidney associated with surgery of the abdominal aorta. Mayo Clin Proc 1979;54:97–103.
55. Moriyasu K, Funami M, Narisawa T, et al. The retroperitoneal approach to aortoiliac surgery associated with a horseshoe kidney: report of a case. Surg Today 1996;26:655–657.
56. Boyle J, Thompson M, Nasim A, et al. Endovascular repair of an inflammatory aortic aneurysm. Eur J Endovasc Surg 1997;13:328–329.

Venous Anomalies Encountered During Abdominal Aortic Surgery

Keith D. Calligaro, M.D.,
Dominic A. DeLaurentis, M.D.,
and Matthew J. Dougherty, M.D.

Reduction in cardiac and pulmonary complications has resulted in improved perioperative morbidity and mortality associated with elective surgery of abdominal aortic aneurysms (AAAs) and aortoiliac occlusive disease.[4] However, during this type of surgery, intraoperative technical misadventure resulting in massive blood loss is still associated with significant complications. Venous anomalies (VAs) encountered during aortic surgery are potential sources of unexpected and significant hemorrhage, especially if the vascular surgeon is unaware of their presence, inexperienced in dealing with them from a technical standpoint, or needs to perform the operation in an emergent manner, as in the case of a ruptured AAA.[1–3, 6, 10, 11] These anomalies primarily involve the left renal vein (LRV) and the inferior vena cava (IVC).

During the past 30 years, our group has had an interest in these anomalies. In this chapter, we review our experience with VAs associated with AAAs and aortic occlusive disease in terms of their embryology, incidence, diagnosis, and management.[10]

Assessment of Venous Anomalies

Patients and Survey Methods

Between January 1, 1967, and December 31, 1996, we performed 1386 abdominal aortic operations. The operations included 792 AAA repairs and 594 surgical procedures for aortoiliac occlusive disease. Data were recorded on index cards until 1989 and on a computerized registry thereafter. VAs documented by preoperative tests such as computed tomography (CT) scan, ultrasonography, or magnetic resonance imaging (MRI) were included in this review only if patients underwent surgery. Patients with VAs discovered during surgery, but who did not have preoperative imaging studies capable of diagnosing these lesions, were included in this report.

Survey Results

Of the 1386 abdominal aortic cases performed during the past 30 years, 39 (2.8%) VAs were encountered intraoperatively: 21 (1.5%) retroaortic left renal veins, 11 (0.8%) circumaortic renal collars, 5 (0.4%) double IVCs, and 2 (0.1%) left-sided or transposed IVCs. Four (10.3%) of the 39 patients with VAs suffered massive intraoperative hemorrhage, and one died of ruptured aneurysm. In all four cases, VAs were unrecognized preoperatively: two VA injuries were associated with ruptured AAAs, and two patients who underwent elective aortic surgery did not have preoperative imaging studies that might have identified them.

Twenty-one patients had retroaortic LRVs. In 19 patients, these veins were recognized intraoperatively or with preoperative CT scans, and inadvertent injury was avoided. In one patient, a retroaortic LRV was not recognized during repair of a ruptured AAA, resulting in venous injury, massive hemorrhage, and death. Another patient with a ruptured AAA was found to have a fistula between the aneurysm and a retroaortic LRV when the aneurysm was opened, producing massive venous bleeding.[7] The venous defect was oversewn from within the aneurysm, and the patient did well. The emergent need for surgery in these patients prohibited obtaining preoperative CT scans.

Eleven patients had circumaortic renal collars identified. In 10 patients, the anomaly was recognized, and no injury occurred. One patient who did not have a preoperative CT scan sustained an injury to the retroaortic component of a renal vein collar that led to massive hemorrhage. This was eventually controlled after division of the infrarenal aorta and suture repair. The patient survived.

Five patients had duplicated IVCs. In four patients, the double IVC was recognized and was not injured. Two of these patients had a small, left-sided IVC that passed anteriorly to the AAA to join the LRV. The left-sided, duplicated vein was ligated below its junction with the LRV. In the two other patients who did not suffer iatrogenic injury, the left-sided segment joined the LRV more laterally, and ligation of the left IVC was unnecessary. The fifth patient had a large AAA, and during mobilization of the aneurysm to gain proximal control, a duplicate IVC located posterior and to the left of the aorta was injured. The laceration was controlled, and the aneurysm was resected without further complications. An ultrasonographic scan had been obtained preoperatively, but it had not detected the duplicate IVC.

Two patients had a left-sided or transposed IVC. In both patients, the VAs were recognized at surgery, and there was no venous injury. Division of these left-sided IVCs was unnecessary, and reconstruction was carried out by gentle retraction.

Embryology

The postcardinal, subcardinal, and supracardinal veins, which are three parallel pairs of embryologic veins, develop into the IVC and renal veins (Fig. 15–1).[3, 11, 13, 16] The postcardinal veins develop in association with the mesonephros dorsal to the aorta and anastomose with the subcardinal veins. The postcardinal veins persist only as the iliac vein bifurcation. The right subcardinal system develops into the suprarenal IVC and a segment of the infrarenal IVC. The supracardinal veins form in a plane dorsal to the aorta and anastomose with the ventral subcardinal system to form a collar of veins that persists. The left supracardinal vein regresses to form a normal infrarenal IVC to the right of the aorta. The ventral part of the circumaortic ring persists, and the dorsal segment regresses to form the normal LRV found anterior to the aorta. These transformations occur during the fourth to eighth week of embryologic development.

The left supracardinal vein may persist, resulting in a double IVC or, if the right supracardinal vein regresses, a single, left-sided IVC. With a double IVC, the LRV typically drains into the left IVC, which then continues cephalad

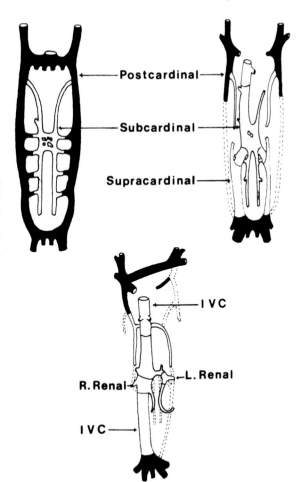

Figure 15-1. Embryology of the abdominal inferior vena cava and renal veins. IVC, inferior vena cava. (From DeLaurentis DA, Savarese RP, Ritchie WGM, Kaplan SM. Venous anomalies encountered in aortic surgery: their preoperative detection by CAT scan and intraoperative management. *In* Veith FJ (ed). Current Critical Problems in Vascular Surgery. St. Louis: Quality Medical Publishing, 1989:284–290.)

to drain into the right IVC. The entire circumaortic ring may persist and form a circumaortic renal collar or, if the ventral portion regresses, a retroaortic LRV.

Operative Experience With Venous Anomalies

VAs adjacent to the abdominal aorta are unusual intraoperative findings but familiar to most vascular surgeons who perform large numbers of aortic operations. The reported incidence of these anomalies depends on whether the figures are based on preoperative, intraoperative, or autopsy findings. In a review of clinical and autopsy series, the incidence of circumaortic renal collars was 1.5% to 8.7%; duplication of the IVC, 2% to 3%; retroaortic LRVs, 2%; and left-sided IVCs, less than 0.5%.[9] Using CT scanning, an incidence of VAs of 1.8% (20 of 1095) was reported.[10] The difference in clinical incidence is partly explained by the higher incidence found by surgeons who resect small aneurysms and surgeons who routinely use a "toe" anastomosis for occlusive disease.

VAs may be discovered during a preoperative evaluation but frequently are discovered incidentally during surgery. These anomalies can be diagnosed using ultrasonography, but they are frequently missed. MRI can be used but is rarely performed before aortic surgery. The anomalies are most commonly and accurately identified using CT scans.[8, 13, 14] CT scans rarely miss these lesions, but the radiologist or surgeon reviewing the studies may not recognize the anomalies or confuse them with paraaortic lymph nodes.

We have an interest in the preoperative and postoperative management of patients undergoing aortic surgery from a cost perspective.[5] In an era of cost containment and third-party payers, an unresolved issue is the role of routine aortography or CT scanning (or both) for patients undergoing AAA repair or operations for aortoiliac occlusive disease. Some type of imaging study that accurately reflects the size of an aneurysm, whether it is CT scan, ultrasonography, or MRI, is routinely performed before elective AAA surgery. Aortography is mandatory before surgery for aortoiliac occlusive disease. However, arteriography is not routinely performed by many vascular surgeons before AAA surgery, and few vascular surgeons routinely obtain CT scans before aortoiliac surgery.[9] An experienced and careful vascular surgeon is rarely caught unaware of these anomalies.

Our strategy for patients requiring elective AAA repair is that poor-risk patients should have both CT scans and arteriography performed preoperatively to identify any unexpected intraabdominal anomalies so that surgery may be planned as carefully and be performed as expeditiously as possible. However, for good-risk patients with otherwise uncomplicated infrarenal aortic aneurysms, we do not obtain CT scans if high-quality ultrasonography was performed, although we generally perform aortography. Some vascular surgeons do not obtain a preoperative arteriogram for patients with AAAs without evidence of renovascular disease, aortoiliac occlusive disease, or chronic mesenteric ischemia, and they are willing to operate based on ultrasonographic results alone.[9] With the availability of spiral CT, the need for arteriography is becoming less common, although expense remains an issue.[12]

In patients requiring surgery for aortoiliac occlusive disease, arteriography is essential to determine optimal inflow and outflow tracts. For poor-risk patients with aortoiliac occlusive disease, the surgeon should consider obtaining a preoperative CT scan to identify intraabdominal anomalies so that the operation may be performed as expeditiously as possible. For most patients who are deemed very high risk, we choose to perform an extraanatomic bypass. Cost containment considerations and the low incidence of VAs prohibit obtaining CT scans for most patients undergoing surgery for aortoiliac occlusive disease. In our hospital, preoperative CT scans are much more commonly obtained before AAA surgery and almost never ordered before surgery for aortoiliac occlusive disease.

When VAs are identified preoperatively, we suggest the following maneuvers to avoid massive venous hemorrhage when performing abdominal aortic

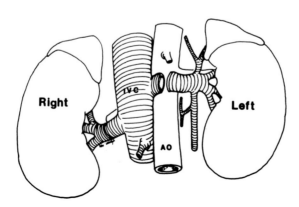

Figure 15–2. Normal left renal vein anatomy. IVC, inferior vena cava; AO, aorta. (From DeLaurentis DA, Savarese RP, Ritchie WGM, Kaplan SM. Venous anomalies encountered in aortic surgery: their preoperative detection by CAT scan and intraoperative management. *In* Veith FJ (ed). Current Critical Problems in Vascular Surgery. St. Louis: Quality Medical Publishing, 1989: 284–290.)

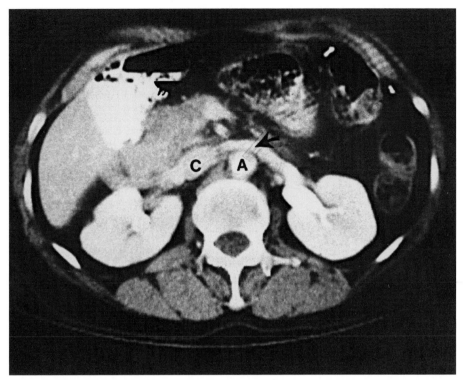

Figure 15–3. Computed tomography image of normal left renal vein *(arrow)*. A, aorta; C, inferior vena cava. (From DeLaurentis DA, Savarese RP, Ritchie WGM, Kaplan SM. Venous anomalies encountered in aortic surgery: their preoperative detection by CAT scan and intraoperative management. *In* Veith FJ (ed). Current Critical Problems in Vascular Surgery. St. Louis: Quality Medical Publishing, 1989:284–290.)

surgery. During exposure of the proximal infrarenal aorta, the LRV should routinely be identified anterior to the aorta (Figs. 15–2 and 15–3). If the LRV is not identified in its normal position, the surgeon should carefully sharply dissect the juxtarenal aorta under direct vision enough to place an anteroposteriorly directed clamp. Although in most circumstances we favor circumferential control of the proximal infrarenal aorta, vertical placement of an aortic clamp proximal to a retroaortic LRV is preferable to avoid inadvertent tearing of the vein. Blunt aortic dissection encircling the aorta to obtain proximal control should never be performed when the LRV is not visualized crossing anterior to the aorta. A retroaortic LRV usually runs caudally to join the IVC (Figs. 15–4 and 15–5). Proximal aortic control can usually be obtained above the visualized retroaortic LRV. In the event the LRV is inadvertently injured, proximal and distal control of the aorta should be obtained, followed by division of the aorta so that the posteriorly located vein can be identified and oversewn.

Even in the presence of an anterior LRV, the surgeon should recognize that a circumaortic renal collar may be present (Figs. 15–6 and 15–7). For this reason, blind posterior dissection of the periaortic tissue should be avoided, but the surgeon should identify the posterolateral aspects of the aorta before circumferential control is obtained. A left renal vein that is adherent to the anterior aorta or a small, anterior LRV should alert the surgeon to the possibility of a circumaortic renal collar. When LRV division is necessary to obtain juxtarenal aortic control, we routinely measure LRV stump pressures to determine if this maneuver is safe and to ensure that venous congestion of the left

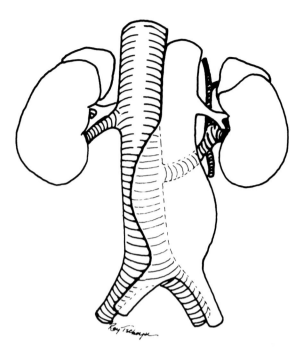

Figure 15–4. Retroaortic left renal vein. This anomalous vein courses obliquely and caudally to join the inferior vena cava posterior to the aneurysm. (From DeLaurentis DA, Savarese RP, Ritchie WGM, Kaplan SM. Venous anomalies encountered in aortic surgery: their preoperative detection by CAT scan and intraoperative management. *In* Veith FJ (ed). Current Critical Problems in Vascular Surgery. St. Louis: Quality Medical Publshing, 1989: 284–290.)

kidney will not result.[7, 15] In one patient who required LRV division, the stump pressure was low and equaled the central venous pressure, which occurs in about three fourths of the cases.[7] After further dissection of the aorta and surrounding tissues, we discovered a circumaortic renal collar with a large retroaortic component that decompressed the anterior part of the vein. Control of the aorta in the presence of this anomaly may be obtained above or below the vein.[2, 3, 10] If the collar is very tight and does not allow safe mobilization for proximal aortic control, the anterior vein may be divided at the confluence with the IVC. Similar to a retroaortic LRV, the posterior component of the collar can course quite caudad and obliquely before joining the IVC. A preoperative CT scan can identify a circumaortic renal collar (see Fig. 15–7).

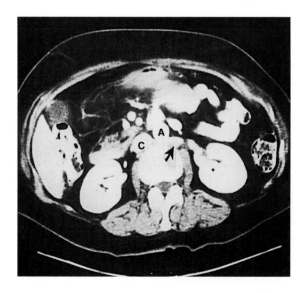

Figure 15–5. Computed tomographic image of retroaortic left renal vein *(arrow)*. A, aorta; C, inferior vena cava. (From DeLaurentis DA, Savarese RP, Ritchie WGM, Kaplan SM. Venous anomalies encountered in aortic surgery: their preoperative detection by CAT scan and intraoperative management. *In* Veith FJ (ed). Current Critical Problems in Vascular Surgery. St. Louis: Quality Medical Publishing, 1989:284–290.)

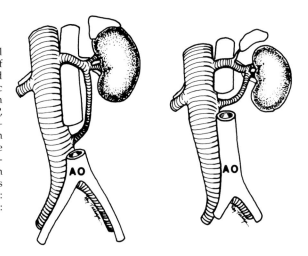

Figure 15-6. Circumaortic renal collar. The posterior portion of the collar can be located cephalad or caudad, similar to a retroaortic left renal vein. AO, aorta. (From DeLaurentis DA, Savarese RP, Ritchie WGM, Kaplan SM. Venous anomalies encountered in aortic surgery: their preoperative detection by CAT scan and intraoperative management. *In* Veith FJ (ed). Current Critical Problems in Vascular Surgery. St. Louis: Quality Medical Publishing, 1989: 284–290.)

A duplicate IVC can be handled by several options, depending on the location of the left-sided cava. If the left side of the system is anterior, the left IVC can be transected below its confluence with the LRV. The portion of the left IVC that crosses the aorta to join the right-sided IVC can then be reflected superiorly. Another technique to manage this anomaly is to transect the left-sided IVC where it crosses the aorta proximal to its junction with the LRV so the LRV can drain into the distal left IVC (Fig. 15–8).

To manage the left-sided or transposed IVC, retraction of the vein to the left and cephalad retraction of the LRV may provide sufficient exposure of the infrarenal aorta. If this maneuver does not produce adequate exposure, a second technique includes transection of the left-sided IVC below the LRV and mobilization of the proximal portion cephalad. However, this may lead to massive, bilateral, lower extremity venous thrombosis and chronic edema. A third choice is to transect the right renal vein close to its junction with the

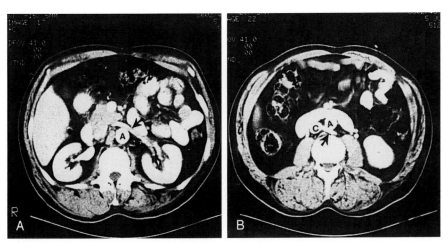

Figure 15-7. *A,* Computed tomography (CT) scan of a circumaortic renal collar: upper portion *(arrow).* Notice the absence of the dorsal segment at this level. A, aorta. *B,* CT scan of a circumaortic renal collar: posterior portion 4 cm below the anterior portion *(arrow).* C, inferior vena cava; A, aorta. (From DeLaurentis DA, Savarese RP, Ritchie WGM, Kaplan SM. Venous anomalies encountered in aortic surgery: their preoperative detection by CAT scan and intraoperative management. *In* Veith FJ (ed). Current Critical Problems in Vascular Surgery. St. Louis: Quality Medical Publishing, 1989:284–290.)

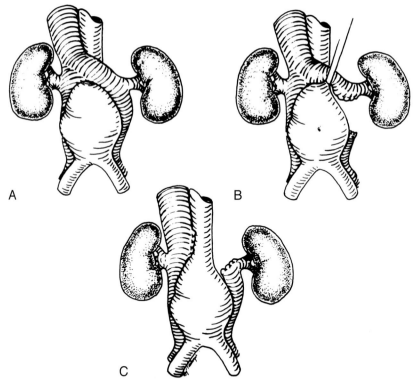

Figure 15–8. For a duplicated inferior vena cava *(upper left)*, the options include division of the left inferior vena cava below its junction with the left renal vein *(upper right)* or division of the left renal vein near its junction with the right inferior vena cava *(lower center)*. (From DeLaurentis DA, Savarese RP, Ritchie WGM, Kaplan SM. Venous anomalies encountered in aortic surgery: their preoperative detection by CAT scan and intraoperative management. *In* Veith FJ (ed). Current Critical Problems in Vascular Surgery. St. Louis: Quality Medical Publishing, 1989:284–290.)

left-sided IVC (Fig. 15–9). The right renal vein in the presence of a transposition of the vena cava usually has the same collateral venous drainage found in the normal LRV system. A left-sided IVC usually is easily diagnosed by a preoperative CT scan (Fig. 15–10).

Conclusions

Our 30-year operative experience with surgery of the abdominal aorta revealed that IVC and LRV anomalies occur in about 2% of cases. Preoperative studies, especially CT and MRI, can accurately identify VAs. However, experienced and careful vascular surgeons can manage well without a preoperative diagnosis of these anomalies. We recommend that any poor-risk patient requiring elective AAA repair and, rarely, poor-risk patients requiring surgery for aortoiliac occlusive disease have a preoperative CT scan. Identification of these anomalies preoperatively should decrease the chance of inadvertent injury and massive bleeding. Patients requiring emergent surgery for ruptured AAAs are more likely to suffer iatrogenic VA trauma because of a lack of time to obtain preoperative diagnostic imaging studies and the urgency to obtain aortic control. Even during these emergent operations the vascular surgeon should be aware of the possibility of these anomalies and make all efforts to identify them intraoperatively. Most VAs are best recognized by

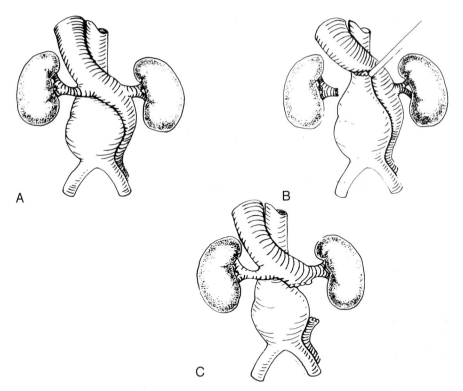

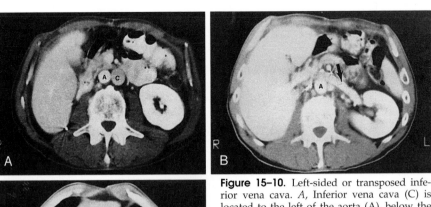

Figure 15–9. Surgical management of a left-sided or transposed inferior vena cava. (From DeLaurentis DA, Savarese RP, Ritchie WGM, Kaplan SM. Venous anomalies encountered in aortic surgery: their preoperative detection by CAT scan and intraoperative management. *In* Veith FJ (ed). Current Critical Problems in Vascular Surgery. St. Louis: Quality Medical Publishing, 1989:284–290.)

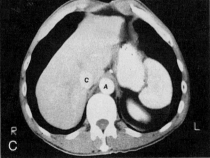

Figure 15–10. Left-sided or transposed inferior vena cava. *A,* Inferior vena cava (C) is located to the left of the aorta (A), below the renal veins. *B,* The left renal vein *(arrow)* joins the inferior vena cava anterior to the aorta (A). *C,* Normal intrahepatic position of the suprarenal inferior vena cava (C). (From DeLaurentis DA, Savarese RP, Ritchie WGM, Kaplan SM. Venous anomalies encountered in aortic surgery: their preoperative detection by CAT scan and intraoperative management. *In* Veith FJ (ed). Current Critical Problems in Vascular Surgery. St. Louis: Quality Medical Publishing, 1989:284–290.)

meticulous dissection of the proximal infrarenal aorta and an increased awareness of their presence.

References

1. Baldridge ED Jr, Canos AJ. Venous anomalies encountered in aortoiliac surgery. Arch Surg 1987;122:1184–1188.
2. Bartle EJ, Pearce WH, Sun JH, Rutherford RB. Infrarenal venous anomalies and aortic surgery: avoiding vascular injury. J Vasc Surg 1987;6:590–593.
3. Brener BJ, Darling RC, Frederick PL, et al. Major venous anomalies complicating abdominal aortic surgery. Arch Surg 1974;108:159–165.
4. Calligaro KD, Azurin DJ, Dougherty MJ, et al. Pulmonary risk factors of elective abdominal aortic surgery. J Vasc Surg 1993;18:914–921.
5. Calligaro KD, Dandura R, Dougherty MJ, et al. Same-day admissions and other cost-saving strategies for elective aortoiliac surgery. J Vasc Surg 1997;25:141–144.
6. Calligaro KD, Savarese RP, DeLaurentis DA. Unusual aspects of aortovenous fistulas associated with ruptured abdominal aortic aneurysms. J Vasc Surg 1990;12:586–590.
7. Calligaro KD, Savarese RP, McCombs PR, DeLaurentis DA. Division of the left renal vein during aortic surgery. Am J Surg 1990;160:192–196.
8. Cory DA, Ellis JH, Bies JR, Olson EW. Case report: retroaortic left renal vein demonstrated by nuclear magnetic resonance imaging. J Comput Assist Tomogr 1984;8:339–340.
9. Couch NP, O'Mahony J, McIrvine A, et al. The place of abdominal aortography in abdominal aortic aneurysm resection. Arch Surg 1983;118:1029–1034.
10. DeLaurentis DA, Savarese RP, Ritchie WGM, Kaplan SM. Venous anomalies encountered in aortic surgery: their preoperative detection by CAT scan and intraoperative management. *In* Veith FJ (ed). Current Critical Problems in Vascular Surgery. St. Louis: Quality Medical Publishing, 1989:284–290.
11. Giordano JM, Trout HH III. Anomalies of the inferior vena cava. J Vasc Surg 1986;3:924–928.
12. Gomes MN, Davros WJ, Zeman RK. Preoperative assessment of abdominal aortic aneurysm: the value of helical and three-dimensional computed tomography. J Vasc Surg 1994;20:367–376.
13. Kellman GM, Alpern MB, Sandler MC, Craig BM. Computed tomography of vena caval anomalies with embryologic correlation. Radiographics 1988;8:533–536.
14. Marincek B, Young SW, Castellino RA. A CT scanning approach to the evaluation of left paraortic pseudotumors. J Comput Assist Tomogr 1981;5:723–727.
15. McCombs PR, DeLaurentis DA. Division of the left renal vein. Am J Surg 1979;138:257–263.
16. Milloy FJ, Anson BJ, Bauldwell EW. Variations in the inferior caval veins and in their renal and lumbar communications. Surg Gynecol Obstet 1962;115:131–142.

Management of Ruptured Abdominal Aortic Aneurysms

Kaj Johansen, M.D., Ph.D.

Ruptured abdominal aortic aneurysm (AAA) is a vascular catastrophe. Associated with an in-hospital mortality rate of approximately 50% that has stubbornly failed to improve over the past three decades, ruptured AAA is the most common lethal vascular surgical problem seen in hospital emergency rooms. This chapter addresses the epidemiology, biophysics, clinical presentation, operative management, expected postoperative complications, and outcome of patients who suffer ruptured AAA and suggests strategies that may improve its morbid outcome.

Epidemiology of Abdominal Aortic Aneurysms

AAA is relatively common, especially in elderly men. Various studies suggest that approximately 2% of an unselected elderly autopsy population have AAAs. Even taking into account improved diagnostic screening, the incidence of AAA has risen threefold in the past 30 years.[1] Risk factors for AAA include advanced age, male gender, prolonged use of cigarettes, and a history of arterial aneurysms at other sites. Patients attending a peripheral vascular surgery clinic have up to a 10% risk for AAA, and one fifth of the first-degree relatives of AAA subjects also themselves may harbor an AAA.

Untreated, most AAAs progressively enlarge, and increasing diameter is associated with a geometrically rising risk of rupture, exsanguination; and death. Approximately one third of AAA patients suffer aneurysmal rupture. The hospital mortality rate for ruptured AAA approximates 50%,[2] but the community mortality rate is even higher. A substantial number of patients die at home or en route to the hospital; several series demonstrate that the overall mortality rate for ruptured AAA may exceed 90%.[3, 4] Ruptured AAA ranks 13th among all causes of death in the United States.[5]

Biophysics of Aneurysm Rupture

Ninety-eight percent of AAAs begin distal to the renal arteries, and this discussion is mostly restricted to infrarenal AAAs. AAA rupture is defined by the presence of extraaneurysmal blood; this usually develops to the left, proximally, and posteriorly in the retroperitoneum in an area devoid of contiguous structures (Fig. 16–1). Rupture presumably occurs when circumferential tensile strength of the aneurysm wall is exceeded by the stresses characterized by the product of the intraluminal pressure and the radius of the aneurysm (ie, Laplace's law). Patients with large AAAs or with hypertension have an increased risk of aneurysmal rupture.

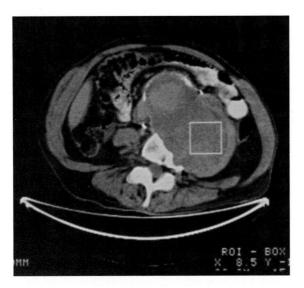

Figure 16–1. Most abdominal aortic aneurysms rupture to the left and posteriorly, as demonstrated by this abdominal computed tomography (CT) scan. The time required to perform such procedures and the necessity to move hemodynamically unstable patients from the emergency department to the CT scanner limit the indications for such studies.

Laplace's relationship describes the factors governing the rupture of idealized thin-walled spherical objects, and data suggest that dimensions other than transverse aneurysmal radius may govern aneurysmal expansion and rupture.[6, 7] Eccentricities in aneurysm morphology (eg, aortic "blebs") may increase rupture risk.[8] Thinning of the arterial wall as the aorta dilates or altered serum levels or ratios of collagenase and elastase[9, 10] may also play a role in aneurysmal expansion and rupture.

Although large aneurysms increasingly become lined with a concentric layer of organized thrombus, no evidence supports the intuition that this inner "layer" reinforces the aneurysm wall and diminishes the likelihood of aneurysmal rupture. The presence of an "inflammatory" component to the aneurysmal wall is not protective; inflammatory AAAs appear to have an equivalent or even greater likelihood of rupture, even though these lesions' walls are often markedly thickened compared with standard bland AAAs.[11]

Clinical Presentation and Diagnosis

Although unruptured AAAs are usually asymptomatic and most patients harboring them are unaware of their presence, aneurysmal rupture is almost universally associated with pain and, if the rupture leads to substantial blood loss, symptoms of hypovolemia (eg, dizziness, syncope). Most AAAs rupture into the left retroperitoneum; accordingly, pain is felt in the left flank, back, or abdomen. Probably because of lumbosacral nerve root irritation, patients may have radicular pain radiating into the left thigh, groin, or scrotum, resulting occasionally in an initial diagnostic impression of ureteral stone. Rupture to the right side of the abdomen occurs only occasionally, as in the case of Albert Einstein.[12] Initial diagnostic efforts may be mistakenly directed toward the biliary tree or other right-sided abdominal structures. Rupture of an AAA into the inferior vena cava, resulting in an aortocaval fistula, may be heralded by symptoms of acute congestive heart failure.[13]

Initial physical findings for patients with ruptured AAAs include hypotension and variable clinical manifestations of hypovolemia, such as pallor, tachycardia, air hunger, anxiety, and sweating. A pulsatile epigastric mass may or not be palpable; especially in the presence of significant hypotension, this finding may be evanescent or absent. The abdomen may be distended and may have diffuse tenderness; outright signs of peritoneal irritation can be seen, although this clinical finding is unusual.

The paramedic or emergency physician is commonly confronted by the clinical scenario of an elderly male patient with truncal pain and some degree of cardiovascular collapse. Although multiple diagnostic possibilities confront the initial caregiver, the most important distinction to make is between myocardial infarction and AAA rupture. In a few patients, this differential diagnosis may be further complicated. For example, the patient with an unruptured AAA may suffer a major myocardial infarction resulting in cardiogenic shock, or the ruptured aneurysm patient may have hypotension resulting in critical coronary insufficiency. Diagnostic studies can assist in distinguishing between these common causes of cardiovascular collapse.

Although absolutely reliable distinctions between patients suffering a myocardial infarction and a ruptured AAA may not be immediately available in the emergency setting, most ruptured AAA patients show clear signs of hypovolemia, with hypotension and skin or mucous membrane evidence of volume loss. Patients with myocardial infarction significant enough to cause shock and cardiovascular collapse are usually hypervolemic, with distended neck veins, rales during auscultation of the lung fields, and a cardiac gallop.

Because physical examination findings and the clinical scenario may be confusing, the use of various imaging techniques may be of substantial diagnostic value. Abdominal computed tomography (CT) scanning and magnetic resonance (MRI) imaging are undoubtedly highly accurate ways for diagnosing AAA.[14, 15] Equivalently favorable sensitivity and specificity accompany diagnosis of AAA rupture.[16] Unfortunately, the time required to obtain even limited abdominal CT scanning or MRI and the requirement that the patient be moved from the emergency suite to another site make these studies unsafe and therefore imprudent. A portable imaging technique that can be brought to the bedside and performed rapidly and simultaneous with resuscitation is needed in this setting.

For more than 15 years, my colleagues and I have used B-mode ultrasonography brought to the bedside in the emergency department for the evaluation of patients thought to harbor a ruptured abdominal aneurysm[17] (Fig. 16–2). As expected, given its excellent sensitivity and specificity for detecting the presence and determining size of uncomplicated AAA,[18, 19] ultrasonography has proved highly effective for making the diagnosis of AAA in the emergency setting. In more than 400 patients studied, with more than 200 AAAs discovered, only one false-negative and no false-positive diagnoses (sensitivity 99.5%, specificity 100%) have been made. Approximately 5% of studies have been nondiagnostic because of massive obesity, intestinal gas, or ascites.[17]

Emergency ultrasonography is not accurate for the diagnosis of acutal AAA rupture. In our experience, the presence of extraaortic blood is not readily discerned during the 2 or 3 minutes allowed for this examination. We have adopted the management posture of immediate laparotomy in patients fitting the appropriate clinical scenario with emergency abdominal ultrasonography positive for AAA. During the past decade, we have successfully diagnosed more than 200 ruptured AAAs and five nonruptured aortic aneurysms (ie, two in patients with coexisting intraabdominal sepsis, two with intraabdominal hemorrhage from solid organ trauma, and one in a patient with a ruptured thoracic aortic aneurysm). We have concluded that emergency abdominal ultrasonography is the optimal diagnostic method for establishing

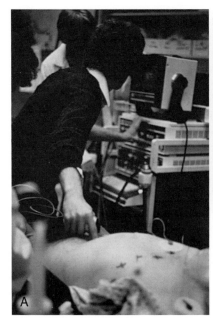

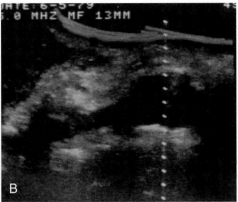

Figure 16–2. *A*, The accuracy, rapidity, and portability of ultrasonography make it ideal as an emergency screening diagnostic examination for patients thought to harbor a ruptured abdominal aortic aneurysm (AAA). *B*, Such studies can identify an AAA but are inaccurate in identifying extravascular blood or a hematoma. Undertaking urgent laparotomy is a clinical decision.

the presence of AAA in a patient whose clinical circumstances suggest an aneurysmal rupture.

Operative Management

Up to 5% of patients with ruptured AAAs are moribund, or they or their families decline operation because of concurrent disease or a prior living will, in which case simple supportive care, such as administration of analgesic and sedative medication, is sufficient.

Most patients who are candidates for operation for ruptured AAAs should be transferred immediately to the operating room and prepared for laparotomy. If the patient is hemodynamically stable, it may be prudent to take a few extra minutes for the anesthesiologists to insert a radial arterial cannula and a central venous pressure introducer sheath (which may later be converted into a Swan-Ganz pulmonary artery catheter). If unstable, the patient may be intubated, paralyzed, and rendered unconscious and amnestic without necessarily undergoing the potentially deleterious cardiac depressant and vasodilatory effects of a general anesthetic. Placement of warming devices[20] and the use of cell-saver[21] and rapid reinfusion[22] equipment is obligatory for the management of these complex and critically ill patients. Anesthetic induction should not be initiated until the operating surgeon is scrubbed and gowned and the patient is prepared and draped from upper chest to midthigh.

A longitudinal, midline abdominal incision is used to obtain entry into the abdomen for proximal aortic control. Chang and colleagues[23] reported success with a left extraperitoneal approach, but this concept lacks intuitive appeal to many surgeons because it exposes and decompresses the usual left retroperitoneal site of aneurysmal rupture. A left thoracotomy approach with clamping of the aorta in an entirely uninvolved area above the diaphragm was popular in the past but has generally been discarded.

The optimal site for control of the aorta is at the aneurysmal neck just distal to the renal arteries. This area is often not immediately visible because it is surrounded by the retroperitoneal hematoma resulting from the aneurysm rupture. If the patient is in shock, the aortic pulse may not be palpable. In this circumstance, gaining access to the supraceliac aorta at the diaphragmatic hiatus offers the most straightforward opportunity for aortic control. The lesser omentum is incised, and the left lobe of the liver is retracted toward the right; similarly, the esophagus at the level of the gastroesophageal junction is retracted to the left. In the middle of the field, obscured by the crura of the diaphragm, is the supraceliac aorta, which can be compressed bluntly against the vertebral column or, if time permits, exposed by incision of the diaphragmatic crura to permit direct placement of an aortic clamp. It is unnecessary to clamp or occlude the aorta immediately if the patient is stable and has a systolic blood pressure greater than 90 mm Hg.

After proximal aortic control is ensured, attention is immediately turned to dissecting the area of the perianeurysmal hematoma to gain infrarenal aortic clamp control. Frequently, a plane appears to have developed between the hematoma and the upper pole of the aneurysm; the operator's hand can dissect bluntly cephalad and dorsally on the aneurysm until the vertebral body is palpated. The orientation of the aneurysm neck is often not straight cephalad to caudad, but rather may course in unusual directions because of the abdominal aorta's tendency to "uncoil" and become ectatic (Fig. 16–3). The neck of the aneurysm should be formally dissected so that clamping is effective and safe.

Extreme care must be taken to avoid damage to the left renal vein or the

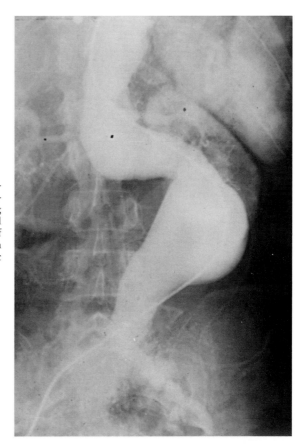

Figure 16–3. The aneurysmal abdominal aorta becomes significantly ectatic. Effective clamping of the "neck" of this aneurysmal aorta would require placement of a clamp in a *coronal* orientation rather than the more anatomic *sagittal* plane.

inferior vena cava. Because of the hematoma in the area, these structures are often not visible, and staying as close to the aneurysm wall and guiding the ends of the vascular clamp with the operator's fingers are crucial aspects to placement of this clamp without damaging these venous structures.[24] If necessary, division and ligation of the left renal vein may aid exposure and is generally well tolerated,[25] although it is not entirely benign.[26]

Hypovolemic patients with ruptured AAAs typically have little backbleeding from the iliacs, and it may not be necessary to expose and control the iliac arteries (thereby sparing the iliac veins from potential trauma). My approach has been to place the proximal infrarenal aortic clamp, open the aneurysm longitudinally, and inspect distally for iliac artery backbleeding after removing the omnipresent mural thrombus. If there is significant backbleeding, it can be controlled by placement of iliac artery clamps or by inflation of balloon-tipped occlusion catheters beyond the iliac artery orifices.

Operation in ruptured AAA patients should be considered one of emergency aortic hemostasis, not of complete vascular reconstruction. Although iliac artery aneurysms and aortic bifurcation atherosclerosis are common, I consider it imprudent to treat nonlethal concurrent disease at the time of operation for a ruptured AAA. Unless the terminal aorta is impenetrably atherosclerotic, there is little indication for placing a bifurcation graft to the iliac or femoral arteries; a tube graft to the terminal aorta suffices in more than 90% of cases (Fig. 16–4).

After longitudinal opening the aneurysm, it is incised dorsally to provide maximum exposure to the proximal aorta for performance of the graft-aorta anastomosis. Taking the time to remove diseased or arteriosclerotic intima from within the aneurysmal sac can provide a better surface on which to suture the aortic prosthesis and makes suturing of backbleeding inferior mesenteric, lumbar, and sacral caudal arteries more straightforward. A woven or albumin- or collagen-impregnated, knitted prosthetic graft is selected appropriate to the size of the proximal aorta. It is sutured, posterior wall first, using 3-0 or 4-0 nonabsorbable suture. In the occasional circumstance of an aneurysmal juxtarenal aorta, every effort is made to place the proximal suture line below the renal arteries. When the aorta is fragile or tenuous, placement of a Teflon felt bolster sandwiching the outside and inside of the anastomosis may occasionally be useful.

Distally, the same approach is adopted. Endarterectomy of the aneurysm sac just proximal to the orifices of the iliac arteries is carried out, with suture

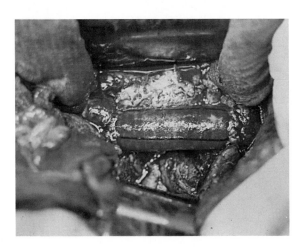

Figure 16–4. Most ruptured abdominal aortic aneurysm repairs can be successfully accomplished by interposition of a tube graft into the infrarenal aorta.

of the distal end of the graft to this area. The bifurcation is rarely aneurysmal, and cutting the aortic prosthesis on the bias usually provides sufficient graft circumference for the distal suture line. Although such an approach seems to risk dissection of the distal intimal plaque into the proximal iliac arteries, such plaque is usually tightly adherent to the underlying media; dissection is extremely uncommon. This approach solves the problem of trying to penetrate the thick plaque of the terminal aorta directly with the suture needle. Placement of bifurcation graft limbs to the proximal iliac arteries is sometimes required because of impenetrable plaque at the aortic bifurcation.

Because the patient usually has not been administered heparin for the operation, it is particularly important to flush the graft free of adherent clot before closing the distal suture line. I have occasionally been forced to open the middle of the graft transversely to remove adherent thrombus before restoring flow distally.

Although contemporary anesthetic practices and monitoring techniques have markedly reduced the incidence of the once-feared "declamping" hypotension that attended restoration of flow after aortic reconstruction,[27] it is nonetheless prudent to warn the anesthesiologist 5 to 10 minutes before completion of the distal anastomosis so that a slightly hypervolemic state, obtained with administration of extra blood and crystalloid, can be achieved at the time of declamping. The complex physiology associated with aortic declamping includes rapid reperfusion of a vasodilated distal arterial circulation and central translocation of large amounts of potassium, metabolic acids, and thrombotic debris, all of which may threaten cardiac irritability after aortic declamping.[27, 28] Gradual reperfusion by partial unclamping of the aortic graft, with close attention to the arterial pressure tracing, is helpful.

After removal of clamps and restoration of flow, hemostasis should be ensured. The groins (which should have been prepared into the field) should be palpated for a pulse. When a pulse is not present, attempts at reopening the aortic graft and passing thrombectomy catheters into the iliac arteries have uniformly been futile. The optimal approach is a rapid exposure of the common femoral artery at the groin and interposition of a unilateral Dacron bypass graft between the aortic tube graft and the femoral artery.

Attention should then be directed to abdominal closure. The first aspect is to reclose the aneurysm wall over the graft to protect against future development of an aortoenteric fistula, which is much more common after emergency aortic repair than after elective reconstruction.[29] Because most ruptured aneurysms are large, it is often possible to construct a flap of aneurysm wall that can be rotated proximally and sutured between the base of duodenum and the proximal aortic-graft suture line,[30] the site where most aortoenteric erosions occur.

The abdomen should then be closed as quickly as possible and the patient conducted to the intensive care unit (ICU). It is commonplace for hypothermia, acidosis, and coagulopathy to have developed and for diffuse bleeding to be present at this point in the operation. On occasion techniques found useful in the trauma setting may be important or even lifesaving in expediting transfer of the patient out of the operating room and to the ICU setting for proper resuscitation (see the following discussion).

Postoperative Care

Initial survivors of ruptured AAAs can be some of the most complex and high-risk patients to be managed in the ICU. The chronic physiologic deficits often present in the elderly are amplified by this condition's superimposition of major blood loss and hypovolemic shock and by the emergency operation with its concomitant massive transfusion, hypothermia, coagulopathy, and acid-base problems.

Stark testimony to the morbid consequences of a ruptured AAA and its immediate management on ultimate outcome was the finding that, among 180 ruptured AAA patients managed during the period 1980 to 1989, only 13% died in the operating room, but 51% of patients admitted postoperatively to the ICU ultimately died there.[31] Although many of those dying in the first 24 hours in the ICU did so because of irreversible complications of intraoperative blood loss, such data suggest that reduction in the excessive mortality rate for ruptured AAA may result from improvements in postoperative critical care rather than intraoperative surgical technique.

This patient population can suffer virtually all the complications that confront the critically ill or injured, including adult respiratory distress syndrome, myocardial infarction or other cardiac problems, and various manifestations of multiple system organ failure. Although a complete discussion of the whole panoply of cardiopulmonary, renal, metabolic, and acid-base problems in such patients is beyond the scope of this chapter, several postoperative complications specific to the ruptured AAA patient warrant discussion, because vigilance to their presence can be lifesaving.

Acute Renal Failure

Acute renal failure, defined by a rise in the creatinine level to greater than 3.0 mg/dL, occurs in up to 40% of patients initially surviving a ruptured AAA.[32] Although acute renal failure was previously considered to be inevitably lethal in this patient population, aggressive dialysis management has made it possible for up to 25% of patients to survive this complication.[33, 34] Numerous studies have demonstrated that preoperative chronic renal insufficiency substantially increases the likelihood of acute renal failure in ruptured AAA patients.[35, 36] Intraoperative administration of mannitol and (if the patient is producing urine) diuretics probably can help mitigate the development of acute renal failure in this setting. Nephrologists may use chronic venovenous hemofiltration for fluid removal postoperatively; early dialysis of patients with acute renal failure may be helpful.[32–34, 37]

Abdominal Compartment Syndrome

The excessive mortality and morbidity rates for patients undergoing operative repair for ruptured AAA reflect the fact that these are elderly, frequently chronically ill patients who *also* are undergoing general anesthesia and major emergency vascular reconstruction simultaneously with a large volume resuscitation. Acute respiratory and renal failure may result from development of the abdominal compartment syndrome. Reported originally in trauma patients,[38, 39] this condition is characterized by excessively high intraabdominal pressures caused by massive visceral edema that compresses the diaphragms, impedes respiratory excursion,[40] and may occlude renal vein outflow, resulting in acute renal failure.[41]

Impressed by the salutary effects of temporary towel clip or synthetic mesh closure of the laparotomy wound in hyperresuscitated trauma victims,[42] my colleagues and I have used a similar approach in selected ruptured AAA patients in whom efforts to close the laparotomy incision would result in unacceptably high intraabdominal pressures.[43] Once in place, these deliberate abdominal wall hernias, composed of polyethylene or Silastic sheeting, can be serially reduced at the bedside. As bowel wall edema diminishes, intraabdominal intestinal domain is regained. The patient can then be electively returned to the operating room for abdominal wall closure, performed primarily or with an elective mesh incisional herniorrhaphy. We have been able to demonstrate a trend toward improved survival for patients so treated compared with those in whom primary laparotomy closure was attempted.[43]

Colonic Infarction

Although colon ischemia is unusual in elective aortic reconstruction, it may occur in up to 60% of patients initially surviving ruptured AAAs.[44-46] Signs suggesting colonic ischemia include early bowel evacuation and blood in the stool, but the sensitivity and specificity of these clinical findings are low.

Early in our very large experience with this entity,[45, 46] we adopted the approach of performing flexible sigmoidoscopy within the first 12 hours after arrival in the ICU following repair of ruptured AAA.[31] If the sigmoidoscopic result is positive (usually demonstrating a diffusely ischemic or necrotic sigmoid colonic mucosa) patients are returned to the operating room for laparotomy. Occasionaly, despite abnormal flexible sigmoidoscopic findings, the sigmoid and descending colon appear normal at the time of laparotomy, and we have left the colon in place, accepting that late colonic stricture formation may occur. If the descending or sigmoid colon is clearly necrotic, it is resected, with stapling of the proximal rectum and an end transverse colostomy and later reconstruction, if warranted.

The splanchnic circulation responds to hypotension with significant vasoconstriction,[47] and we had originally proposed that colonic infarction after ruptured AAA resulted from prolonged shock.[45] However, Meissner's[46] subsequent case-control study of 25 ruptured AAA patients who had developed colonic infarction, compared with 25 others who had not, revealed that the most specific predictor of colonic ischemia was intraoperative administration of α-adrenergic pressor agents. We attempt to avoid using these agents as much as possible and are even more vigilant regarding the development of this complication in patients in whom their administration has been required.

Pulmonary Embolism

Most vascular surgery patients are at low risk for venous thromboembolism (VTE), probably because of the heparin that virtually all of them are administered early in their hospital course. However, ruptured AAA patients seem to be at substantial risk of developing this complication. Such patients are elderly, hospitalized, and immobilized for substantial periods, and they usually are not anticoagulated during emergency aortic reconstructive procedures. As a consequence, VTE may occur in a substantial proportion of this patient population, significantly prolonging hospitalization and sometimes resulting in death.[48]

Parallels between ruptured aneurysm and major trauma have been drawn several times in this chapter, and the risk of VTE provides a further basis for this analogy. Victims of major trauma are recognized to be at substantial risk for VTE,[49] and strategies such as early mobilization, prophylactic subcutaneous heparin administration,[50] duplex scan surveillance of the proximal veins of the lower extremities,[51] and consideration of "prophylactic" vena caval filter insertion[52] are considered in the trauma setting. Although untested in the ruptured AAA population, these may be prudent strategies to consider for this high-risk, VTE-prone patient population.

Outcome

Predictors of Outcome

The overall hospital mortality rate for ruptured AAAs has remained at about 50% for the past three decades.[2] Factors such as the degree of cardiovascular decompensation, adequacy of prehospital resuscitation, time since rupture occurred, and time that transfer to the hospital consumed all play a role in patient survival.[53] For example, although two series[24, 54] of patients with ruptured AAAs reported from Houston had hospital mortality rates of only 15% and 23%, most of these patients had been admitted previously to the emergency room of at least one hospital, and only a few patients were in shock at the time of ultimate hospitalization. Naturally, withholding intervention until all but the most stable and resilient patients remain results, in Darwinian fashion, in excellent outcomes.[54]

In Seattle, King County, WA, where a highly sophisticated prehospital resuscitation and transport system, the Seattle/King County Medic-1,[55] has been in place for more than two decades, all individuals who suffer cardiovascular collapse are resuscitated at the scene and transported to a single receiving hospital by highly trained fire department paramedics. As a consequence, the unanticipated autopsy finding of retroperitoneal hemorrhage from ruptured AAA in elderly patients who died of cardiovascular collapse, commonly underdiagnosed elsewhere,[56] has become virtually nonexistent in Seattle and King County (Donald Reay, M.D., personal communication 1990). The fact that virtually all ruptured AAA patients in our series[31] had prehospital blood pressures <90 mm Hg suggests that the consequences of an excellent prehospital system will be that most ruptured AAA patients will no longer die at home, rather being delivered alive but moribund to the hospital. It is little surprise that hospital mortality has risen to 70% in this circumstance.[31] These data suggest that optimizing prehospital, intraoperative, and ICU care appears to improve the overall community survival rate for ruptured AAA from between 10% and 15% to about 30%. This probably approaches the optimal outcome that can be anticipated for ruptured AAAs.

Several studies have evaluated large series of ruptured AAA patients to discern individual predictors of survival.[36, 57, 58] A particularly useful analysis was carried out by Wakefield and colleagues.[36] From a large series of ruptured AAA patients managed at the University of Michigan, these investigators identified several factors that predicted mortality. These predictors were further broken down into patient- or disease-related factors and contrasted with those that might be influenced by physician intervention.

Patient-related predictors of ruptured AAA mortality included prior active heart disease, hypertension, renal dysfunction (creatinine greater than 3.0 mg/dL), flank ecchymosis, or hematocrit less than 33%. Intraoperative variables potentially reparable by appropriate and timely care included operating time longer than 400 minutes, prolonged hypotension, blood loss greater than 11 L, crystalloid administration greater than 7 L, transfusion exceeding 17 units, hypotension at the completion of the case, and intraoperative cardiac arrest. Timely, technically adept operative management clearly plays a role in outcome following ruptured AAA.

Late Outcomes

Most outcome analyses emphasize operative survival (ie, 30-day mortality), but some have looked at late outcomes for patients surviving ruptured AAAs. Although a successful *elective* repair of an AAA returns the patient to the survival curve of the age-matched control population, the overall consequences after rupture of an AAA remain dismal. Those who initially survive operation for ruptured AAAs have an actuarial 9-year decrement in long-term life span.[60]

Most patients who suffer aneurysmal rupture die, and in the era of skilled prehospital transport, an ever increasing number of such patients can be retrieved, resuscitated, and delivered—frequently moribund—to hospital emergency rooms, resulting in lengthy and extraordinarily costly hospitalization. For example, calculations by Munoz[61] suggest expenditures in excess of $300,000 per life saved after a ruptured AAA. Pasch and colleagues[62] suggested that $50 million (in 1984 dollars) could be saved if patients at risk for ruptured AAA could be identified and operated on electively.

Improving Outcome

Significant controversy has arisen about issues such as the setting in which ruptured AAA patients should be treated (ie, community hospital or transfer to a major receiving hospital), who should perform such procedures (ie, general surgeons or vascular specialists), and whether adequate data exist to identify patients for whom operative repair is futile and should be abandoned.

Ouriel[63] suggested that outcomes after ruptured AAAs are better when operative management is carried out by vascular specialists. However, it is possible that the time spent to transfer such patients to a major medical center where the specialists are located may neutralize the outcome benefit.[64] I am firmly convinced that transfer of ruptured AAA patients to an institution with level I trauma capabilities and readily available operating rooms can optimize outcome for these critically ill patients.

My group[31] have observed that certain clinical features predict a lethal outcome with such certainty after ruptured AAA that their presence may warrant abandoning the operation. Others[66-68] have disagreed, some vociferously.[69] Although such factors as preoperative cardiac arrest, age greater than 80 years, female gender, and massive blood loss have been associated with death of more than 90% of ruptured AAA patients who have any one of these features,[31, 65, 66] an occasional patient survives. The threshold at which one considers intervention futile remains more ideologic or philosophic than clinical.[70]

Hospital management of critically ill patients with ruptured AAA has failed to keep pace with the general improvement in outcome after elective repair of AAA (now well under 5% operative mortality) or with advances in prehospital resuscitation or transport. It is likely that an unacceptably high toll will continue to be paid by patients who undergo repair of AAA after rupture. The intuitive worth of screening programs for populations at risk for AAA and of repairing aneurysms electively before rupture has been confirmed both by a mathematical model[35] and by a prospective randomized trial.[71]

References

1. Bengtsson H, Bergqvist D, Sternby NH. Increasing prevalence of abdominal aortic aneurysms: a necropsy study. Eur J Surg 1992;158:19–23.

2. Gloviczki P. Ruptured abdominal aortic aneurysms. *In* Rutherford RB (ed). Vascular Surgery, 4th ed. Philadelphia: WB Saunders, 1995.

3. Johansson G, Swedenborg J. Ruptured abdominal aortic aneurysms: a study of incidence and mortality. Br J Surg 1986;73:101–103.

4. Ingoldby CJH, Wujanto R, Mitchell JE. Impact of vascular surgery on community mortality from ruptured aortic aneurysms. Br J Surg 1986;73:551–553.

5. United States Public Health Service. Vital Statistics of the United States, vol II. Mortality, Part A. Department of Health and Human Service, publication number (PHS) 87-101. Washington, DC: U.S. Government Printing Office, 1987.

6. Inzoli F, Boschetti F, Zappa M, et al. Biomechanical factors in abdominal aortic aneurysm rupture. Eur J Vasc Surg 1993;7:667–674.

7. Elger DF, Blackketter DM, Budwig RS, Johansen K. The influence of shape on the stresses in model abdominal aortic aneurysms. J Biomed Eng 1996;118:326–332.

8. Hunter GC, Leong SC, Yu GSM, et al. Aortic blebs: possible site of aneurysm rupture. J Vasc Surg 1989;10:93–99.

9. Zarins CK, Runyon-Hass A, Zatina MA, et al. Increased collagenase activity in early aneurysmal dilatation. J Vasc Surg 1986;3:238–246.

10. White JV, Haas K, Phillips S, et al. Adventitial elastolysis is a primary event in aneurysm formation. J Vasc Surg 1993;17:371.

11. Crawford JL, Stowe CL, Safi HJ, et al. Inflammatory aneurysms of the aorta. J Vasc Surg 1985;2:113–118.

12. Cohen JR, Graver LM. The ruptured abdominal aortic aneurysm of Albert Einstein. Surg Obstet Gynecol 1990;170:455.

13. Gilling-Smith GL, Mansfield AO. Spontaneous abdominal arteriovenous fistulae: report of eight cases and review of the literature. Br J Surg 1991;78:421.

14. Todd GJ, Nowygrod R, Benvenisty A, et al. The accuracy of CT scanning in the diagnosis of abdominal and thoracoabdominal aortic aneurysms. J Vasc Surg 1991;13:302–310.

15. Petersen MJ, Cambria RP, Kaufman JA, et al. Magnetic resonance angiography in the preoperative evaluation of abdominal aortic aneurysms. J Vasc Surg 1995;21:891–899.

16. Weinbaum FI, Dubner S, Turner JW, Pardees JG. The accuracy of computed tomography in the diagnosis of retroperitoneal blood in the presence of abdominal aortic aneurysm. J Vasc Surg 1987;6:11–16.

17. Shuman WP, Hastrup W, Kohler TR, et al. Suspected leaking abdominal aortic aneurysm: use of sonography in the emergency room. Radiology 1988;168:117–119.

18. Lederle FAA, Walker JM, Reinke DB. Selective screening for abdominal aortic aneurysms with physical examination and ultrasound. Arch Intern Med 1988;148:1753–1756.

19. Thomas P, Shaw J, Ashton H, et al. Accuracy of ultrasound in a screening programme for abdominal aortic aneurysms. J Med Screen 1994;1:3–6.

20. Farrara A, MacArthur JD, Wright HK, et al. Hypothermia and acidosis worsens coagulopathy in patients requiring massive transfusion. Am J Surg 1990;160:515–521.

21. Tawes RL, Scribner RG, DuVall TB, et al. The cell-saver and autotransfusion: an underutilized resource in vascular surgery. Am J Surg 1986;152:105–110.

22. Satiani B, Fried SJ, Zeeb P, et al. Normothermic rapid volume replacement in traumatic hypovolemia. Arch Surg 1987;122:1044–1050.

23. Chang BB, Shah DM, Paty PSK, et al. Can the retroperitoneal approach be used for ruptured abdominal aortic aneurysms? J Vasc Surg 1990;11:326–330.

24. Crawford ES, Saleh SA, Babb JW, et al. Infrarenal abdominal aortic aneurysms: factors influencing survival after operation over a 25-year period. Ann Surg 1981;193:699–706.

25. Szilagyi DE, Elliott JP, Berguer R. Temporary transection of the left renal vein: a technical aid in aortic surgery. Surgery 1969;65:32–34.

26. AbuRahma AF, Robinson PA, Boland JP, Lucente FC. The risk of ligation of the left renal vein in resection of abdominal aortic aneurysm. Surg Gynecol Obstet 1991;173:33–36.

27. Gelman S, McDowell H, Varner PD, et al. The reason for cardiac output reduction after aortic cross-clamping. Am J Surg 1988;155:578–584.

28. Falk JL, Rackow EC, Blumenberg R, et al. Hemodynamic and metabolic effects of abdominal aortic cross-clamping. Am J Surg 1981;142:174–180.

29. Moulton S, Adams M, Johansen KH. Aortoenteric fistula: a seven-year urban experience. Am J Surg 1986;151:607–611.

30. Hertzer NR. A rotated aneurysm cuff for separation of aortic graft and duodenum. Surg Gynecol Obstet 1978;147:84–85.

31. Johansen K, Kohler TR, Nicholls SC, et al. Ruptured abdominal aortic aneurysm. The Harborview experience. J Vasc Surg 1991;13:240–247.

32. Powers SR. Renal failure after ruptured aneurysm. Arch Surg 1975;110:1069–1075.

33. Tromp-Meesters RC, van der Graaf Y, Vos A, Eikelboom BC. Ruptured aortic aneurysm: early postoperative prediction of mortality using an organ system failure score. Br J Surg 1994;81:512–516.

34. Gordon AC, Pryn S, Collin J, et al. Outcome in patients who require renal support after surgery for ruptured abdominal aortic aneurysm. Br J Surg 1994;81:836–838.

35. Cronenwett JL, Katz DA. Cost-effectiveness of early surgery for small abdominal aortic aneurysms. J Vasc Surg 1993:18:538–539.

36. Wakefield TW, Whitehouse WM, Wu S, et al. Abdominal aortic aneurysm rupture: statistical analysis of factors affecting outcome of surgical treatment. Surgery 1982;91:586–596.
37. Yagi N, Paganini EP. Acute dialysis and continuous renal replacement: the emergence of new technology involving the nephrologist in the intensive care setting. Semin Nephrol 1997;17:306–320.
38. Smith PC, Tweddell JS, Bessey PQ. Alternative approaches to abdominal wound closure in severely injured patients with massive visceral edema. J Trauma 1992;32:16–20.
39. Bendahan J, Coetzee CJ, Papagiaopoulos C, Muller R. Abdominal compartment syndrome. J Trauma 1995;38:152–153.
40. Obeid F, Saba A, Fath J, et al. Increases in intra-abdominal pressure in critically ill patients. Crit Care Med 1989;17:1118–1121.
41. Cullen DJ, Coyle JP, Teplick R, Long MC. Cardiovascular, pulmonary, and renal effects of massively increased intra-abdominal pressure in critically ill patients. Crit Care Med 1989;17:118–121.
42. Howdieshell TR, Yeh KA, Hawkins MS, Cué JI. Temporary abdominal wall closure in trauma patients: indications, technique, and results. World J Surg 1995;119:154–158.
43. Oelschlager BK, Boyle EM, Johansen K, Meissner MK. Delayed abdominal closure in the management of ruptured abdominal aortic aneurysms. Am J Surg 1997;172:411–415.
44. Maupin GE, Rimar SD, Villalba M. Ischemic colitis following abdominal aortic reconstruction for ruptured aneurysm: a 10-year experience. Am Surg 1989;55:378–380.
45. Bandyk DF, Florence MG, Johansen KH. Colon ischemia accompanying ruptured abdominal aortic aneurysm. J Surg Res 1981;30:297–303.
46. Meissner M, Johansen K. Colon infarction after ruptured aortic aneurysm. Arch Surg 1992;127:979–985.
47. Fry RE, Huber PJ, Ramsey KL, Fry WJ. Infrarenal aortic occlusion, colonic blood flow, and the effect of nitroglycerine afterload reduction. Surgery 1984;95:479–486.
48. Barnett MG, Peterson GJ. Deep venous thrombosis and pulmonary embolism following repair of ruptured abdominal aortic aneurysm. Presented at the Ninth Non-Invasive Diagnosis of Vascular Disease Symposium; St. Louis, MO, March 29, 1995.
49. Shackford SR, Davis JW, Hollingsworth-Fridlund P, et al. Venous thromboembolism in patients with major trauma. Am J Surg 1990;159:365–371.
50. Geerts WH, Jay RM, Code KI, et al. A comparison of low-dose heparin with low-molecular-weight heparin as prophylaxis against venous thromboembolism after major trauma. N Engl J Med 1996;335:701–707.
51. Brasel KJ, Borgstrom DC, Weigelt JA. Cost-effective prevention of pulmonary embolus in high-risk trauma patients. J Trauma 1997;42:456–460.
52. Rodriguez JL, Lopez JM, Proctor MC, et al. Early placement of prophylactic vena caval filters in injured patients at high risk for pulmonary embolism. J Trauma 1996;40:797–802.
53. Johansen K. Ruptured abdominal aortic aneurysm: how should recent outcome studies impact on current practice? Semin Vasc Surg 1995;8:163–167.
54. Lawrie GM, Morris GC, Crawford ES, et al. Improved results of operation for ruptured abdominal aortic aneurysms. Surgery 1979;85:483–488.
55. Cobb LA, Alvarez H, Copass MK. A rapid response system for out-of-hospital cardiac emergencies. Med Clin North Am 1976;60:283–289.
56. McFarlane MJ. The epidemiologic necropsy for abdominal aortic aneurysm. JAMA 1991;26:2085–2088.
57. Donaldson MC, Rosenberg JM, Buckman CA. Factors affecting survival after ruptured abdominal aortic aneurysm. J Vasc Surg 1985;2:564–570.
58. Johnston KW. Ruptured abdominal aortic aneurysm: six-year follow-up of a multicenter prospective study. Canadian Society for Vascular Surgery Aneurysm Study Group. J Vasc Surg 1994;19:888–900.
59. Magee TR, Scott DJ, Dunkley A, et al. Quality of life following surgery for abdominal aortic aneurysm. Br J Surg 1992;79:1014–1016.
60. Aune S, Amundsen SR, Evjensvold J, Trippestad A. Operative mortality and long term relative survival of patients operated on for asymptomatic abdominal aortic aneurysm. Eur J Vasc Endovasc Surg 1995;9:293–298.
61. Munoz E, Kassau MA, Chang JB. Surgonomics: the costs of ruptured abdominal aortic aneurysm. Angiology 1988;38:830–837.
62. Pasch AR, Ricotta JJ, May AG, et al. Abdominal aortic aneurysm: the case for elective resection. Circulation 1984;70(suppl 1):1–4.
63. Ouriel K, Geary K, Green RM, et al. Factors determining survival after ruptured aortic aneurysm: the hospital, the surgeon, and the patient. J Vasc Surg 1990;11:493–496.
64. Meyer AA, Ahlquist RE Jr, Trunkey DD. Mortality from ruptured abdominal aortic aneurysm: a comparison of two series. Am J Surg 1986;152:27–33.
65. Rohrer MJ, Cutler BS, Wheeler HB. Long term survival and quality of life following ruptured abdominal aortic aneurysm. Arch Surg 1988;123:1213–1217.
66. Harris LM, Faggioli GL, Fiedler R, et al. Ruptured abdominal aortic aneurysms: factors affecting mortality rates. J Vasc Surg 1991;14:812–816.
67. Gloviczki P, Pairolero PC, Mucha P Jr, et al. Ruptured abdominal aortic aneurysms: repair should not be denied. J Vasc Surg 1991;15:851–859.

68. McCready RA, Siderys HA, Pittman JN, et al. Ruptured abdominal aortic aneurysms in a private hospital: a decade's experience (1980–89). Ann Vasc Surg 1993;7:225–228.
69. Crawford ES. Ruptured abdominal aortic aneurysm: an editorial. J Vasc Surg 1991;13:348–350.
70. Schneiderman LJ, Jecker NS, Jonsen AR. Medical futility: its meaning and ethical implications. Ann Intern Med 1990;112:949–954.
71. Scott RAP, Wilson NM, Ashton HA, et al. Influence of screening on the incidence of ruptured abdominal aortic aneurysm: 5-year results of a randomized controlled study. Br J Surg 1995;82:1066–1070.

Aortic Ligation and Aneurysm Exclusion as Treatment Options for Abdominal Aortic Aneurysms

Jamal J. Hoballah, M.D., and
John D. Corson, M.B., Ch.B.

Conventional surgical treatment for an infrarenal abdominal aortic aneurysm (AAA) involves replacement of the aneurysmal aortic segment with an in-line aortic bypass graft.[21, 59, 66] This procedure can be performed effectively using a transabdominal or retroperitoneal approach.[49] After establishing proximal and distal control, the aneurysmal sac is opened; the contained, laminated thrombus is removed; backbleeding lumbar arteries and the inferior mesenteric artery are controlled; and an appropriate-sized aortic prosthesis is implanted. The redundant aneurysmal wall is then wrapped around the implanted prosthetic graft to prevent direct contact of the graft with the bowel to minimize late enteric complications.

The benefits of conventional surgical treatment of large AAAs were initially reported by Szilagyi in 1966.[69] This standardized procedure has stood the test of time and is associated with a low perioperative mortality rate and minimal late complications (Table 17–1). Higher perioperative mortality rates can be anticipated for patients with multiple medical comorbidities or persons with more extensive aneurysmal disease, necessitating suprarenal clamping and visceral artery revascularization.[18, 25, 40, 66]

Because the mortality rate associated with ruptured aneurysms continues to be extremely high,[44, 72] elective aortic replacement remains the most effective method of preventing aneurysmal rupture and its consequences. However,

Table 17–1.
Mortality of Elective Infrarenal Abdominal Aortic Aneurysm Replacement

Year	Author	Experience	Patients	Operative Mortality (%)
1989	Green[28]	Single center	379	2.1
1989	Leather[49]	Single center	299	3.7
1990	Golden[26]	Single center	500	1.6
1992	Cambria[12]	Single center	202	2.0
1991	AbuRahma[1]	Multi-center	332	3.6
1994	Baron[5]	Multi-center	457	4.4
1996	Wen[72]	Multi-center	5492	3.8
1996	Kazmers[44]	Multi-center	3419	4.9
1992	Hannan[29]	Population based	1397	7.2
1994	Katz[43]	Population based	8185	7.3

From Rutherford RB (ed). Seminars in Vascular Surgery. Vascular Surgery, vol 2. Philadelphia: WB Saunders, 1995:1038.

when the operative risk is comparable to the risk of rupture, the value of aneurysm replacement becomes questionable. This is especially true in the management of a patient with a relatively small aneurysm or an individual with limited life expectancy because of other medical conditions.

To reduce the operative risk, the patient's overall medical condition must be optimized preoperatively. This may involve measures such as adjustments of cardiac medications and fluid balance, enhancement of the pulmonary status, or even coronary revascularization. If, despite all attempts to ameliorate any correctable medical problems, a patient is still considered to be unable to tolerate a conventional surgical approach for aneurysm replacement, one option is to deny that person an elective surgical procedure.

Alternative, less stressful surgical procedures have been sought for such high-risk patients to avert death from aneurysm rupture. In this chapter, we review the alternative surgical methods available for treatment of AAAs to determine whether such therapy has any role in the modern management of aortic aneurysmal disease.

Historical Perspective

Extremity aneurysms were traditionally treated by incision and cautery (ie, "knife and fire"). The Greek physician Antyllus first described the surgical management of extremity aneurysmal disease in 200 AD.[23] Instead of using the customary therapy, he advocated proximal and distal arterial ligation, followed by incision with evacuation of the aneurysmal contents and packing of the cavity. He cautioned against the resection of the aneurysm sac. Such ligation therapy, however, often resulted in extremity gangrene. The arterial ligatures frequently eroded into the vessel, causing exsanguination. Because of these problems, primary amputation became a favored method for treating large arterial aneurysms of the extremities.

In 1785, Hunter first demonstrated that distal extremity gangrene was less likely to develop if the proximal arterial ligation was performed in a fashion to maintain the collateral circulation.[34] In 1817, Cooper treated a huge external iliac aneurysm that had eroded through the skin of a young man by ligating the aorta proximal to its bifurcation.[15] Unfortunately, the patient died 3 days later.

The first reported successful aortic ligation for the treatment of aortic aneurysmal disease was performed in 1923 by Matas in a young woman with a ruptured syphilitic aneurysm of the aortic bifurcation.[51] Matas placed cotton ligatures just proximal and distal to the aneurysm. This patient lived 17 months after surgery and died of a cause unrelated to her aneurysm surgery. Despite this success, surgeons remained wary of using such techniques for aortic aneurysms because of the consequences of interrupting blood flow to the lower half of the body and the problem of erosion.

Other methods of surgical therapy continued to be developed and used.[4] Some of these methods attempted to induce thrombosis by introducing foreign materials such as horse hair or wire into the aneurysm.[30, 35, 46, 54] Other methods attempted unsuccessfully to externally reinforce and strengthen the aneurysm wall with cellophane or fascia lata in an effort to prevent aneurysm expansion and rupture.[6, 20]

The start of the modern era of surgical treatment of aortic aneurysmal disease was in 1944, when Alexander and Byron[3] resected a thoracic aortic aneurysm resulting from coarctation in a 19-year-old college student. The aorta proximal and distal to the aneurysm was ligated. Although the continuity of the aorta could not be reestablished, the patient had a good recovery, except for persistent headaches and hypertension. Later in 1944, Crafoord[17] of Sweden was the first to succeed in reconstructing the aorta by end-to-end anastomosis after resection of an aortic coarctation. In 1947, Schumaker[67] performed the first successful resection of a thoracic aortic aneurysm. He was able to perform a primary end-to-end aortic anastomosis. In 1951, Dubost[22] was the first surgeon to replace an infrarenal AAA using an aortic thoracic homograft harvested 3 weeks earlier. Unfortunately, the aortic homografts developed aneurysmal changes with time and later required replacement.

The current method of aortic replacement was described by Crech,[19] who warned against resection of the aortic aneurysm. The work of Voorhees and other pioneers resulted in the development of durable prosthetic grafts for aortic replacement.[71]

Treatment of High-Risk Patients

The definition of a high-risk patient was vague and poorly standardized until 1992, when the joint council of the Society for Vascular Surgery and the International Society for Cardiovascular Surgery[33] convened a panel of experts to categorize the medical risks of patients undergoing elective aneurysm replacement. This panel grouped the patients into four categories: low risk, minimal risk, moderate risk, and high risk (Table 17–2).

Categorization as a high-risk patient does not necessarily imply that the patient is a not a candidate for conventional surgical therapy. The predicted mortality rate for high-risk patients was 8% to 30%, compared with 3% to 8% for moderate-risk patients. Because of the overlap, a patient who may be viewed as a poor surgical candidate by one surgeon may be considered an acceptable candidate by another surgeon. Moreover, high-risk patients are not all equally sick, and the probability of a poor outcome after aneurysm replacement is not necessarily the same for all high-risk patients. For example, a patient whose cardiac, pulmonary, and renal conditions are all in the high-risk category could be expected to do worse than the patient who has only one high-risk condition.

Careful patient selection plays a major role in achieving good results. This may explain why the mortality risk for aneurysm replacement in high-risk patients is reported to exceed 60% in some centers[25] but is similar to that for the general population in others.[32] Excellent monitoring, skilled perioperative management, and an experienced vascular team are key components in obtaining good results in treating high-risk patients.[29] The longevity of high-risk patients probably is limited even without surgery because of their comorbidities or the aneurysm disease. Any decision regarding the management of such patients should be the result of a collaborative discourse among the patient, his or her family, the surgeon, and the anesthetist. This decision often depends on the size of the aneurysm, the presence or absence of symptoms, and the extent of the comorbid conditions affecting the patient.

Experience with aneurysm replacement in the octogenarian population indicates that physiologic rather than chronologic age should determine whether a patient is an appropriate candidate for conventional aneurysm replacement.[31, 39] The comorbid medical problems associated with old age are responsible for the poor results in some elderly patients rather than old age alone.

Despite a low ejection fraction, a patient can undergo standard aneurysm replacement successfully. Although no large studies have addressed the re-

Table 17–2.
Medical Risk Categorization: Elective Aneurysm Repair

Risk	Level 0 (Low Risk)	Level I (Minimal Risk)	Level II (Moderate Risk)	Level III (High Risk)
Age (yr)	<75	75–80	85–90	>90
Cardiac	No CAD	CAD: mild stable angina or remote MI, negative coronary angiogram, normal cardiac stress test, LVEF <50% but >30%	CAD: stable angina or remote MI, mild to moderate lesions on coronary angiogram, small reperfusion defects on radionuclide scan, LVEF <30% but >20%	CAD: unstable angina, significant areas of myocardium at risk based on coronary angiogram or radionuclide scans, LVEF <20%, recent CHF
Pulmonary	Normal function	COPD: able to carry out normal activities of daily life	COPD: moderate to severe pulmonary dysfunction	COPD: requiring home oxygen, FEF <20% of predicted
Renal	Normal function	Mild renal dysfunction, creatinine <2 mg/dL	Renal dysfunction, creatinine 2–3.5 mg/dL	Chronic dialysis, creatinine >3.5 mg/dL
Hepatic*				Biopsy-proven cirrhosis with ascites
Abdominal*				Diffuse retroperitoneal fibrosis
Predicted mortality rate	0%–1%	1%–3%	3%–8%	8%–30%

CAD, coronary artery disease; CHF, congestive heart failure; COPD, chronic obstructive pulmonary disease; LVEF, left ventricular ejection fraction; MI, myocardial infarction; FEF, forced expiratory flow.
*Data from Hollier LH, Taylor LM Jr, Ochsner J. Recommended indications for operative treatment of abdominal aortic aneurysm. J Vasc Surg 1992;15:1046.

sults of aortic replacement in patients with left ventricular ejection fractions less than 20%, some data are available for ejection fractions lower than 35%. McCann and Wolfe[53] reported a 5% perioperative mortality rate after aortic aneurysm replacement in a group of 19 patients with ejection fractions less than 35%. This finding was not significantly different from the rate for patients with ejection fractions greater than 35%. Some surgeons have reported the use of intraoperative aortic balloon counterpulsation simultaneously in selected patients with low ejection fractions undergoing standard AAA replacement procedures.[32] Others have used a temporary axillofemoral bypass to prevent sudden hemodynamic stresses on the heart during aortic clamping. Even a patient with the myocardium at risk can successfully undergo aortic aneurysm replacement.

In our experience at the University of Iowa with routine preoperative cardiac evaluation using thallium scans, several patients were identified as having reversible reperfusion defects and were also found to have nonreconstructable coronary artery disease based on cardiac catheterization. Twelve of these patients underwent successful aneurysm replacement. In some patients with symptomatic or very large aneurysms and severe reconstructable coronary disease, coronary artery bypass grafting and AAA replacement could be performed as a combined procedure.

Although chronic renal failure is an independent risk factor for increased morbidity, aortic aneurysm replacement can be carried out electively in such individuals with planned perioperative dialysis and appropriate renal revascularization in carefully selected patients. Cohen and colleagues[14] showed that patients with serum creatinine values less than 4 mg/dL can undergo elective aneurysm replacement without additional morbidity.

The incidence of major pulmonary complications after aortic replacement is 2% to 8%. However, Robison and associates[60] showed that, in a group of 17 patients considered to be extremely high-risk patients because of pulmonary disease, the overall incidence of postoperative pulmonary complications was 22%. Most patients ultimately did well, and the surgeons concluded that chronic obstructive pulmonary disease alone need not preclude appropriate surgical intervention when required for aortic aneurysm replacement. The use of epidural anesthesia can be useful in the postoperative period to allow painless deep breathing and pulmonary physiotherapy. The proponents of AAA replacement through a retroperitoneal approach contend that this method is preferential for patients with pulmonary comorbidities. The prospective randomized trials comparing the transabdominal with the retroperitoneal approach do not support this claim.[11, 68]

Obesity is often cited as a significant risk factor. One possible explanation is that overweight patients are considered more prone to develop pulmonary and venous thrombotic complications than nonobese patients. The procedure can be technically more demanding in this group of patients. We have operated successfully on morbidly obese patients, preferentially using a retroperitoneal approach that facilitates the aneurysm procedure.

Many patients who could be classified as high risk can still undergo a successful conventional infrarenal aortic aneurysm replacement, especially if treated by a skilled team in a large institution. However, the idea that no patient is too frail to undergo conventional aortic aneurysm replacement procedure is unrealistic. The patient who suffers from several poorly controlled comorbid medical conditions cannot be expected to undergo a conventional aortic aneurysm replacement without a high probability of a perioperative mortality.

Alternative Procedures

To avoid an unacceptably high perioperative mortality rate for high-risk patients, surgeons have sought less stressful alternatives to a conventional surgical aortic aneurysm replacement.

Blaisdell[9] recommended proximal aortic ligation as definitive treatment for an infrarenal aortic aneurysm in high-risk individuals. His favorable experience with the use of axillofemoral bypasses to revascularize the lower extremities in high-risk patients with aortoiliac occlusive disease encouraged him to try a similar approach in a high-risk patient with an aortic aneurysm. He staged the procedure by first performing an axillobifemoral bypass under light, general anesthesia. Four weeks later, he excluded the aorta from the main bloodstream by placing ligatures proximally at the neck of the aneurysm and distally on the common iliac arteries. When he tried this procedure in another patient, spontaneous thrombosis of the AAA occurred after placement of the axillobifemoral bypass, which he attributed to the presence of competitive flow. Ligation was considered unnecessary in this patient and was not performed.

Because aneurysmal thrombosis was presumed to protect against future aneurysm rupture, other surgeons sought other techniques to induce aneurysm thrombosis. Outflow occlusion was tried in selected patients by ligating the distal external iliac arteries after performing the femoral anastomoses of the axillobifemoral bypass. Because aortic aneurysm thrombosis occurred in most of these cases, procedures involving proximal aortic ligation of the aneurysm neck, which required general anesthesia and laparotomy, were less frequently performed.

Berguer[7, 8] used another technique to induce thrombosis. He exteriorized the external iliac arteries and injected thrombin into the aneurysm. As it became apparent that external iliac artery ligation alone did not routinely result in aortic aneurysmal thrombosis because of the continued patency of the hypogastric arteries, the inferior mesenteric artery, or the lumbar arteries, Leather and Karmody[48] refined their nonresective technique and ligated, in appropriate patients, the common iliac arteries through a retroperitoneal approach using a left flank or bilateral small flank incisions. Residual patent vessels maintaining aneurysm blood flow were occluded by transcatheter embolization techniques, using materials such as Bucrylate, thrombin, pledgets, coils, and occlusive balloons.[27, 62] The concept of inducing aortic aneurysm thrombosis without ligating the aorta at the level of the aneurysm neck was appealing and was embraced by several surgeons. However, Kwaan and associates[46, 47] continued to advocate total exclusion of the aneurysm achieved by ligating the infrarenal aorta at the aneurysm neck, the common iliac arteries, and other patent tributaries such as the inferior mesenteric and lumbar arteries.

As the interest in the newer, nonresective therapies widened, they were used more liberally. Although such approaches were anticipated to reduce the perioperative mortality of high-risk patients, several studies indicated that these nonresective procedures were associated with unacceptably high mortality rates.[13, 36, 64] Alarming reports of delayed aortic aneurysm rupture after nonresective therapy began to appear in the literature.[45, 58, 63, 64]

Corson and coworkers[16] devised another method for the treatment of infrarenal aortoiliac aneurysm disease. This method used a modification of the standard retroperitoneal approach for abdominal aortic replacement. The aneurysmal sac is not opened in the modified method. The aorta is clamped and transected proximally for an end-to-end anastomosis, and the upper end of the aneurysm is oversewn or stapled. Distal to the aneurysm, the vessels are ligated, and the graft is anastomosed at the level of the aortic bifurcation or to the iliac or femoral arteries, depending on the extent of the aneurysmal occlusive disease. This procedure was referred to as *in situ management of AAA* (ISMAA). Corson and coworkers[16] believed that the retroperitoneal approach might be better tolerated in high-risk patients.

Three nonresective methods have evolved:

1. Aortic exclusion by proximal and distal ligation combined with an axillobifemoral bypass (Fig. 17–1)
2. Induced aortic thrombosis without proximal aortic ligation combined with axillobifemoral bypass (Fig. 17–2)
3. Retroperitoneal aortic exclusion and distal ligation with placement of an in-line, aortic bypass graft (ie, ISMAA) (Fig. 17–3)

When evaluating alternative therapeutic modalities, the following questions must be addressed:

1. Does aortic aneurysm thrombosis protect against future aortic rupture?
2. Which nonresective therapy should be used and when?
3. Which patients are candidates for nonresective therapy?
4. What are the morbidity, mortality, and survival rates associated with these procedures?
5. Does the late rupture rate depend on the procedure used?

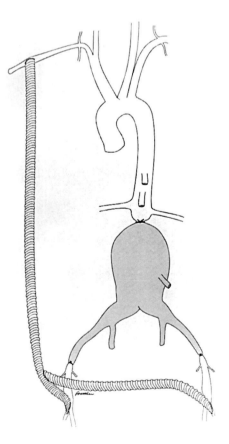

Figure 17–1. The external iliac arteries are ligated just above the origin of the circumflex iliac vessels to preserve collateral flow. If the internal iliac arteries are patent, they are ligated through a retroperitoneal approach. (From Corson JD, Hoballah JJ. Is there a role for abdominal aortic aneurysm exclusion or induced thrombosis? Semin Vasc Surg 1995; 8:155–162.)

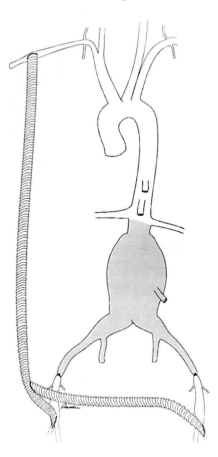

Figure 17-2. The significant difference between total aneurysm exclusion and the induced aneurysm thrombosis procedure is that the infrarenal aorta is ligated just above the origin of the aneurysmal disease in the total aneurysm exclusion. (From Corson JD, Hoballah JJ. Is there a role for abdominal aortic aneurysm exclusion or induced thrombosis? Semin Vasc Surg 1995;8:155–162.)

Figure 17-3. The bypass lies well in the retroperitoneum and is posterior to and parallel to the decompressed aneurysm sac. (From Corson JD, Hoballah JJ. Is there a role for abdominal aortic aneurysm exclusion or induced thrombosis? Semin Vasc Surg 1995;8:155–162.)

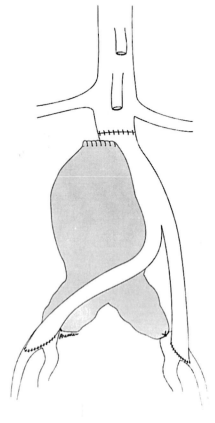

6. What is the incidence of incomplete aneurysmal sac thrombosis after occlusion of the aortic outflow vessels?

Treatment Results

Induced Aneurysm Thrombosis

The incidence of incomplete aortic aneurysm thrombosis after external iliac artery ligation alone is hard to determine from the available literature. After occlusion of the external and internal iliac arteries without proximal aortic ligation, aortic thrombosis develops in most patients. In Karmody's[42] series of 60 patients treated by this method, 42 patients (70%) developed aortic aneurysm thrombosis within 72 hours. Aortic thrombosis was clinically determined by the disappearance of expansile aortic pulsations. Ultrasonographic and radionuclide aortic flow studies were used to confirm thrombosis of the aneurysm. Later in the series, the radionuclide flow studies were replaced by enhanced computed tomographic (CT) studies.

The incidence of aneurysm thrombosis after total exclusion achieved by adding proximal aortic ligation is higher. This incidence can be determined from Blumenberg's[10] and Shah's[65] reports on ISMAA patients. In Blumenberg's series, staple exclusion of abdominal aneurysms and aortic bypass were performed in 100 consecutive patients. Ultrasonographic studies confirmed that 87.2% of the aneurysms were thrombosed at 6 months and 90% at 1 year. At 5 years, all living patients showed thrombosis of the excluded aneurysms. No aneurysm rupture occurred during the study period. Shah and colleagues[65] also studied the fate of the aneurysmal sac after total exclusion with ultrasonography. After ligation of the aortic aneurysm proximally and distally in 330 patients, all aneurysmal sacs developed thrombosis, except in two individuals who were receiving anticoagulation therapy.

Operative Mortality

The lowest operative mortality rate reported after induced aneurysm thrombosis without proximal ligation was reported by Karmody and associates.[42] Their reported operative mortality rate was 7%, and the patient survival rate was 50% at 30 months. However, prohibitively high operative mortality rates were reported in other series. Schwartz and coworkers[64] reported an operative mortality rate of 31% and a survival rate of only 23% at 12 months. Cho and associates[13] reported a mortality rate of 80% in their limited experience with five patients.

Lynch and colleagues[50] polled 120 active members of the North American chapter of the International Society of Cardiovascular Surgery regarding their experience with nonresective AAA procedures. The pooled data from 113 responding surgeons were analyzed. The collected data for induced aneurysm thrombosis without proximal ligation revealed an operative mortality rate of 34%.[50] This was significantly higher than the operative mortality rate (5.1%) in the pooled data for aortic exclusion procedures with proximal and distal ligation ($P = .000001$) and compared favorably with Kwaan's data.

The mortality rate for the ISMAA procedure was 2.8%, as reported by Corson and coworkers[16] and 4% as reported by the research groups of Shah[65] and Blumenberg.[10] In these series, low- and high-risk patients were included. The mortality rate of the ISMAA procedure for high-risk patients has not yet been defined by these studies.

Morbidity

A variety of complications have been reported after the use of the various nonresective procedures. Some of these complications result from pelvic ischemia when blood flow to both hypogastric vessels is interrupted. Complications include buttock claudication, paraplegia, vasculogenic impotence, and mesenteric ischemia. In the 5.5-year Albany experience with induced aneurysm thrombosis, no pelvic ischemic complications were reported.

Additional complications after induced aortic thrombosis may develop because of proximal propagation of the aortic thrombus, causing renal failure and visceral ischemia.[46] A rare reported complication was abscess formation.[24] Disseminated intravascular coagulopathy occurred when thrombin was directly injected into the aneurysm to induce thrombosis.[64] Additional morbidity involving the use of nonresective therapy in association with an extraanatomic bypass is the failure of such conduits. Initial results with axillofemoral bypasses were discouraging.[57] Almost 30% of axillobifemoral bypass grafts occlude during the first year after implantation.[37, 38, 61] However, higher patency rates have been achieved, possibly because of the use of externally supported bypass grafts in association with long-term anticoagulation.[41, 70] Improved long-term, secondary patency rates can generally be achieved in aneurysmal patients who tend to have good distal runoff. However, the overall results are less satisfactory than those achieved with an in-line aortic bypass graft.

The morbidity of the ISMAA procedure is relatively low. In the large series reported by Shah and colleagues,[65] nonfatal complications were reported for only 6% of the patients. None of these complications were directly related to aortic aneurysm exclusion. The aortic bypass patency rate was 98% at 5 years. In the series by Blumenberg and coworkers,[10] major pulmonary complications occurred in 17% of patients. However, reintubation was necessary in only 2%. Acute renal failure occurred in 8%, but dialysis was not required for any of these patients. However, acute renal failure might have contributed to the multisystem organ failure and death of one patient (1%). Postoperative myocardial infarction occurred in 4% and gastrointestinal complications occurred in 2%. One of the latter complications resulted from partial strangulation of the colonic wall through a defect in the peritoneum and was related to the retroperitoneal approach. The other was caused by ischemic colitis that involved the entire colon and ultimately resulted in the patient's death.

Before performing a nonresective procedure, a preoperative angiogram and CT scan are necessary to reduce morbidity. The angiogram is needed to assess the visceral circulation, and the CT scan is used to determine the extent of the aneurysmal disease.

Aortic Rupture

Aortic rupture can occur despite attempts to induce aortic aneurysm thrombosis, whether the aorta proximal to the aneurysm was ligated or left undisturbed.[45, 50, 58, 63, 64] The incidence of rupture is lowest when proximal ligation is performed. Kwaan[47] treated 40 patients using this method, and none developed an aortic rupture during the follow-up period. The pooled data collected by Lynch and coworkers[50] revealed a rupture rate of 3.3% for 118 patients who underwent an exclusion procedure involving proximal and distal ligation as recommended by Kwaan.[47] The pooled data also revealed that the incidence of rupture for the 88 patients treated by induced thrombosis alone without proximal ligation was 20%. This is markedly different from the 5% incidence of aneurysm rupture reported by the Albany group.[42] One possible explanation for the difference in results is that the incidence of rupture may depend on whether aortic thrombosis has been achieved. In the Albany experience, the incidence of aortic thrombosis was carefully documented, and further radiologic interventions were required to induce thrombosis in 17 of the 60 patients treated by this method.

Karmody and associates[42] suggested that the cause of rupture in some patients was the result of an inaccurate assessment of aortic thrombosis, implying that rupture would not develop if thrombosis definitely occurred. However, several reports have shown that the aorta can rupture despite appropriate documentation of aortic aneurysm thrombosis. In Lynch's pooled data,[50] rupture occurred in four patients despite documented aneurysm thrombosis.

Several theories have been offered to explain the failure of rupture protection after a nonresective procedure. The mechanism of rupture may vary with the nonresective procedure used. If aneurysmal thrombosis has been attempted by outflow occlusion without proximal ligation, and thrombosis did not occur, no rupture protection could be expected, and the risk of rupture could be increased because of the higher outflow resistance. When rupture occurred after documented aneurysm thrombosis, the site of the rupture was usually seen at the junction between the normal aorta and the proximal aneurysm.[56, 58, 63] This finding demonstrates that the aortoaneurysmal junction is not protected from rupture by aneurysm thrombosis. Kwaan[47] favored the total exclusion procedure because it allowed complete isolation of the aneurysm and protected the weakened aortoaneurysmal junction from rupture.

Rupture of the aneurysmal sac after thrombosis using the exclusion method should be rare based on the experience with the ISMAA method. When the data from Shah's series[65] and Blumenberg's series[10] are combined, only 2 of 380 patients had nonthrombosed aneurysms and had evidence of rupture at follow-up assessments that necessitated intervention. Both patients were receiving anticoagulation therapy. If aneurysm thrombosis does not develop early after total exclusion, additional attempts at inducing thrombosis should be made to decrease the chance of rupture.

Endovascular Technology

Developments in endovascular technology have allowed placement of a bypass graft into the aortic lumen through a femoral or iliac insertion site.[52, 55] Self-expanding or balloon-expandable devices are used to anchor the bypass graft to the arterial wall proximally and distally. Although this application of endovascular technology is still in its infancy and being investigated, it shows the feasibility of placing a tube or bifurcated graft from within the arterial lumen in selected aortic aneurysm patients with favorable anatomy.

This innovative approach is not complication free. Some patients may require conversion to an open procedure. Aortic aneurysms can rupture after an apparently successful endovascular stent graft procedure. Such complications have been reported when a seal is not achieved between the endoprosthesis and the aortic wall. In the presence of an endoleak, blood flow persists in the aneurysmal sac. For this type of therapy to be successful, problems with stent migration and sealing must be overcome. The effect of backbleeding into the aneurysm sac through lumbar vessels or the inferior mesenteric artery also must be further evaluated.

Most surgeons would agree that a high-risk patient with an asymptomatic small aneurysm could be best monitored by serial imaging studies. The upper limit of size at which this can be done safely will be better defined by data from ongoing prospective studies such as the Aneurysm Detection and Management (ADAM) and the United Kingdom Small Aneurysm Studies. Current management of a high-risk patient with a very large or symptomatic aortic aneurysm remains a dilemma. If the patient is suffering from only one high-risk comorbid condition, he or she is probably best served by a conventional aneurysm replacement procedure. However, if the patient has several comorbidities and a decision has been made to intervene, aortic exclusion using the ISMAA procedure is a reasonable option. Another option is to refer the patient to a center with endovascular aortic aneurysm replacement capabilities. However, such an option may not be immediately available, especially for a symptomatic patient, or the patient may not be anatomically suitable for placement of a stented graft. Very-high-risk patients who are not suitable for a stent graft may be considered for aortic ligation and extraanatomic bypass grafting.

The aorta is amenable to laparoscopic dissection.[2] With the continued progress of laparoscopic surgery, the aortic exclusion procedure could be further simplified. The aorta and the iliac arteries could be exposed and stapled laparoscopically, eliminating the need for the limited laparotomy required for ligating these vessels. This potential form of therapy remains investigational.

Conclusions

Induced aortic aneurysm thrombosis without proximal ligation provides the least protection of the nonresective therapies against aortic rupture. This technique has no role in the management of infrarenal AAAs. The addition of proximal aortic ligation excludes the aneurysm from the axial circulation and provides adequate protection from rupture. This procedure has low perioperative morbidity and mortality rates and may still have a role in the management of a symptomatic and very-high-risk patient with unfavorable anatomy for an endovascular stent graft procedure. With the continued development and progress of endovascular methods for replacing abdominal aneurysms, the need for and use of nonresective surgical techniques should diminish.

References

1. Abu Rahma AG, Robinson PA, Boland JP, et al. Elective resection of 332 abdominal aortic aneurysms in a southern West Virginia community during a recent 5 year period. Surgery 1991;109:244.
2. Ahn SS, Hiyama DT, Rudkin GH, et al. Laparoscopic aortobifemoral bypass. J Vasc Surg 1997;26:128.
3. Alexander J, Byron FX. Aortectomy for thoracic aneurysms. JAMA 1944;126:1139.
4. Bahnson HT. Definitive treatment of saccular aneurysms of the aorta with excision of the sac and aortic suture. Surg Gynecol Obstet 1953;96:382.
5. Baron JF, Mundler O, Bertrand M, et al. Dipyridamole-thallium scintigraphy and gated radionuclide angiography to assess cardiac risk before abdominal aortic surgery. N Engl J Med 1994;330:663.
6. Bergan JJ, Yao JST. Modern management of abdominal aortic aneurysms. Surg Clin North Am 1974;54:175.
7. Berguer R, Feldman AJ, Karmody AM. Intravascular thrombosis of abdominal aortic aneurysm in high-risk patients. Vasc Diagn Ther 1981;1:24.
8. Berguer R, Schneider J, Wilner HI. Induced thrombosis of inoperable abdominal aortic aneurysm. Surgery 1978;84:425–429.
9. Blaisdell FW, Hall AD, Thomas AN. Ligation treatment of an abdominal aortic aneurysm. Am J Surg 1965;109:560.
10. Blumenberg RM, Skudder PA Jr, Michael LG, et al. Retroperitoneal nonresective staple exclusion of

abdominal aortic aneurysms: clinical outcome and fate of the excluded abdominal aortic aneurysms. J Vasc Surg 1995;21:623.

11. Cambria RP, Brewster DC, Abbott WM, et al. Transperitoneal versus retroperitoneal approach for aortic reconstruction: a randomized prospective study. J Vasc Surg 1990;11:314.

12. Cambria RP, Brewster DC, Abbott WM, et al. The impact of selective use of dipyridamole-thallium scans and surgical factors on the current morbidity of aortic surgery. J Vasc Surg 1992;15:43–50.

13. Cho SI, Johnson WC, Bush HL, et al. Lethal complications associated with nonresective treatment of abdominal aortic aneurysms. Arch Surg 1982;117:1214.

14. Cohen JR, Mannick JA, Couch NP, Whittemore AD. Abdominal aortic aneurysm repair in patients with preoperative renal failure. J Vasc Surg 1986;3:867.

15. Cooper A. Case of ligature of the aorta, part I. *In* Cooper and Travis Surgical Essays, vol 83. James Webster, Philadelphia, 1821:83–103.

16. Corson JD, Chang BB, Shah DM, et al. Extraperitoneal aortic bypass with exclusion of the intact infrarenal aortic aneurysm: a preliminary report. J Cardiovasc Surg (Torino) 1987;28:274.

17. Crafoord C, Nylin G. Congenital coarctation of the aorta and its surgical treatment. J Thorac Surg 1945;14;347.

18. Crawford ES, Salch SA, Babb JW, et al. Infrarenal abdominal aortic aneurysm: factors influencing survival after operation over a 25-year period. Ann Surg 1981;193:699.

19. Crech O. Endoaneurysmorrhaphy and treatment of aortic aneurysm. Am Surg 1966;164:935.

20. Dale WA. The beginnings of vascular surgery. Surgery 1974;76:849.

21. Darling RC, Brewster DC. Elective treatment of abdominal aortic aneurysms. World J Surg 1980;4:661.

22. Dubost C. First successful resection of an aneurysm of an abdominal aorta with restoration of the continuity by a human arterial graft. World J Surg 1982;6:256.

23. Friedman SG. A History of Vascular Surgery. Mt. Kisco, NY: Futura Publishing, 1989.

24. Gale ME, Kiser LC, Cho SI. Abscess in the aorta following nonresective treatment of an abdominal aortic aneurysm. J Comput Assist Tomogr 1982;6:635.

25. Gardner RJ, Gardner HL, Tarnay TJ, et al. The surgical experience and one- to 16-year follow-up of 277 abdominal aortic aneurysms. Am J Surg 1978;135:226.

26. Golden MA, Whittemore AD, Donaldson MC, et al. Selective evaluation and management of coronary artery disease in patients undergoing repair of abdominal aortic aneurysm: a 16 year experience. Ann Surg 1990;212:415.

27. Goldman ML, Sarrafizadeh MA, Philip PK, et al. Bucrylate embolization of the distal abdominal aorta: an adjunct to non-resective therapy of abdominal aortic aneurysms. AJR 1980;135:1195.

28. Green RM, Ricotta JJ, Ouriel K, et al. Results of supraceliac aortic clamping in difficult elective resection of infrarenal abdominal aortic aneurysm. J Vasc Surg 1989;9:124.

29. Hannan EL, Kilburn H, O'Donnell JF, et al. A longitudinal analysis of the relationship between in-hospital mortality in New York State and the volume of abdominal aortic surgeries performed. Health Serv Res 1992;27:517–542.

30. Hicks GL, Rob C. Abdominal aortic aneurysm wiring: an alternative method. Am J Surg 1976;131:664.

31. Hoballah JJ, Martinasevic M, Chalmers RTA, et al. Management of infrarenal abdominal aortic aneurysms in the elderly: "the geriatric abdominal aortic aneurysm." Int J Angiol 1997;5:222.

32. Hollier LH, Reigel MM, Kamzier FJ, et al. Conventional repair of AAA in high risk patients: a plea for abandonment of nonresective treatment. J Vasc Surg 1986;3:712.

33. Hollier LH, Taylor LM Jr, Ochsner J. Recommended indications for operative treatment of abdominal aortic aneurysms. J Vasc Surg 1992;15:1046.

34. Home E. An account of Mr. Hunter's method of performing the operation for popliteal aneurysm [letter to Dr. Simmons]. London Med J 1786;7:391 [reprinted in Med Classics 1939;40(suppl 4):449].

35. Hunner G. Aneurysm of the aorta treated by the insertion of a permanent wire and galvanism (Moore-Corradi method) with a report of 5 cases. Bull Johns Hopkins Hosp 1900;11:263.

36. Inahara T, Geary GL, Mukherjee D, et al. The contrary position to the nonresective treatment for abdominal aortic aneurysm. J Vasc Surg 1985;2:42.

37. Johnson WC, LoGerfo FW, Vollman RW, et al. Is axillobilateral femoral graft an effective substitute for aortic-bilateral iliac/femoral graft? An analysis of ten years' experience. Ann Surg 1977;186:123.

38. Johnson WC, Squires JW. Axillo-femoral (PTFE) and infrainguinal revascularization (PTFE and umbilical vein). J Cardiovasc Surg 1991;32:344.

39. Johnston KW, Scobie TK. Multicenter prospective study of nonruptured abdominal aortic aneurysms. I. Population and operative management. J Vasc Surg 1988;7:69.

40. Johnston KW. Multicenter prospective study of nonruptured abdominal aortic aneurysms. II. Variables predicting morbidity and mortality. J Vasc Surg 1989;9:437.

41. Kalman PG, Hosang M, Cina C, et al. Current indications for axillounifemoral and axillofemoral bypass grafts. J Vasc Surg 1987;5:828.

42. Karmody AM, Leather RP, Goldman M, et al. The current position of non-resective treatment for abdominal aortic aneurysm. Surgery 1983;94:591.

43. Katz DJ, Stanley JC, Zelenock GB. Operative mortality rates for intact and ruptured abdominal aortic aneurysms in Michigan: an eleven-year experience. J Vasc Surg 1994;19:804–817.

44. Kazmers A, Jacobs L, Perkins A, et al. Abdominal aortic aneurysm repair in Veterans Affairs medical centers. J Vasc Surg 1996;23:191.

45. Kwaan JHM, Dahl RK. Fatal rupture after successful surgical thrombosis of an abdominal aortic aneurysm. Surgery 1984;95:235.

46. Kwaan JHM, Khan RJ, Connolly J. Total exclusion technique for the management of abdominal aortic aneurysms. Am J Surg 1983;146:93.
47. Kwaan JHM. Rupture after nonresective treatment of abdominal aortic aneurysm [letter]. Surgery 1985;97:249.
48. Leather RP, Shah D, Goldman M, et al. Nonresective therapy of abdominal aortic aneurysms. Arch Surg 1979;144:1402.
49. Leather RP, Shah DM, Kaufman JL, et al. Comparative analysis of retroperitoneal and transperitoneal aortic replacement for aneurysm. Surg Gynecol Obstet 1989;168:387.
50. Lynch K, Kohler, TR, Johansen K. Nonresective therapy for aortic aneurysm: results of a survey. J Vasc Surg 1986;4:469.
51. Matas R. Aneurysm of the abdominal aorta at its bifurcation into the common iliac arteries. Ann Surg 1940;112:909.
52. May J, White GH, Yu W, et al. Endoluminal grafting of abdominal aortic aneurysm: causes of failure and their prevention. J Endovasc Surg 1994;1:44.
53. McCann RL, Wolfe WG. Resection of abdominal aortic aneurysm in patients with low ejection fractions. J Vasc Surg 1989;10:240.
54. Moore CH, Murchison D. On a new method of procuring the consolidation of fibrin in certain incurable aneurysms. Med Chir Trans (London) 1884;47:129.
55. Parodi JC, Palmaz JC, Barone HD. Transfemoral intraluminal graft implantation for abdominal aortic aneurysms. Ann Vasc Surg 1991;5:491.
56. Pevec WC, Holcroft JW, Blaisdell FW. Ligation and extraanatomic arterial reconstruction for the treatment of aneurysms of the abdominal aorta. J Vasc Surg 1994;20:629.
57. Ray LI, O'Connor JB, Davis CC, et al. Axillofemoral bypass: a critical reappraisal of its role in the management of aortoiliac occlusive disease. Am J Surg 1979;138:117.
58. Ricotta JJ, Kirshner RL. Case report: late rupture of a thrombosed abdominal aortic aneurysm. Surgery 1984;95:753.
59. Rob C. Extraperitoneal approach to the abdominal aorta. Surgery 1963;51:87–89.
60. Robison JG, Beckett WC, Mills JL. Aortic reconstruction in high-risk pulmonary patients. Ann Surg 1989;210:112.
61. Rutherford RB, Patt A, Pearce WH. Extra-anatomic bypass: a closer view. J Vasc Surg 1987;6:437.
62. Savarese RP, Rosenfeld JC, DeLaurentis DA. Alternatives in the treatment of abdominal aortic aneurysms. Am J Surg 1981;142:226.
63. Schanzer H, Papa MC, Miller CM. Rupture of surgically thrombosed abdominal aortic aneurysm. J Vasc Surg 1985;2:278.
64. Schwartz RA, Nighols WK, Silver D. Is thrombosis of the infrarenal aortic aneurysm an acceptable alternative? J Vasc Surg 1986;3:448.
65. Shah DM, Chang BB, Paty PS, et al. Treatment of abdominal aortic aneurysm by exclusion and bypass: an analysis of outcome. J Vasc Surg 1991;13:15.
66. Shepard AD, Scott GR, Mackey WC, et al. Retroperitoneal approach to high risk abdominal aortic aneurysm. Arch Surg 1996;121:444.
67. Schumacker HB Jr. Coarctation and aneurysm of the aorta. Report of a case treated by excision and end-to-end suture of aorta. Ann Surg 1948;127:655.
68. Sicard GA, Freeman MB, Vander Woude JC, Anderson CB. Comparison between the transabdominal and retroperitoneal approach for reconstruction of the infrarenal abdominal aorta. J Vasc Surg 1987;5:19.
69. Szilagyi DE, Smith RF, DeRosso FJ, et al. Contribution of abdominal aortic aneurysmectomy to prolongation of life. Ann Surg 1966;164:678.
70. Taylor LM, Moneta GL, McConnell D, et al. Axillofemoral grafting with externally supported polytetrafluoroethylene. Arch Surg 1994;129:588.
71. Voorhees AB, Jaretski A, Blakemore AH. The use of tubes constructed from vinyon N cloth in bridging arterial defects. Ann Surg 1952;135:332.
72. Wen SW, Simunovic M, Williams JI, et al. Hospital volume, calendar age, and short term outcomes in patients undergoing repair of abdominal aortic aneurysms: the Ontario experience, 1988–92. J Epidemiol Commun Health 1996;50:207.

Prevention and Treatment of Complications of Abdominal Aortic Aneurysm Surgery

Prevention of Sigmoid and Pelvic Ischemia During Abdominal Aortic Aneurysm Surgery

James M. Seeger, M.D.

Rich collateral connections within the pelvis and among the pelvic, visceral, and lower extremity circulations limit the risk of ischemia of the distal colon and pelvic organs (ie, rectum, distal spinal cord, buttocks, and perineum) when direct blood supply to these organs is interrupted during aortic reconstruction. However, clinically significant colonic ischemia has occurred in as many as 2% of patients undergoing elective aortic reconstruction,[1-3] and buttock, perineal, and distal spinal cord ischemic injuries also have occurred after aortic surgery.[4-10] The mortality rate associated with buttock and perineal ischemia or colonic infarction is 80% or higher, and distal spinal cord ischemia usually results in irreversible paraplegia. Colonic and pelvic collateral perfusion is not always adequate when direct blood flow to the pelvic organs is interrupted, and ensuring adequate colonic and pelvic perfusion is the key to prevention of the devastating consequences of pelvic ischemia after aortic reconstruction.

Colonic and Pelvic Collateral Circulation

Understanding the relationships among the superior mesenteric artery, the inferior mesenteric artery, the hypogastric arteries, and the profunda femoris arteries (Fig. 18–1) is essential in preventing colonic and pelvic ischemia and its associated complications. Collateral pathways for inferior mesenteric artery perfusion include connections between the superior mesenteric artery and the inferior mesenteric artery through the meandering artery and the marginal artery of Drummond and connections between the hypogastric arteries and the inferior mesenteric artery through the hemorrhoidal arteries. The meandering artery and the marginal artery of Drummond arise from the left branch of the middle colic artery and connect to the inferior mesenteric artery through the left colic artery. The meandering artery is the most hemodynamically important of these two collateral arteries, and when large (Fig. 18–2), it is a vital collateral pathway for perfusion of the sigmoid colon in the presence of inferior mesenteric artery occlusion or for the small bowel when superior mesenteric artery disease exists.

The contribution of the hypogastric arteries to the perfusion of the sigmoid colon appears limited in the face of acute inferior mesenteric artery occlusion.[11] However, when chronic inferior mesenteric artery occlusion is present, the hypogastric arteries can provide critical blood supply to the sigmoid colon, as shown by the occurrence of colonic ischemia with interruption of

223

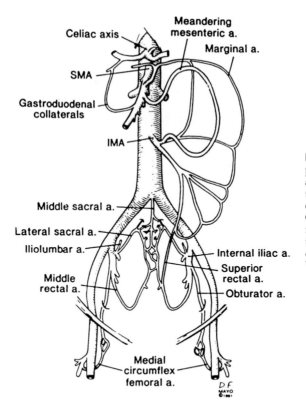

Figure 18–1. Important collateral pathways for the sigmoid colon and pelvis. IMA, inferior mesenteric artery; SMA, superior mesenteric artery. (From Bergman RT, Gloviczki P, Welch TC, et al. The role of intravenous fluorescein in the detection of colon ischemia during aortic reconstruction. Ann Vasc Surg 1992;6:74–79.)

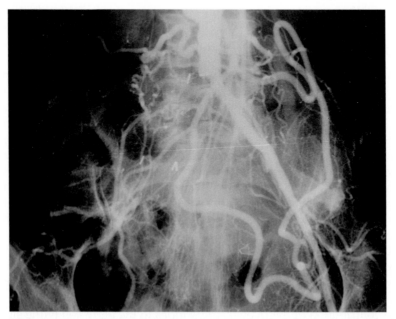

Figure 18–2. Large, meandering mesenteric artery connecting the inferior mesenteric and superior mesenteric arteries. With significant superior mesenteric artery disease, retrograde perfusion through the meandering mesenteric artery can be important for small bowel and right colon perfusion.

antegrade hypogastric artery blood flow during aortobifemoral bypass. The hypogastric arteries also provide the blood supply for the sacral plexus and the distal spinal cord through the iliolumbar and lateral sacral arteries, although the contribution to the distal spinal cord blood supply from the hypogastric arteries is usually limited. However, when the arteria radiculomedullaries (ARM, artery of Adamkiewicz) is occluded or arises abnormally high, the blood supply to the spinal cord from the hypogastric arteries can become critical. In the presence of bilateral hypogastric artery occlusion, buttock and perineal perfusion can be maintained by collateral perfusion from the medial circumflex femoral artery, a branch of the profunda femoris artery, through its connection with the obturator artery, a terminal branch of each hypogastric artery. Distal spinal cord perfusion also can be maintained by this collateral pathway.

Connections between the superior mesenteric artery and the inferior mesenteric artery allow adequate perfusion of the sigmoid colon, the pelvis, and ultimately the distal spinal cord in the face of inferior mesenteric artery or hypogastric artery occlusion. Alternatively, the hypogastric arteries can provide blood supply to the left colon during inferior mesenteric artery occlusion and to the distal spinal cord when the ARM is occluded. Buttock, perineal, and possibly distal spinal cord perfusion can be maintained from the deep femoral artery during hypogastric artery occlusion. Ligation of a patent inferior mesenteric artery, occlusion of one or both hypogastric arteries, interruption or injury to the meandering artery, or failure to revascularize the profunda femoris artery can therefore result in colonic, pelvic, or distal spinal cord ischemia.

Colon Ischemia After Aortic Reconstruction

In 1954, Moore[12] described the first case of ischemic colitis after aortic reconstruction, which occurred in a patient who had ligation of the inferior mesenteric artery and both hypogastric arteries during repair of an abdominal aortic aneurysm. Subsequently, the incidence of clinically significant ischemic colitis has been 1% to 2% after elective aortic reconstructive procedures[1-3] and up to 32% for patients surviving repair of ruptured abdominal aortic aneurysms.[13] Prospective studies using colonoscopy have found evidence of ischemic colonic mucosa in 7% to 35% of patients undergoing elective aortic procedures[14] and in up to 60% of patients who survive ruptured aortic aneurysms.[15]

The morbidity and mortality of colonic ischemia after aortic reconstruction depends on the degree of colonic ischemic injury. When only mucosal ischemia is present, symptoms are generally mild (eg, limited diarrhea), and supportive therapy results in full recovery. When ischemic injury involves the entire bowel wall, symptoms are more severe (eg, significant bloody diarrhea, abdominal pain), and subsequent healing of the injured area may result in colonic stricture. Systemic sepsis with resultant distant organ (eg, pulmonary, renal) injury may develop despite an intact bowel wall, and when the ischemic injury to bowel wall is irreversible, perforation occurs, killing 80% to 100% of the affected patients.[16, 17]

Colonic ischemia after aortic reconstruction is primarily caused by ligation of a patent inferior mesenteric artery in the face of inadequate collateral perfusion to the left colon from the superior mesenteric artery and/or the hypogastric arteries.[17] Less common causes include atheroembolization to the left colon during aortic dissection and significant hypotension during the aortic procedure or in the postoperative period. The inferior mesenteric artery is found to be patent in approximately 50% of patients undergoing elective aortic reconstruction,[18] and the 1% to 2% incidence of clinically significant ischemic colitis demonstrates that colonic collateral blood flow is adequate to prevent left colon ischemia after ligation of patent inferior mesenteric arteries in most patients.

Clinical predictors of inadequate collateral perfusion to the sigmoid colon include previous colon resection,[19] previous pelvic irradiation for prostate or other types of pelvic cancer,[20] and occlusion of both hypogastric arteries.[4] All of these problems can interrupt collateral blood supply from the superior mesenteric artery or hypogastric arteries to the left colon, as can operative injury of the meandering artery or marginal artery of Drummond, usually from excessive traction by a mechanical retractor. However, ischemic colitis can occur after ligation of a patent inferior mesenteric artery despite the absence of these predictors of postoperative ischemic colitis. Assessment of the adequacy of collateral blood flow to the left colon is essential before ligation of a patent inferior mesenteric artery.

Several methods of intraoperative assessment of the adequacy of inferior mesenteric artery collateral blood flow have been developed (Table 18–1). Ernst and colleagues[21] introduced the use of inferior mesenteric artery stump pressure measurements in 1978 and reported that ligation of a patent inferior mesenteric artery was safe during aortic reconstruction when the inferior mesenteric artery stump pressure was more than 40 mm Hg or the inferior mesenteric artery to systolic pressure ratio was greater than 0.4. Hobson and associates[22] reported use of intraoperative Doppler ultrasonography to assess blood flow to the bowel in 1976 and recommended that a patent inferior mesenteric artery should be reimplanted when no Doppler signal could be detected in the mesentery or on the anti-mesenteric border of the left colon after inferior mesenteric artery ligation. In 1986, Fiddian-Green and coworkers[23] reported that a colonic mucosal pH of 6.86, measured using a rectal tonometer, was a strong predictor of postoperative ischemic colitis, and in 1988, Ouriel and colleagues[24] recommend reimplantation of a patent inferior mesenteric artery when arterial pulsatility and transcolonic oxygen saturation determined using a sterile pulse oximeter probe were abnormal. In 1992, Bergman and coworkers[25] found that an abnormal colonic fluorescein pattern after inferior mesenteric artery ligation was associated with postoperative ischemic colitis, but a normal pattern indicated that a patent inferior mesenteric artery could be safely ligated.

Good results have been reported with use of each of the described methods of assessment of the adequacy of colonic collateral blood flow, but each technique can be difficult to use and subject to some degree of variability. Intraoperative assessment of the adequacy of colonic collateral perfusion is done at a time when cardiac output and intravascular volume probably are

Table 18–1.
Intraoperative Detection of Colonic Ischemia

Method	Assessment
Inferior mesenteric artery stump pressure	<40 mm Hg (mean)
Doppler flow in colonic mesentery	Absence of flow signal
Photoplethysmography	Loss of pulsatile flow
Tonometric measurement of colonic mucosal pH	pH <6.86
Intravenous fluorescein	Abnormal fluorescein pattern

optimal, and none of these techniques can predict whether collateral blood flow to the left colon will be adequate if postoperative mesenteric vasoconstriction occurs in response to hypovolemia or hypotension.

Reimplantation of all patent inferior mesenteric arteries is an alternative approach to this problem. At the University of Florida, we have adopted a policy of routine reimplantation of patent inferior mesenteric arteries and have found this to be an effective method of eliminating transmural colonic infarction after aortic reconstruction.[18] A total of 151 patients underwent aortic reconstruction between April 1986 and May 1989. When all patent inferior mesenteric arteries were reimplanted, no patient developed postoperative colonic infarction due to ischemia (Table 18–2). Contrasting results were found for 186 patients undergoing aortic reconstruction between July 1982 and March 1986. When patent inferior mesenteric arteries were selectively ligated based on intraoperative bowel inspection, colonic mesenteric Doppler signals, and inferior mesenteric stump pressures, the incidence of colonic infarction after aortic reconstruction was 2.7% and the postoperative mortality rate due to ischemic colitis was 1.6%. Zelenock and associates[26] also found that reimplantation of patent inferior mesenteric arteries or aggressive attempts at ensuring adequate pelvic blood supply during aortic reconstruction resulted in no transmural colonic ischemia and a 3.4% incidence of colonic mucosal ischemia for 100 prospectively studied patients. In a previous series of 318 patients undergoing aortic reconstruction, colonic ischemia or infarction had accounted for 39% of postoperative deaths. On the basis of these results, Zelenock and colleagues[26] concluded that aggressive attempts at ensuring the adequacy of colonic blood supply were associated with a decreased incidence of ischemic colitis, colonic infarction, and operative deaths after aortic reconstruction, similar to our conclusions at the University of Florida.[18]

Arguments against routine reimplantation of patent inferior mesenteric arteries include the possibility of increased bleeding from the additional anastomosis and potential complications associated with the extra time added to the aortic reconstruction procedure. We have not documented increased bleeding when routine reimplantation of patent inferior mesenteric arteries has been done, and the extra time for this additional anastomosis (approximately 15 minutes) has not adversely affected our results. Because neither our study nor Zelenock's study were randomized, prospective studies, it cannot be stated that routine reimplantation of patent inferior mesenteric arteries is superior to selective ligation of patent arteries after careful, objective assessment of the adequacy of collateral blood flow to the left colon. However, since instituting the policy of routine reimplantation of patent inferior mesenteric arteries at the University of Florida in 1986, no patient undergoing an elective aortic reconstructive procedure has developed transmural ischemic colitis, and mucosal ischemic colitis has only occurred in patients found to

Table 18–2.
Effects of Selective and Routine Reimplantation of Patent Inferior Mesenteric Arteries in 337 Elective Aortic Reconstructions

Result	Selective IMA Ligation (%)	Routine IMA Reimplantation (%)
Transmural colonic ischemia	2.7%	0%
Death from bowel ischemia	1.6%	0%
Death from multiple systems organ failure	2.7%	1.3%

have chronically occluded inferior mesenteric arteries at the time of the aortic reconstruction.

Pelvic Ischemia After Aortic Reconstruction

Interruption of the pelvic blood supply and its collateral network can result in ischemic injury of the buttocks, perineum, rectum, and distal spinal cord. Acute occlusion of both hypogastric arteries has resulted in buttock necrosis, rectal ischemia, impotence, and neurologic deficits.[4, 27] Acute occlusion of only one hypogastric artery has led to unilateral buttock claudication[4, 5] and to unilateral sacral plexus injury in rare cases.[5] Because of the extensive collateral connections among the pelvic, mesenteric, and profunda femoris arteries, this problem is uncommon. Multiple studies have demonstrated that bilateral hypogastric ligation for pelvic bleeding in younger patients is relatively well tolerated,[28–30] and Marin and coworkers[31] showed that acute occlusion of both hypogastric arteries during endovascular aneurysm repair also appears to be well tolerated. However, the development of pelvic ischemia after aortic reconstruction is unpredictable, the consequences are dire and irreversible, and the mortality rate associated with pelvic ischemia after aortic reconstruction is 50% to 100%.[4, 5]

Preservation of pelvic perfusion is best accomplished by maintaining direct blood flow to at least one of the hypogastric arteries. During repair of infrarenal abdominal aortic aneurysms that extend into the common iliac arteries, pelvic perfusion can be best preserved by maintaining direct flow into the hypogastric arteries using an aortoiliac bypass to the iliac artery bifurcation. In contrast, retrograde flow to the hypogastric arteries after bypass to the femoral level is less reliable and has been associated with postoperative colonic infarction or pelvic ischemia from acute thrombosis of the bypassed external iliac artery.

During repair of aortoiliac occlusive disease, when direct flow into the hypogastric arteries through a patent distal aorta and patent common iliac arteries exists, pelvic perfusion can be maintained by using an end-to-side proximal anastomosis for an aortobifemoral bypass. Although O'Connor and associates[32] demonstrated that 67% of the bypassed, patent distal aortic and iliac segments had occluded by 1 year, postoperative pelvic ischemia has not been reported using this approach. When one or both hypogastric arteries must be ligated for aneurysmal disease, when both hypogastric arteries are occluded, or when the hypogastric arteries are patent but not in continuity with the infrarenal aorta, pelvic perfusion should be maintained by reimplantation of patent inferior mesenteric arteries and by ensuring unobstructed blood flow into the profunda femoris arteries.

Iliopoulos and colleagues[33] demonstrated a significant pressure decrease in proximally occluded hypogastric arteries with ipsilateral external iliac artery occlusion, but occlusion of the contralateral hypogastric artery resulted in only a modest reduction in hypogastric artery pressure. Unobstructive, antegrade perfusion of the ipsilateral profunda femoris artery should be maintained even when only one hypogastric artery must be ligated. When pelvic blood flow through these collateral networks can be ensured, direct bypass to proximally occluded hypogastric arteries using a separate bypass graft is rarely necessary, although this is occasionally the only way to ensure adequate pelvic perfusion (Fig. 18–3).

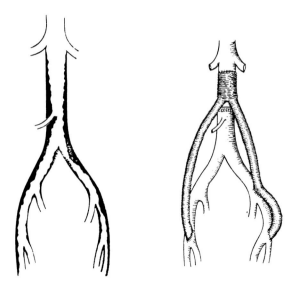

Figure 18–3. A simple technique for maintaining direct perfusion of the hypogastric arteries during aortobifemoral bypass with end-to-end proximal anastomosis. (Adapted from Cronenwett JL, Gooch JB, Garrett HE. Internal iliac artery revascularization during aortofemoral bypass. Arch Surg 1982;117:838–839.)

Spinal Cord Ischemia After Aortic Reconstruction

The blood supply to the spinal cord is segmental and only seven to eight radicular branches reach the spinal cord to perfuse the anterior spinal artery (Fig. 18–4).[34] The cervical portion of the spinal cord between C1 and T1 to T2 is richly supplied by radicular branches from the vertebral and costocervical arteries. In contrast, the midthoracic portion of the spinal cord between T2 and T8 is supplied by a single radicular artery arising at the level of T7, and the lumbar portion of the spinal cord below T9 is supplied by the ARM. The ARM arises between T9 and T12 in 75% of cases, between T5 and T8 in 15%, and between L1 and L2 in 10%.[34] Thus, the ARM is at risk during 10% of infrarenal aortic reconstructions. The blood supply to the sacral roots and plexus is from the iliolumbar and lateral sacral branches of the hypogastric arteries[9] (Fig. 18–5), and these arteries also supply collateral blood flow to the distal spinal cord, particularly when the ARM arises above T9.

Distal spinal cord injury during infrarenal aortic reconstruction traditionally was thought to be caused by damage to the ARM when that artery arises from below the origin of the renal arteries, an uncommon and unpredictable event. Szilagyi[35] suggests that, based on the incidence of the ARM arising from the infrarenal aorta, paraplegia should occur in 1 of 400 patients after repair of infrarenal abdominal aortic aneurysms and 1 of 5000 patients after infrarenal aortic reconstruction for occlusive disease. The incidence of this complication appears to be significantly lower than this prediction, suggesting that collateral blood supply in some patients is sufficient to maintain spinal cord perfusion when the ARM is occluded. The association between distal spinal cord injury after infrarenal aortic reconstruction and ischemic colitis, buttock ischemia, and an end-to-end proximal anastomosis[4, 8, 9] for aortic grafting further demonstrates the role of pelvic ischemia in this problem (Table 18–3).

This assumption is supported by several case reports. In the seven cases described by Picone and colleagues,[8] five developed spinal cord ischemia

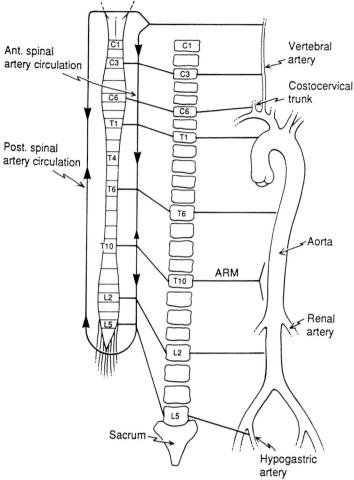

Figure 18–4. Components of the spinal cord blood supply. (From Chaikof EL, Salam AA. Neurologic complications of abdominal aortic reconstruction. *In* Ernst CB, Stanley JC (eds). Current Therapy in Vascular Surgery, ed 3. St. Louis: Mosby–Year Book, 1995:279.)

after hypogastric devascularization, and three also had gluteal and colonic ischemia. In the case report by Salam and coworkers,[10] spinal cord ischemia developed in a patient who had previously had a colonic resection when antegrade hypogastric blood flow was interrupted. Although spinal cord injury after infrarenal aortic reconstruction cannot entirely be prevented, the risk of this devastating complication can be reduced by avoiding pelvic ischemia. Spinal cord ischemia was not seen in a series of more than 700 elective aortic reconstructions done at the University of Florida,[36] and this may be related to our aggressive maintenance of pelvic perfusion by inferior mesenteric artery and hypogastric artery reconstruction.

Conclusions

Maintenance of adequate distal colonic and pelvic perfusion is essential in limiting ischemic complications to the left colon, rectum, perineum, buttocks, and distal spinal cord during and after infrarenal aortic reconstruction. Because of the numerous connections between the colonic and pelvic blood vessels, reconstruction of patent inferior mesenteric arteries and hypogastric

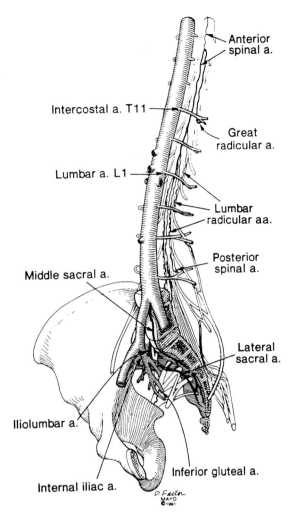

Figure 18–5. Blood supply of the distal spinal cord and lumbosacral roots and plexus. (From Gloviczki P, Cross SA, Stanson AW, et al. Ischemic injury to the spinal cord or lumbosacral plexus after aortoiliac reconstruction. Am J Surg 1991;162:131–136.)

arteries allows maintenance of adequate perfusion to the left colon and pelvic organs. Direct reconstruction of the inferior mesenteric artery and one or both hypogastric arteries has been most satisfactory in maintaining adequate pelvic perfusion, but reliance on retrograde flow through diseased external iliac

Table 18–3.
Pelvic Ischemia After Aortic Reconstruction—Selected Case Reports

	Reconstruction	Complications	Outcome
Case 1*	AAA repair with right CIA and left EIA anastomosis	Left leg paralysis and left buttock ischemia	Left EIA repair, resolved buttock ischemia
Case 2*	Aorta to right CFA and left EIA	Left buttock claudication and impotence	Left IIA repair, resolved buttock claudication and impotence
Case 3†	Aorta to right EIA and right to left fem-fem	Paralysis and colon ischemia	Colon ischemia resolved

AAA, abdominal aortic aneurysm; CIA, common iliac artery; CFA, common femoral artery; EIA, external iliac artery; IIA, internal iliac artery; fem-fem, femoral-femoral bypass.
*From Paty PKS, Shah DM, Chang BB, et al. Pelvic ischemia following aortoiliac reconstruction. Ann Vasc Surg 1994;8:204–206.
†From Salam AA, Sholkamy SM, Chaikof EL. Spinal cord ischemia after abdominal aortic procedures: Is previous colectomy a risk factor? J Vasc Surg 1993;17:1108–1110.

arteries has been associated with significant complications. Adherence to the principle that sigmoid colon and pelvic perfusion must be ensured after aortic reconstruction limits the risk of ischemic injury to the colonic and pelvic organs after infrarenal aortic repair.

References

1. Johnson WC, Nasbeth DC. Visceral infarction following aortic surgery. Ann Surg 1963;86:65–73.
2. Young JR, Humphries AW, Dewolfe VG, Lefevre FA. Complications of abdominal aortic surgery: II. Intestinal ischemia. Arch Surg 1963;86:51–59.
3. Papadopoulos CD, Mancini HW, Marino WM Jr. Ischemic necrosis of the colon following aortic aneurysmectomy. J Cardiovasc Surg 1974;15:949–500.
4. Iliopoulos JI, Howanitz PE, Pierce GE, et al. The critical hypogastric circulation. Am J Surg 1987;154:671–675.
5. Paty PKS, Shah DM, Chang BB, et al. Pelvic ischemia following aortoiliac reconstruction. Ann Vasc Surg 1994;8:204–206.
6. Merkel FK, Najarian JS. Rest pain of the buttock after aortofemoral bypass procedure. Am J Surg 1971;121:617–619.
7. Ferguson LRJ, Bergin JJ, Conn J Jr, et al. Spinal ischemia following abdominal aortic surgery. Ann Surg 1975;81:276–272.
8. Picone AL, Green RM, Ricotta JR, et al. Spinal cord ischemia following operations on the abdominal aorta. J Vasc Surg 1986;3:94–103.
9. Gloviczki P, Cross SA, Stanson AW, et al. Ischemic injury to the spinal cord or lumbosacral plexus after aortoiliac reconstruction. Am J Surg 1991;162:131–136.
10. Salam AA, Sholkamy SM, Chaikof EL. Spinal cord ischemia after abdominal aortic procedures: is previous colectomy a risk factor? J Vasc Surg 1993;17:1108–1110.
11. Iliopoulos JI, Pierce GE, Hermreck AS, et al. Hemodynamics of the inferior mesenteric arterial circulation. J Vasc Surg 1990;11:120–126.
12. Moore SW. Resection of the abdominal aorta with defect replaced by homologous graft. Surg Gynecol Obstet 1954;99:745–747.
13. Bandyk DE, Florence MG, Johansen KH. Colon ischemia accompanying rupture of the abdominal aortic aneurysm. J Surg Res 1981;30:297–303.
14. Fry PD. Colonic ischemia after aortic reconstruction. Can J Surg 1988;31:162–164.
15. Hagihara PF, Ernst TC, Griffen WO. Instance of ischemic colitis following abdominal aortic reconstruction. Surg Gynecol Obstet 1979;149:571–573.
16. Kim MW, Hurdahl SA, Dang CR, et al. Ischemic colitis after aortic aneurysmectomy. Am J Surg 1983;145:392–394.
17. Ernst CB. Prevention of intestinal ischemia following abdominal aortic reconstruction. Surgery 1983;96:102–106.
18. Seeger JM, Coe DA, Kaelin LD, et al. Routine reimplantation of patent inferior mesenteric arteries limits colon infarction after aortic reconstruction. J Vasc Surg 1992;15:635–641.
19. Brewster DC, Franklin DP, Cambria RP, et al. Intestinal ischemia complicating abdominal aortic surgery. Surgery 1991;109:447–454.
20. Israeli D, Dardik H, Wolodiger F, et al. Pelvic radiation therapy as a risk factor for ischemic colitis complicating abdominal aortic reconstruction. J Vasc Surg 1996;23:706–709.
21. Ernst CB, Hagihara PF, Daugherty ME, et al. Inferior mesenteric artery stump pressure: a reliable index for safe IMA ligation during abdominal aortic aneurysmectomy. Ann Surg 1978;187:641–646.
22. Hobson RW, Wright DB, Rich NM. Assessment of colonic ischemia during aortic surgery by Doppler ultrasound. J Surg Res 1976;20:231–235.
23. Fiddian-Green RG, Amelin PM, Herrmann JB. Prediction of the development of sigmoid ischemia on the day of aortic operations. Arch Surg 1986;121:654–660.
24. Ouriel K, Fiore WM, Geary JE. Detection of a colonic ischemia during aortic procedures: use of an interoperative photoplethysmographic technique. J Vasc Surg 1988;7:5–9.
25. Bergman RT, Gloviczki P, Welch TJ, et al. The role of intravenous fluorescein in the detection of colon ischemia during aortic reconstruction. Ann Vasc Surg 1992;6:74–79.
26. Zelenock GB, Strodel WE, Knoll JA, et al. A prospective study of clinically and endoscopically documented colonic ischemia in 100 patients undergoing aortic reconstructive surgery with aggressive colonic and direct pelvic revascularization, compared with historic controls. Surgery 1989;106:771–780.
27. Queral LA, Whitehouse WM Jr, Flinn WR, et al. Pelvic hemodynamics after aortoiliac reconstruction. Surgery 1979;86:799–809.
28. Burchell RC. Internal iliac artery ligation: hemodynamics. Obstet Gynecol 1964;24:737–739.
29. Bao ZM. Ligation of the internal iliac arteries in 100 in cases as a hemostatic procedure during suprapubic prostatectomy. J Urol 1980;124:578.
30. Evans S, McShane P. The efficacy of internal iliac artery ligation of obstetric hemorrhage. Surg Gynecol Obstet 1985;160:250–253.
31. Marin ML, Veith FJ, Cynamon J, et al. Interventional internal iliac artery occlusion to facilitate

endovascular repair of aortoiliac aneurysms and occlusions. Presented at the 25th Annual Meeting of the Society of Clinical Vascular Surgery; Naples, FL, March 1997.

32. O'Connor SE, Walsh DB, Zwolak RM, et al. Pelvic blood flow following aortobifemoral bypass with proximal end-to-side anastomosis. Ann Vasc Surg 1992;6:493–498.
33. Iliopoulos JI, Hermreck AS, Thomas JH, et al. Hemodynamics of the hypogastric arterial circulation. J Vasc Surg 1989;9:637–642.
34. Lazorthes G, Jouaze A, Zadeh JO, et al. Arterial vascularization of the spinal cord. J Neurol Surg 1971;38:253–262.
35. Szilagyi DE. A second look at the etiology of spinal cord damage in surgery of the abdominal aorta. J Vasc Surg 1993;17:1111–1113.
36. Huber TS, Harward TRS, Flynn TC, et al. Operative mortality rates after elective infrarenal aortic reconstructions. J Vasc Surg 1995;22:287–294.

Prevention and Treatment of Spinal Cord Ischemia Associated With Aortic Aneurysm Repair

Roy Greenberg, M.D., and Kenneth Ouriel, M.D.

Paralysis or paraplegia is one of the most dreaded complications of aortic surgery. The incidence ranges from 0% to 30%, depending on the extent of the procedure. [1-3] The complication usually appears as the patient awakens from anesthesia; however, a subset of patients have delayed deficits that occur up to 21 days after surgery. The dysfunction can range from a mild somatosensory loss to complete flaccid paralysis.

Despite marked advances in the technical aspects of surgery and overall patient care, the problem persists, particularly because of its complexity. The various effects of ischemia on the spinal cord are relatively ill defined and consequently have caused much controversy. Animal models lack clinical applicability because of differences in the causes of ischemia and because of anatomic disparities. Surgical devices, pharmacologic agents, radiologic screening, and anesthetic innovations have been tested, alone and in combination, without proof of superiority of one technique over another. The molecular mechanisms of neurologic cell death illustrate the multifactorial nature of the injury. Factors affecting the incidence of spinal cord ischemia, methods of detecting impending deficits, surgical options to improve intraoperative spinal cord blood flow, and pharmacologic agents modifying the biochemical response to ischemia are important considerations and merit discussion.

Molecular Mechanisms of Spinal Cord Ischemia

Cell death in the ischemic spinal cord occurs in two phases. The first phase comprises the ischemic insult and resulting biochemical defects. The second phase is initiated by reperfusion of the previously oxygen-deprived segment, with subsequent microcirculatory failure.

Acute Hypoxic Injury

The effects of acute ischemia on the spinal cord are multifactorial and selective. Spinal motor neurons are more vulnerable to an ischemic insult than other cell populations,[4] although the mechanism of this selective vulnerability is not well understood. The size of an infarct depends on the severity and duration of reduced blood flow.[5] Cellular metabolism quickly changes from aerobic to anaerobic pathways, and without the aid of the tricarboxylic acid cycle, pyruvate is converted to lactate. The lactate accumulates in the intracellular space, extracellular space, and the cerebrospinal fluid (CSF), resulting in a relative acidosis. Continued metabolic demands diminish glucose and deplete the cell of high-energy phosphate bonds. These biochemical changes have been demonstrated in many animal models and subsequently correlated in human subjects undergoing thoracoabdominal aneurysm repair.[6, 7]

The relative lack of intracellular oxygen and glucose eventually reaches a critical level that induces a series of reactions, culminating in neuronal cell death. The sequence begins with the reduction of high-energy substrate bonds in the gray matter, followed by loss of neuronal activity. Anoxic depolarization of neurons releases excitatory amino acids, prostaglandins, and oxygen free radicals.[8] Excessive release of excitatory amino acids are paramount to the development of a positive feedback cycle resulting in cell death that extends beyond the zone of ischemia. Glutamate is the primary excitatory amino acid transmitter of the spinal cord.[9] Aspartate is believed to have similar effects. Toxic levels of glutamate and aspartate can develop rapidly and activate N-methyl-D-aspartate (NMDA) receptors and non-NMDA receptors. These trigger a calcium influx, with subsequent modulation of calcium-dependent second messenger systems. This results in the production of many agents, including prostaglandin$_{2\alpha}$ thromboxane A_2, and prostaglandin I_2. The combination of elevated intracellular calcium and metabolic products of arachadonic acid results in smooth muscle constriction, increasing microvascular resistance and ischemia. The process culminates in cellular membrane destruction.[3, 9, 10] This theory is supported by extensive laboratory work and some elaborate clinical correlates.[6, 7, 11] Blockade of NMDA and non-NMDA glutamate receptors showed various degrees of neuroprotection in animal models of reversible spinal cord ischemia.[12–15]

Histopathologically, acute ischemic damage can be categorized by depth of injury and types of neurons involved. In rats, reversible injuries manifest as scatted neuronal cell death in the gray matter intermediate zone (rexed lamina VII) and the dorsomedial part of the dorsal horn. The development spastic or flaccid paraplegia is heralded by extensive motor neuron loss distributed between rexed laminae III and VII.[9] These observations marry the anatomic blood supply with a predicted picture of ischemic damage. The central gray matter relies heavily on microvascular blood supply. Distanced from the named blood vessels, with a higher cellular and mitochondrial density than the surroundimg white matter, the gray matter requires a larger amount of oxygen-rich blood supply. These observations explain why the central gray matter is the initial area of neuronal cell death, and under conditions of ischemia, this is probably one of the earliest sites of hypoxic free radical generation.[11]

Leukocytes have been implicated as causative agents in the sequence of events resulting in neuronal cell death, although most cases examined have been cerebrovascular accidents. Few studies have examined the acutely ischemic spinal cord. Nevertheless, two mechanisms have been proposed for leukocyte-induced damage. One involves microvascular occlusion by adhesion of activated leukocytes to various exposed endothelial ligands. The second is leukocyte infiltration of the cerebrospinal tissues with release of cytotoxic and inflammatory agents.[16] Blocking the activation of leukocytes, blocking their binding sites (CD11/CD18) with monoclonal antibodies, or inducing an absolute leukocyte depletion holds potential for improving neurologic results in thoracoabdominal aortic surgery.[16, 17]

Reperfusion Injury

Reperfusion of the spinal cord initiates the second phase of injury. The multifactorial nature of the injury includes vasospasm from the release of arachadonic acid metabolites, tissue swelling in a confined space, generation of oxygen free radicals, and cytoxic destruction of cells by leukocytes or macrophages.[2]

Activation of the coagulation and inflammatory cascades occurs in most injuries. Tissue factors are released during the ischemic event and cause membrane decomposition. The metabolic products of the arachadonic acid cascade are predominately vasospastic. Activation of the coagulation cascade results in thrombin generation and fibrin formation.[18] The combination of these actions causes microcirculatory obstruction and, combined with endothelial swelling and interstitial edema, results in the "no-reflow" phenomenon.

The generation of oxygen free radicals in part results from transformation of intracellular enzymes such as xanthine oxidase to the oxidase form instead of the dehydrogenase. In the presence of oxygen, brought about by reperfusion, reactive free radicals are generated. Oxygen free radicals are toxic metabolites of molecular oxygen and represent intermediate states of its electrochemical reduction to water. They include the superoxide anion, hydrogen peroxide, and the hydroxyl radical.[2] These metabolites are thought to induce neuronal cell death through lipid peroxidation. Lipid peroxidation is a self-perpetuating process that spreads in a circumferential pattern, recruiting undamaged neurons and resulting in irreversible injury.[19] Membrane lipid breakdown releases additional excitatory amino acids, which cause calcium influx, further collapse of the microcirculation, and neuronal death.[11]

Anatomy of Spinal Circulation

The spinal cord is supplied by three major arterial sources: the anterior spinal artery and the two posterolateral spinal arteries. The anterior spinal artery supplies most of the gray matter and the anterior aspect of the white matter. The posterior spinal arteries supply the dorsal columns and posterior aspect of the white matter[20–22] (Fig. 19–1).

Occlusion of the anterior spinal artery results in a syndrome characterized by paralysis, sphincter dysfunction, and decreased pain and temperature sensation; vibratory and proprioception, supplied by the posterior spinal artery, remain intact. Significant differences exist between the anterior and posterior circulations of the spinal cord. The posterior spinal arteries are continuous throughout the length of the cord and are supplied by approximately 12 dorsal medullary arteries. In contrast, the anterior spinal artery receives blood in a more segmental fashion, usually from five to eight radicular arteries.[23] These radicular arteries vary in number and location. Two to three radicular arteries originate in the thorax, and two to three arise from the lumbar region.[22]

The most prominent radicular artery was described by Adamkiewicz in 1882,[24] and is known as the artery of Adamkiewicz, arteria radiculomedullaries magna, and the great radicular artery (GRA). The GRA can arise anywhere from T8 to L3 but originates between T9 and T12 in 75% of patients. The internal thoracic, long thoracic arteries, intercostal arteries, scapular arteries, proximal radicular arteries, and erectae spinae arteries also provide collateral flow to the anterior spinal cord.[25] Nevertheless, Wadouh and colleagues[26] documented a 72% rate of paraplegia after isolated GRA ligation in pigs.

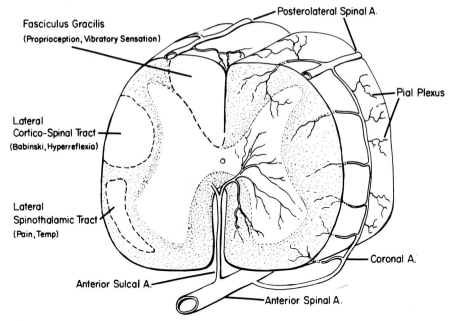

Figure 19–1. Details of the terminal division of the blood supply of the spinal cord. (From Szilagyi D, Hageman J, Smith R, Elliot J. Spinal cord damage in surgery of the abdominal aorta. Surgery 1978;83:38–56.)

Unlike most arteries in the human body, the diameter of the anterior spinal artery increases as the vessel progresses distally. Svensson and colleagues [27] used baboons to demonstrate that the anterior spinal artery had a mean diameter of 0.27 mm at the site of entry of the GRA, but more caudally, the diameter increased to 0.744 mm. Basic hemodynamic principles suggest that vascular resistance to retrograde flow is high. The lower thoracic spinal cord largely depends on antegrade flow below the level of the GRA, a postulate supported by the work of Fried and coworkers.[28] They found that ligation of the anterior spinal artery above the GRA was unlikely to cause paraplegia in monkeys, but paraplegia was common if the artery was interrupted below the GRA.[28]

Localization of the Great Radicular Artery

The location of the GRA is a critical issue in the evaluation of the risk of paraplegia after aortic surgery. Selective spinal arteriography was developed by Dichiro and colleagues in 1967.[29] Much controversy has arisen regarding the necessity of preoperative angiography to localize the GRA and guide reimplantation.[26, 30, 31] The success of localization attempts largely depends on the skill of the angiographer. Savader and associates[30] were able to localize the GRA in 65% of 57 patients. However, the frequency of neurologic complications or mortality of patients with angiographically identifiable GRAs was not different from those of patients with unidentified arteries.[30] When assessing the need for preoperative localization, the risks of a contrast load, pseudoaneurysm formation, and potential for embolization and paraplegia must be weighed against the marginal benefit obtained.

Collateral Circulation

Disease in the region of the GRA promotes the formation of collateral channels to the anterior spinal cord. This collateral circulation is commonly seen in patients with large thoracoabdominal aneurysms or congenital coarctation of the aorta. The cervical spinal cord has multiple collateral connections and is well protected from development of an ischemic neuronal injury.[32] The upper thoracic cord also receives adequate collateral flow from the vertebral arteries. The lower thoracic cord, however, has a poor collateral supply and the highest risk for ischemic injury. The distal spinal cord circulation relies on a marginal network of collateral channels, including the lumbar, iliolumbar, and lateral sacral arteries. The patency of the hypogastric and pelvic circulation is crucial for distal spinal cord perfusion. This supply becomes clinically significant in patients with aortic dissections and patients with concomitant infrarenal or multiple aneurysms.[21]

The adequacy of collateral circulation is best demonstrated by comparing patients undergoing correction of an aortic coarctation, typically having a well-developed collateral circulation, with those suffering from acute traumatic aortic rupture and having notably poor collateral flow. The relative incidence of paraplegia in these two groups is drastically different, 0.41% and 19.2%, respectively.[33] Consequently, the chronicity of aortic pathology protects against development of paraplegia.[1]

Determinants of Spinal Cord Ischemia

Aneurysmal Anatomy and Hemodynamics

The extent and cause of the aneurysm has substantial impact on the postoperative incidence of neurologic insult. The Crawford classification of aneurysms is commonly used when categorizing the frequent of complications (Fig. 19–2).[1, 32] The highest incidence (28%) of paraplegia is associated with class II aneurysms. Classes I, III, and IV are associated with paraplegia incidences of 10%, 3%, and 2%, respectively.[1] The risk of paraplegia appears to be closely linked to the length of aorta over which the spinal arterial supply is disrupted.

The hemodynamics of flow during resection also influences outcome. The relationship between the aortic crossclamping and intercostal vessels can alter the normal direction of flow in both collaterals and the anterior spinal artery. A "spinal steal" is thought to occur when the orifice of the GRA is in the excluded aortic segment and allowed to backbleed while the proximal anastomosis is constructed.[3] Flow in this situation is probably derived from antegrade flow through the anterior spinal artery. In the setting of mild ischemia, the spinal cord itself becomes a high-resistance bed, forcing blood through the lower-resistence conduit of the excluded aortic segment. The enlarging diameter of the distal anterior spinal artery discourages retrograde flow from the lumbar segment, and inadequate oxygenation of the lower thoracic cord results. Bleeding intercostals should be oversewn rapidly or temporarily occluded as soon as the aneurysm is opened to prevent spinal steal from occurring.

Duration of Aortic Crossclamping

The most influential factor affecting paraplegia risk is the clamp time. In 1910, Carrel[34] experimentally described a safe aortic crossclamp time of 10 to

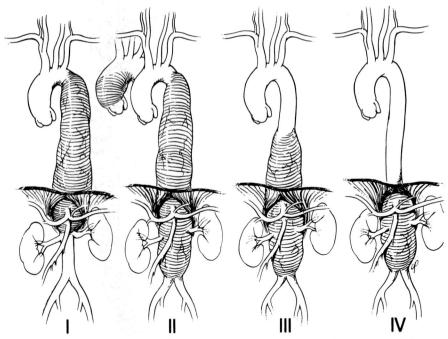

I   II   III   IV

Figure 19–2. Crawford classification of thoracoabdominal aneurysms. (From Shenaq S, Svensson L. Paraplegia following aortic surgery. J Cardiothorac Vasc Anesth 1993;7:81–94.)

15 minutes. Many series subsequently showed that clamp times of less than 20 to 30 minutes are rarely associated with paraplegia.[10, 35, 36] Animal studies show that aortic crossclamping for more than 60 minutes uniformly results in paraplegia.[37, 38] Clamp times of more than 50 to 60 minutes in humans are also believed to place the patients at very high risk for paraplegia.[39, 40] Returning to the example of traumatic aortic rupture, Katz and colleagues[40] correlated the duration of crossclamping with the probability of paraplegia. The period between 20 and 50 minutes of aortic clamping resulted in a linear rise in the risk of paraplegia. This interval probably represents the time during which interventions used to improve spinal cord perfusion or prevent neurologic demise are influential.[25] This is best demonstrated in Figure 19–3.

Some contemporary clinical series have been unable to associate increasing

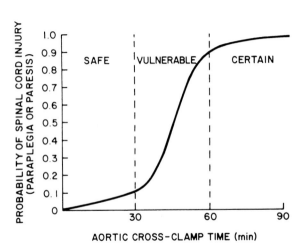

Figure 19–3. Time of aortic crossclamping in high-risk patients correlated with probability of spinal cord injury. (From Svensson L, Loop F. Prevention of spinal cord ischemia in aortic surgery. *In* Yao JT (ed). Arterial Surgery. New York: Grune & Stratton, 1988: 273–285.)

duration of clamp time with the incidence of spinal cord ischemia.[41, 42] The issue of clamp time is clouded by the cause of disease, the variable use of perfusion adjuncts, differences in surgical technique, and experience at different centers. Unquestionably, rapid thoracoabdominal aneurysm repair is in the patient's best interest. It is difficult to evaluate the true effects of clamp time on the risk of paraplegia without the impossible elimination of other variables. A risk-benefit judgment must be made for each patient with regard to the use of perfusion adjuncts to improve spinal cord flow.

Effects of Proximal Aortic Hypertension

Placement of the proximal aortic crossclamp alters in the patient's normal physiologic state. The dramatic drop in distal aortic pressure influences metabolism of the entire lower body. The simple placement of an aortic crossclamp reduces the spinal cord blood flow to 8% to 12% of the control value in rodent models.[8] Svensson and colleagues[27] obtained similar results in the baboon model, which more closely approximates human anatomy. Concomitant with the diminished spinal cord blood flow is proximal aortic hypertension. Profound proximal aortic hypertension alters blood flow to the coronary and cerebral systems. This effect has been implicated as the causative factor of left heart strain, increased cerebrospinal fluid pressure, and disorders of the cerebral autoregulatory system.

Management of proximal aortic hypertension is controversial. Powerful vasodilating agents or hypovolemic hypotension are commonly utilized. Caution should be emphasized when attempting to control the hypertension. Dropping the proximal aortic pressures has a variable effect on spinal cord perfusion. The effect of mixed arteriovenous dilators in this setting are potentially dangerous.[43–45] The loss of central nervous system autoregulation, diminished collateral flow arising from the arch vessels,[8] and the further drop in distal aortic pressures[46] have been associated with the use of vasodilators. This information led others to use techniques of partial exsanguination to treat this phenomenon.[46] Theoretically maintaining a distal aortic pressure without distal vasodilation and eliminating the alteration of the cerebral and spinal autoregulatory mechanisms.[47]

Detection of Spinal Cord Ischemia

Patterns of hypoxic damage largely depend on the regional variations in oxygen use and arterial supply. The effects of hypoxia and impending neurologic damage are defined by the basic cellular physiology of normal nerve function and on impulse generation and conduction. With diminished oxygen delivery, reflexive mechanisms enable nervous tissue to improve oxygen extraction. A marked reduction of blood supply resulting in neuronal dysfunction should alter impulse generation and conduction. Knowledge of typical patterns of damage is generally based on a combination of animal models and clinical studies. The intraoperative measurement of neurologic dysfunction may be the first warning sign of permanent neurologic injury. However, the excessive number of variables relating to the development of paraplegia preclude any surgeon, regardless of skill, from uniformly preventing neurologic demise. It is hoped that with specific intraoperative monitoring devices, a directed approach can be taken to resolve acute reversible neurologic ischemia and diminsh the incidence of paraplegia.

Somatosensory evoked potentials (SEPs) are typically generated by bilateral stimulation of posterior tibial nerves. The impulses are conducted through the dorsal column, and the amplified cortical response is measured and averaged over time. The SEP is then expressed as a tracing with two major parameters: latency and amplitude.[48] Evoked potentials do not follow surface pathways as electroencephalographic recordings do. Consequently, they are more resistant to the depressant effects of anesthetics and major sedatives.[49] SEP monitoring is only useful in the setting of a distal perfusion adjunct and with a surgeon who is committed to alter the repair technique based on the SEP readings (Fig. 19–4).[50]

Ischemia can manifest as an increase in latency or a decrease in the amplitude of the response. Changes in these variables occur with ischemia and progress to SEP loss if the ischemia persists.[50] The changes in response can be classified with regard to the intraoperative modifications required and can be grouped into four different categories of SEP response. The first response occurs when no distal aortic perfusion adjunct is used. The characteristic changes involve decreased amplitude and increased latency, with progression to complete loss of conduction 8 to 9 minutes after aortic clamping. This response implies a poor collateral bed and suggests that the surgeon should rapidly institute distal aortic perfusion. The second type has unchanged SEPs after aortic clamping in the presence of a distal perfusion device. This response indicates that critical intercostal arteries or other collateral circulation are not in the excluded segment and are being adequately perfused. The third change involves the loss of SEPs in the presence of distal aortic perfusion. This response indicates that critical collateral circulation exists in the excluded aortic segment and suggests that the surgeon should rapidly reimplant the excluded collaterals. The final response involves fading of SEP tracing over 30 to 50 minutes when the distal aortic perfusion is lower than 60 mm Hg. In this situation, adjustment of the distal flow or rapid completion of the anastomoses are the only available options.[48]

Despite theoretical benefits, the use of SEPs has some problems. SEP recording sites must cover areas at risk during specific clinical procedures.[49] This poses certain clinical problems. First, the SEP is a measure of posterior column function, not a direct measurement of anterior spinal artery flow. Peripheral nerve ischemia alters the SEPs, but it is possible to differentiate peripheral nerve ischemia from spinal cord ischemia. In the setting of a crossclamped aorta without distal perfusion adjuncts, spinal cord ischemia develops within 3 to 4 minutes, whereas peripheral nerve ischemia results in changes after 20 minutes.[48] The loss of SEP because of peripheral nerve ischemia negates further monitoring. In the setting of a bypass procedure requiring femoral artery cannulation, the side cannulated usually has abnormal SEPs, depending on the degree of collateral circulation. The effects of hypothermia, anesthetics, and hypotension on nerve conduction also are

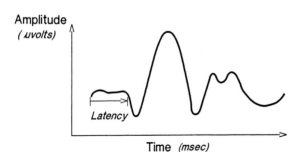

Figure 19–4. Typical somatosensory evoked potential depicting latency and amplitude. (From Marini C, Cunningham J. Issues surrounding spinal cord protection. *In* Karp R, Laks H, Wechsler A (eds). Adv Cardiac Surg. St. Louis: Mosby–Year Book, 1993: 89–107.)

variable. The placement of stimulators in the epidural space has been described in an attempt to eliminate aspects of peripheral nerve ischemia.[51]

The difficulties with SEP result in a fair number of false-positive and false-negative measurements, and despite an unchanged SEP tracing, paraplegia can still occur.[52] A prospective randomized trial was performed by Crawford's group,[1] comparing patients for whom SEPs and selective distal perfusion were used with a group for whom these adjuncts were not used. No statistical difference in complication rates was found for the two groups.[53] The investigators concluded that paraplegia occurs equally for patients with distal perfusion adjuncts and those for whom the clamp and sew technique has been used.[32]

Motor evoked potentials have been evaluated as an alternative to SEP monitoring. SEPs are a measure of the dorsal column function; therefore, the primary blood supply is through the posterior spinal arteries. However, the anterior horn cells along the motor tracts are more sensitive to ischemia.[54] This information led to the development of motor evoked potentials, which are measured after direct stimulation of the motor cortex or through epidural electrodes and measurements of the muscle action potentials over the anterior tibialis or thenar muscles. Responses can also be recorded from the epidural space or a peripheral nerve.[55] The amplitude and latency are measured in a fashion similar to that for SEPs. A reduction of the amplitude to 25% or less of baseline was considered an indicator of spinal cord ischemia.[55] Motor evoked potentials have some advantages. Peripheral nerve ischemia does not affect the measurement, and the anterior spinal artery distribution is being monitored instead of the posterior circulation.[50] Because this is a more direct measurement of anterior spinal cord flow, there are fewer false-negative results compared with SEPs.[55] The disadvantages include the potential for causing a seizure[32] and difficulty with maintaining a low-level, stable neuromuscular blockade using pharmocologic agents.[55]

Prevention of Spinal Cord Ischemia

Reimplantation of Intercostal and Lumbar Arteries

Reattachment of intercostal or lumbar arteries is another heavily debated aspect of aortic surgery. It would seem logical that, if most of the blood supply to the lower thoracic and lumbar cord is generated from a intercostal arteries arising between T8 and L1, these intercostals should be identified and reanastomosed. However, reanastomosis of intercostal vessels is time consuming and thus adds to the duration of crossclamp time. Some surgeons believe that reimplantation of intercostals has no influence on the development of paraplegia,[35] but reconstruction of a noncritical region has been associated with increased risk of injury.[56]

Studies using baboons have demonstrated that the normal lumbar blood flow in the lumbar spinal cord drops from 15 to 20 mL/100 g tissue/min to 1.8 mL/100 g tissue/min after a clamp time of 60 minutes. Further quantification demonstrated that blood flow equal to or exceeding 10 mL/100 g tissue/min does not result in an ischemic insult. Flows less than 4 mL/100 g tissue/min result uniformly in paraplegia.[27]

Spinal cord blood flow cannot be quantified in humans. Consequently, many clinicians advocate the use of SEPs or motor evoked potentials to guide reimplantation decisions. However, these are not as specific or accurate as desired. Some groups rely on preoperative arteriographic localization techniques to identify the critical intercostal and lumbar arteries.[30, 31, 57]

Several clinical series have looked at intercostal reimplantation. In Crawford's[1] evaluation of 605 patients, reimplantation was not a significant predictor of paraplegia. Schepens[58] evaluated the use of SEPs to determine the necessity of intercostal artery reimplantation. Like Crawford, he found no relationship between intercostal artery reimplantation and paraplegia. Shiiya[59] reported a significant decrease in the risk of delayed paraplegia with reimplantation of critical intercostals as determined by SEPs. Svensson and coworkers[60] found a diminished incidence of paraplegia when patent intercostals were reattached in a prospective study of 99 patients. Svensson observed, however, that the risk of paraplegia was markedly diminished in patients with few or no patent intercostals, regardless of the specific type of therapy.

The presence of many variables confounds studies looking at specific issues sounding the causes and prevention of spinal cord ischemia. The question of critical segment reimplantation is related to the risk of increasing crossclamp time duration, the potential for increased hemorrhage, the amount of operative and postoperative blood flow, and the long-term blood supply to the spinal cord.

A potentially promising technique was described by Svensson and colleagues.[60] It involves injection of hydrogen-saturated saline into the exposed intercostal orifices. A platinum electrode is placed in the intrathecal space, and the current created is measured. This technique was shown to be accurate and safe,[60] providing a relatively rapid (5.8 minute average measurement time) intraoperative assessment of collateral flow to the spinal cord.

The surgical technique of reimplantation varies. The cuffs of the intercostal arteris can be cut into Carrel patches and directly reimplanted into the graft. This may result in multiple anastomoses, increasing operative time and risk of bleeding, but this method is commonly used when one or two intercostals are being implanted. Alternatively, the graft can be beveled to include a long portion of the posterior aortic wall containing the intercostal ostia. Late follow-up of these patients occasionally demonstrated dilation of the residual aortic wall.[60] Interposition grafts can be placed from the intercostal orifices to the aortic graft. Sequential unclamping of the graft and moving the clamp distally as additional anastomoses are completed may increase the risk of thrombosis of the intercostals from thromboembolism within the aortic graft because of inadequate outflow through the intercostal vessels alone.[60]

The pelvic circulation is of particular importance in complicated distal aortic surgery. Although data are scarce because of the rarity of paraplegia in isolated infrarenal aneurysms, attempts should be made to preserve the patency of the hypogastric vessels. Reimplanation of the inferior mesenteric artery should also be given consideration.

Cerebrospinal Fluid Drainage

Placement of the proximal aortic crossclamp increases intracranial pressure, which has been implicated in the development of paraplegia by diminishing the normal perfusion gradient between the distal aorta and the spinal cord.[37, 38] The physiologic mechanism correlating proximal aortic hypertension with the rise in CSF pressure is elusive. Evidence suggests that CSF pressure more closely correlates with central venous pressure and does not necessarily relate to the proximal aortic pressure.[61] As CSF pressure increases in response to increasing central venous pressure, it may eventually exceed cerebrovascular venous pressure. Arterial pressures are not affected, but the venous capacitance rises in the beds of the dural space, resulting in even higher CSF pressures.[61] Spinal cord perfusion is determined by the difference between mean arterial pressure in the spinal cord blood supply and the interstitial cord pressure. Perfusion decreases with increasing CSF pressures, a premise used to justify CSF drainage in an effort to improve spinal cord perfusion pressure.

Several animal models have been evaluated to explore this phenomenon, but significant interspecies differences have complicated the interpretation of various experiments and made it difficult to apply the experimental data to human subjects. CSF drainage in the dog was found to have a protective effect on the spinal cord.[62] In the pig model, this was not the case.[26] Baboon studies have shown some benefit, but only with the addition of intrathecal papaverine.[63] Despite the prevalence of anecdotal reports and small series favoring CSF drainage, only one prospective, randomized study has been conducted. In a trial of 98 patients, Crawford and colleagues[36] found no significant difference in paraplegia incidence between the spinal cord drainage group and controls.[36] Critics of the study state that the drainage protocol was too restrictive, allowing only *intraoperative* drainage with a maximum drainage volume of only 50 mL.[47, 64] Many clinical protocols require monitoring and drainage of CSF for up to 48 hours. The subject remains heavily debated.

Hypothermia

Hypothermia can potentially increase the tolerance of the spinal cord to a hypoxic insult. A dramatic reduction in ATP, energy charge, and glucose level, with a rise in lactate, after normothermic spinal cord ischemia was observed in rabbits. Hypothermic ischemia had little effect on lactate but did significantly preserve the cellular energy charge and reduce the rate of the decline of ATP and glucose concentrations. The release of excitatory amino acids was diminished in this model.[6] The metabolic rate and associated oxygen demand of brain tissue was reduced by 6% for each 1°C the core temperature is lowered.[64] This correlates with the observation that CSF lactate concentrations in humans diminished significantly with hypothermic perfusion compared with normothermic situations.[7] The benefits of hypothermia in reducing the risk of paraplegia must be balanced with the increased risk of hemorrhage induced by temperature effects on the coagulation mechanisms.

Surface cooling to 25 to 30°C, direct perfusion cooling by infusing cooled lactated Ringer's solution or blood into an excluded segment of the descending thoracic aorta, selective cooling by infusion of 5°C saline into the subarachnoid space, or profound systemic hypothermia with cardiopulmonary bypass are all potential methods of achieving hypothermia.[3]

Bleeding, cardiac arrhythmias, and other complications have essentially eliminated the use of surface cooling and limited the use of systemic cooling to special circumstances such as congenital defects or replacement of the ascending aorta and arch vessels. Selective cooling through epidural perfusion appears to hold great promise. Wisselink and colleagues[64] demonstrated that, by circulating 5°C fluid in the CSF of dogs, the spinal cord was completely protected from injury, compared with a 100% paraplegia rate for controls. Serious technical difficulties are often encountered when attempting to use epidural, subdural, or subarachnoid spinal cord cooling.[64, 65] These difficulties have delayed the development of a usable device for safe epidural cooling. Consequently, the only viable method of spinal cord cooling has been perfusion of open collateral segements in the excluded aortic segment with normal saline solution or Ringer's lactate. This technique has diminished the incidence of paraplegia.[66]

Distal Aortic Perfusion

Many mechanisms are employed to increase distal aortic perfusion. The premise that distal aortic perfusion will result in retrograde flow into non-excluded intercostals and lumbars is primarily based on experimental models.[63, 67] Theoretically, distal aortic perfusion increases spinal cord blood flow and minimizes metabolic derangements, resulting from aortic crossclamping. However, improvement in distal aortic flows may correlate well with improved lumbar cord flow but do not equate with lower thoracic cord flow.[56] The complexity of the systems, increased operative time, and potential for emboli argue against the use of distal perfusion adjuncts. It is unlikely that any randomized, prospective trial will be able to prove the superiority of distal perfusion over the clamp and sew technique.

The history of the development of distal aortic perfusion devices provides some insights into the difficulties we face in clinically comparing the techniques. Cardiopulmonary bypass was initially employed for complicated aneurysms. Hemorrhagic complications occurred with the use of systemic anticoagulation necessary to prevent thrombosis in the bypass circuit. Heparin-bonded shunts were developed to avoid the need for systemic anticoagulation. However, the inability to control distal aortic flows and the small diameter of the shunts prompted the use of partial bypass circuits. Although it is possible encounter enthusiasm from individual surgeons, no prospective, randomized studies support the use of any distal perfusion adjunct or the efficacy of one technique over another.

Cardiopulmonary bypass theoretically provides perfusion of the unclamped segments of the aorta at a controlled flow rate. The ability to systemically cool the patient, manage potentially malignant cardiac arrhythmias, and quickly induce hypothermic circulatory arrest are also potentially helpful. However, the need to systemically anticoagulate the patient can result in significant increases in morbidity and mortality. Up to one third of patients operated on for thoracoabdominal aneurysms died of hemorrhage.[33, 35, 39] Suture line dehiscence has also been associated with the use of partial bypass techniques requiring anticoagulation.[68]

The development of the tridecylmethylammonium chloride–heparin-bonded shunt in 1972 by Gott[69] eliminated the need for systemic anticoagulation. Two sizes are available: 7 and 9 mm. The internal diameters are 5 and 6 mm, respectively.[32] The 9-mm shunt is equivalent to approximately 7% of the cross-sectional area of the descending aorta; consequently, flow through the shunt rarely exceeds 50% of cardiac output and pressure gradients across the shunt are often in excess of 60 mm Hg.[25] It would seem foolish to chose the smaller shunt.[35] The use of this shunt was strongly supported by the work of Verdant and associates[70] in 1988. Verdant's group[70] reported the use of the Gott shunt in 173 patients, with a mean clamp time of 37 minutes and no cases of paraplegia. Other surgeons found shunts to be most useful when short segments of aorta are excluded, as in type III aneurysms and traumatic aortic rupture.[40] Unfortunately, many problems have been cited with the use of shunts, including the ease of shunt dislodgment, embolization, stroke, death, and hemorrhage.[71] The use of an axillo-femoral bypass performed before clamping may serve as an excellent alternative to shunting. Although the concept is appealing, the use of shunts has not been clinically proven to decrease the incidence of paraplegia or mortality.[33, 42, 72, 73]

The ability to provide distal aortic flow without systemic anticoagulation is the primary advantage of the partial bypass techniques. Control of distal flow rates and management of proximal aortic hypertension without hypovolemia are also benefits. Cannulation can be done from the pulmonary veins, left atrium, or descending aorta to the femoral artery or distal aorta. The mesenteric and renal arteries can be selectively cannulated after the aorta is open. Increased neurologic complications probably result from thromboembolism.[25] Partial distal perfusion often increases the distal aortic pressures but not to preclamp levels. To ensure adequate distal pressures, an excessive amount of blood may have to be drained from the heart, resulting in poor left heart function and hypotension proximal to the clamps. This may cause reversal of flow in collateral channels and stagnation of blood in the watershed area of the spinal cord.[25] The literature evaluating the efficacy of partial bypass techniques in humans is sparse. Meta-analyses have repeatedly demonstrated no benefit over the clamp and sew technique.[25, 35, 42, 74]

Distal perfusion techniques will never be universally used in thoracoabdominal aneurysm repair. The risks of neurologic injury, atheroemboli, hemorrhage, and increased operative time may preclude it. Patient variables may determine the true risk of paraplegia rather than surgical technique.[35] It is likely that this controversy will not be resolved and that surgeon preference will prevail for years to come.

Pharmacologic Therapy

The use of pharmacologic agents to protect the spinal cord during ischemia is an appealing concept to surgeons because of the complexity of distal perfusion techniques. Pharmacologic protection of the spinal cord is directed at the basic mechanisms involved in ischemic injury, including aberrant calcium fluxes, vasoconstrictor and platelet-aggregating prostanoids, and oxygen free radical–induced lipid peroxidation.[11]

Calcium-induced smooth muscle contraction is hypothesized to induce vasoconstriction, compounding the effects of the already diminished blood flow. Prevention of initial calcium ion fluxes was attempted by modifying the excitatory amino acid release with the use of baclofen, but this treatment remains experimental.[10] Despite the lack of clinical efficacy in the stroke model,[10] calcium channel antagonists[11, 75] and papaverine[63] have been used experimentally to limit spinal cord injury. Results have been variable, possibly because the dose of the agents has been limited for fear of systemic hypotension. Papaverine was used clinically after noticing its powerful vasodilatory effect on intracranial cerebrovasculature during spasm induced by subarachnoid hemorrhage. Intrathecal injection of papaverine after lumbar drainage in baboons decreased the risk of paraplegia.[63] The effects of papaverine do not appear to be limited to vasodilation of the anterior spinal artery. Increased mitochondrial calcium uptake, diminished nucleotide breakdown, and prevention of hypoxanthine entry are also related to the use of papaverine and may be causally related to spinal cord protection.[76]

Increased concentration of intracellular calcium results in the activation of calcium-dependent membrane phospholipids, particularly phospholipase. This results in the accumulation of metabolites of the arachadonic acid pathway, including $PGF_{2\alpha}$ and thromboxane A_2. With this in mind, cyclooxygenase inhibitors and specific thromboxane synthetase antagonists were tested experimentally, but results were disappointing.[11] Nitric oxide, an endogenous vaso-dilator synthesized by endothelial and neuronal cells, plays a neuroprotective role in spinal ischemia. Reports demonstrate a positive dose-response relationship between inhibition of nitric oxide synthesis and ischemic neuronal death.[77] In an effort to limit microvascular thrombosis, tissue factor pathway inhibitor was evaluated. This factor X_a–dependent inhibitor of coagulation was shown to have some promise in an experimental model.[18] Other agents directed at limiting microvascular stasis have been beneficial. Despite the fact that leukotriene-induced neutrophil aggregation is increased in ischemic injury,[16] evaluation of immunologic aggregate antagonists yielded no benefit.[17]

The generation of oxygen free radicals is potentially the most dangerous of all the ischemic mechanisms, in part because of the self-perpetuating nature of lipid peroxidation and cell membrane destruction. Retardation of this vicious cycle holds promise. Hall and coworkers[11] found that pretreatment with vitamin E and selenium maintained spinal cord blood flow to near-preinjury levels in an ischemic cat model. Conflicting results regarding the use of superoxide dismutase have observed.[78] Other free radical scavengers have been used successfully to protect neural tissue from reperfusion injury.[79] Steroids have a membrane-stabilizing effect and inhibit complement activation and neutrophil aggregation. Methylprednisolone is commonly used in blunt spinal cord trauma and has been hypothesized to have a similar effect on ischemic neurologic injury during thoracoabdominal aneurysm repair.[23] Naloxone had similar effects.[80] The combination of thiopental, a membrane stabilizer, and hypothermia dramatically improved neurologic outcome from spinal cord ischemia in the rabbit model.[81]

Conclusions

Spinal cord injury occurs during the period of aortic clamping and hypoperfusion, during the reperfusion that follows, or from contrived ischemia secondary to insufficient reestablishment of flow through important arterial branches to the spinal cord. Distal aortic perfusion with a variety of shunts and left heart bypass have been explored to prevent ischemia. Preoperative angiographic identification of the spinal cord arterial supply and reimplantation of important intercostal branches may decrease the risk of paraplegia, but results are guarded. SEPs and motor evoked potentials have been employed to define the patients best served by distal aortic perfusion during aortic clamping. Cooling of the spinal cord has been used to lessen ischemic injury, and drainage of spinal fluid has been used to improve arterial perfusion. Search continues for pharmacologic agents to protect the spinal cord from injury.

Despite the wealth of investigations in the protection of the spinal cord during and after major aortic surgery, no single modality has been clearly documented as efficacious. In the absence of compelling data, the most appropriate means of achieving an acceptable rate of paraplegia rests on the performance of a technically proficient repair by an operator well versed in thoracoabdominal aortic surgery.

References

1. Crawford E, Crawford J, Safi H, et al. Thoracoabdominal aortic aneurysms: preoperative and intraoperative factors determining immediate and long-term results of operation in 605 patients. J Vasc Surg 1986;3:389–404.
2. Wisselink W, Nguyen J, Becker M, et al. Ischemia-reperfusion injury of the spinal cord:

the influence of normovolemic hemodilution and gradual reperfusion. Cardiovasc Surg 1995;3:399–404.

3. Kouchoukos N, Rokkas C. Descending thoracic and thoracoabdominal aortic surgery for aneurysm or dissection: how do we minimize the risk of spinal cord injury. Semin Thorac Cardiovasc Surg 1993;5:47–54.

4. Sakurai M, Aoki M, Abe K, et al. Selective motor neuron death and heat shock protein induction after spinal cord ischemia in rabbits. J Thorac Cardiovasc Surg 1997;113:159–164.

5. Kwun BD, Vacanti F. Mild hypothermia protects against irreversible damage during prolonged spinal cord ischemia. J Surg Res 1995;59:780–782.

6. Allen B, Davis C, Osborne D, Karl I. Spinal cord ischemia and reperfusion metabolism: the effect of hypothermia. J Vasc Surg 1994;19:332–340.

7. Drenger B, Parker S, Frank S, Beattie C. Changes in cerebrospinal fluid pressure and lactate concentrations during thoracoabdominal aortic aneurysm surgery. Anesthesiology 1997;86:41–47.

8. Taira Y, Marsala M. Effect of proximal arterial perfusion pressure on function, spinal cord blood flow, and histopathologic changes after increasing intervals of aortic occlusion in the rat. Stroke 1996;27:1850–1858.

9. Marsala M, Sorkin L, Yaksh T. Transient spinal cord ischemia in the rat: characterization of spinal cord blood flow, extracellular amino acid release, and concurrent histopathological damage. J Cereb Blood Flow Metab 1994;14:604–614.

10. Rothman S, Olney J. Glutamate and the pathophysiology of hypoxic-ischemic brain damage. Ann Neurol 1986;19:105–111.

11. Hall E, Wolf D. A pharmacological analysis of the pathophysiological mechanisms of posttraumatic spinal cord ischemia. J Neurosurg 1986;64:951–961.

12. von Euler M, Seiger A, Holmberg L, Sundstrom E. NBQX, a competitive non-NMDA receptor antagonist, reduces degeneration due to focal spinal cord ischemia. Exp Neurol 1994;129:163–168.

13. Madden K, Clark W, Zivin J. Delayed therapy of experimental ischemia with competitive N-methyl-D-aspartate antagonist in rabbits. Stroke 1993;24:1068–1071.

14. Follis F, Miller K, Scremin O, et al. NMDA receptor blockade and spinal cord ischemia due to aortic crossclamping in the rat model. Can J Neurolog Sci 1994;21:227–232.

15. Bowes M, Swanson S, Zivin J. The AMPA antagonist LY293558 improves functional neurological outcome following reversible spinal cord ischemia in rabbits. J Cereb Blood Flow Metab 1996;16:967–972.

16. Clark W, Walsh C, Briley D, Brace C. Neutrophil adhesion in central nervous system ischemia in rabbits. Brain Behav Immun 1993;7:63–69.

17. Forbes A, Slimp J, Winn R, Verrier E. Inhibition of neutrophil adhesion does not prevent ischemic spinal cord injury. Ann Thorac Surg 1994;58:1064–1068.

18. Koudsi B, Chatman D, Ballinger B, et al. Tissue factor pathway inhibitor protects the ischemic spinal cord. J Surg Res 1996;63:174–178.

19. Ueno T, Furukawa K, Katayama Y, et al. Spinal cord protection: development of a paraplegia-preventive solution. Ann Thorac Surg 1994;58:116–120.

20. Svensson L, Klepp P, Hinder R. Spinal cord anatomy of the baboon: comparison with man and implications for spinal cord blood flow during thoracic aortic cross-clamping. S Afr J Sur 1986; 24:32–34.

21. Picone A, Green R, Ricotta J, et al. Spinal cord ischemia following operations on the abdominal aorta. J Vasc Surg 1986;3:94–103.

22. Szilagyi D, Hageman J, Smith R, Elliot J. Spinal cord damage in surgery of the abdominal aorta. Surgery 1978;83:38–56.

23. Gharagozloo F, Larson J, Dausmann M, et al. Spinal cord protection during surgical procedures on the descending thoracic and thoracoabdominal aorta. Chest 1996;109:799–809.

24. Adamkiewicz A. Die Blutgefasse des Menschlichen Ruckernmarkes. I. Theil Die Gefasse der Ruckenmarksubstanz. Sitzungsb Akad Wissensh Wien Math Naturw Klass 1882;84:469.

25. Svensson L, Loop F. Prevention of spinal cord ischemia in aortic surgery. In Yao JST (ed). Arterial Surgery; New York: Grune & Stratton, 1988:273–285.

26. Wadouh F, Lindemann E, Arndt C, et al. The arteria radicularis magna anterior as a decisive factor influencing spinal cord damage during occlusion. J Thorac Cardiovasc Surg 1984;88:1–10.

27. Svensson L, Rickards E, Coull A, et al. Relationship of spinal cord blood flow to vascular anatomy during thoracic aortic cross-clamping and shunting. J Thorac Cardiovasc Surg 1986;91:71–78.

28. Fried L, Di Chiro G, Doppman J. Ligation of major thoraco-lumbar spinal cord arteries in monkeys. J Neurosurg 1969;31:608–614.

29. Dichiro G, Doppman J, Omemaya A. Selective arteriography of arteriovenous aneurysms of spinal cord. Radiology 1967;88:1065–1077.

30. Savader S, Williams G, Trerotola S, et al. Preoperative spinal artery localization and its relationship to postoperative neurologic complications. Radiology 1993;189:165–171.

31. Bachet J, Guilmet D, Rosier J, et al. Protection of the spinal cord during surgery of thoracoabdominal aortic aneurysms. Euro J Cardiothorac Surg 1996;10:817–825.

32. Shenaq S, Svensson L. Paraplegia following aortic surgery. J Cardiothorac Vasc Anesth 1993;7:81–94.
33. von Oppell U, Dunne T, De Groot M, Zilla P. Spinal cord protection in the absence of collateral circulation: meta-analysis of mortality and paraplegia. J Card Surg 1994;9:685–691.
34. Carrel A. On the experimental surgery of the thoracic aorta and the heart. Ann Surg 1910;52:83.
35. Livesay L, Cooley D, Ventemiglia R, et al. Surgical experience in descending thoracic aneurysmectomy with and without adjuncts to avoid ischemia. Ann Thorac Surg 1985;39:37–46.
36. Crawford E, Svensson L, Hess K, et al. A prospective randomized study of cerebrospinal fluid drainage to prevent paraplegia after high-risk surgery on the thoracoabdominal aorta. J Vasc Surg 1990;13:36–46.
37. Blaisdell F, Cooley D. The mechanism of paraplegia after temporary thoracic aortic occlusion and its relationship to spinal fluid pressures. Surg 1962;51:351–355.
38. Miyamoto K, Ueno A, Wada T, et al. A new and simple method of preventing spinal cord damage following temporary occlusion of the thoracic aorta by draining the cerebrospinal fluid. J Cardiovasc Surg 1960;1:188–203.
39. Jex R, Schaff H, Piehler J, et al. Early and late results following repair of dissection of the descending aorta. J Vasc Surg 1986;3:226–237.
40. Katz N, Blackstone E, Kirklin J, et al. Incremental risk factors for spinal cord injury following operation for acute traumatic aortic transection. J Thorac Cardiovasc Surg 1981;81:669–674.
41. Hollier L, Symmonds J, Pairolero P, et al. Thoracoabdominal aortic aneurysm repair: analysis of postoperative morbidity. Arch Surg 1988;123:871–875.
42. Crawford E, Rubio P. Reappraisal of adjuncts to avoid ischemia in the treatment of aneurysms of the descending aorta. J Thorac Cardiovasc Surg 1973;66:693–704.
43. Marini C, Grubbs P, Toporoff B, et al. Effect of sodium nitroprusside on spinal cord perfusion and paraplegia during aortic cross-clamping. Ann Thorac Surg 1989;47:379–383.
44. Gelman S, Reves J, Fowler K, et al. Regional blood flow during cross-clamping of the thoracic aorta and infusion of sodium nitroprusside. J Thorac Cardiovasc Surg 1983;85:287–291.
45. Laschinger J, Owen J, Rosenbloom N, et al. Detrimental effects of sodium nitroprusside on spinal cord motor tract perfusion during thoracic aortic cross-clamping. Surg Forum 1987;38:195–196.
46. Wolszyn T, Marini C, Coons M, et al. Partial exsanguination effectively controls proximal hypertension and protects the spinal cord during thoracic aortic cross-clamping. Surg Forum 1989;1989:193–195.
47. Uceda P, Basu S, Robertazzi R, et al. Effect of cerebrospinal fluid drainage and/or partial exsanguination on tolerance to prolonged aortic cross-clamping. J Card Surg 1994;9:631–637.
48. Cunningham JJ, Laschinger J, Merlin H, et al. Measurement of spinal cord ischemia during operations upon the thoracic aorta. Ann Surg 1982;196:285–296.
49. Prior P. The rationale and utility of neurophysiological investigations in clinical monitoring for brain and spinal cord ischemia during surgery and intensive care. Comput Methods Programs Biomed 1996;51:13–27.
50. Marini C, Cunningham J. Issues surrounding spinal cord protection. *In* Karp R, Laks H, Wechsler A (eds). Advances in Cardiac Surgery. St. Louis: Mosby–Year Book, 1993:89–107.
51. Kaschner A, Sandman W, Larkamp H. Percutaneous flexible bipolar epidural neuroelectrode for spinal cord stimulation. J Neurosurg 1984;60:1317–1319.
52. Lesser R, Raudzens P, Luder H, et al. Postoperative neurologic deficits may occur despite unchanged intraoperative somatosensory evoked potentials. Ann Neurol 1986;19:22–25.
53. Crawford E, Mizhari E, Hess K, et al. The impact of distal aortic perfusion and somatosensory evoked potential monitoring on prevention of paraplegia after aortic operation. J Thorac Cardiovasc Surg 1988;95:357–367.
54. Agnew W, McCreery D. Considerations of safety in the use of extracranial stimulation for motor-evoked potentials. Neurosurgery 1987;20:143–147.
55. de Haan P, Kalkman C, de Mol B, et al. Efficacy of transcranial motor-evoked myogenic potentials to detect spinal cord ischemia during operations for thoracoabdominal aneurysms. J Thorac Cardiovasc Surg 1997;113:87–101.
56. Svensson L, Patel V, Robinson M, et al. Influence of preservation or perfusion of intraoperatively identified spinal cord blood supply on spinal motor evoked potentials and paraplegia after aortic surgery. J Vasc Surg 1991;13:355–365.
57. Kieffer E, Richard T, Chiras J, et al. Preoperative spinal cord arteriography in aneurysmal disease of the descending thoracic and thoracoabdominal aorta: preliminary results in 45 patients. Ann Vasc Surg 1989;3:34–46.
58. Schepens M, Boezeman E, Hamerlijnck R, et al. Somatosensory evoked potentials during exclusion and reperfusion of critical aortic segments in thoracoabdominal aortic aneurysm surgery. J Card Surg 1994;9:692–702.
59. Shiiya N, Yasuda K, Matsui Y, et al. Spinal cord protection during thoracoabdominal aneurysm repair: results of selective reconstruction of the critical segmental arteries guided by evoked spinal cord potential monitoring. J Vasc Surg 1995;21:970–975.
60. Svensson L, Hess K, Coselli J, Safi H. Influence of segmental arteries, extent, and artiofemoral bypass on postoperative paraplegia after thoracoabdominal aortic operation. J Vasc Surg 1994;20:255–262.

61. Paino G, Gewertz B. Mechanism of increased cerebrospinal fluid pressure with thoracic aortic occlusion. J Vasc Surg 1990;11:695–701.
62. Bower T, Murray M, Gloviczki P, et al. Effects of thoracic aortic occlusion and cerebrospinal drainage on regional spinal cord blood flow in dogs: correlation with neurologic outcome. J Vasc Surg 1989;9:135–144.
63. Svensson L, Von Ritter C, Groeneveld H, et al. Cross-clamping of the thoracic aorta: influence of aortic shunts, laminectomy, papaverine, calcium channel blockers, allopurinol, and superoxide dismutase on spinal cord blood flow and paraplegia in baboons. Ann Surg 1986;204:38–47.
64. Wisselink W, Becker M, Nguyen J, et al. Protecting the ischemic spinal cord during aortic clamping: the influence of selective hypothermia and spinal cord perfusion pressure. J Vasc Surg 1994;19:788–796.
65. Malatova Z, Vanicky I, Galik J, Marsala M. Epidural perfusion cooling protects against spinal cord ischemia in rabbits. Mol Chem Neuropathol 1995;25:81–96.
66. Coles J, Wilson G, Sima A, et al. Intraoperative management of thoracic aortic aneurysms: exprimental evaluation of perfusion cooling of the spinal cord. J Thorac Cardiovasc Surg 1983;85:292–299.
67. Laschinger J, Cunningham J, Nathan I, et al. Experimental and clinical assessment of the adequacy of partial bypass in maintenance of spinal cord blood flow during operation of the thoracic aorta. Ann Thorac Surg 1986;36:417–426.
68. DeBakey M. The treatment of acute traumatic rupture of the aorta. Ann Surg 1976;184:308–316.
69. Gott V. Heparinized shunts for thoracic vascular operations [editorial]. Ann Thorac Surg 1972;14:219.
70. Verdant A, Page A, Cossette R, et al. Surgery of the descending aorta: spinal cord protection with the gott shunt. Ann Thorac Surg 1988;46:147–154.
71. Crawford E, Fenstermacher J, Richardson W, Sandiford F. Reappraisal of adjuncts to avoid ischemia in treatment of thoracic aortic aneurysms. Surg 1970;67:182.
72. Molina J, Cogordan J, Einzigs, et al. Adequacy of ascending aorta–descending aorta shunt during cross-clamping of the thoracic aorta for prevention of spinal cord ischemia. J Thorac Cardiovasc Surg 1985;90:126–136.
73. Svensson L, Antunes M, Kinsley R. Traumatic rupture of the thoracic aorta: A report of 14 cases and a review of the literature. S Afr Med J 1985;67:853–857.
74. Najafi H, Javid H, Hushang J, et al. Descending aortic aneurysmectomy without adjuncts to avoid ischemia. Ann Thorac Surg 1980;30:326–335.
75. Rhee R, Gloviczke P, Cambria R, et al. The effects of nimodipine on ischemic injury of the spinal cord during thoracic aortic cross-clamping. Int Angiol 1996;15:153–161.
76. Imai S, Kitagawau T. A comparison of the differential effects of itroglycerine, nifedipine, and papaverine on contractures induced in vascular and intestinal smooth muscle by potassium and lanthanum. Jpn J Pharmacol 1981;31:193–199.
77. Yezierski R, Liu S, Ruenes G, et al. Neuronal damage following intraspinal injection of a nitric oxide synthase inhibitor in the rat. J Cereb Blood Flow Metab 1996;16:996–1004.
78. Novelli G, Melani M, Consales G, Paternostro E. Antioxidant drugs in cerebral and spinal ischemia. Minerva Anestesiol 1994;60:543–546.
79. Francel P, Long B, Malik J, et al. Limiting ischemic spinal cord Injury using a free radical scavenger 21-aminosteroid and/or cerebrospinal fluid drainage. J Neurosurg 1993;79:742–751.
80. Archer C, Wynn M, Hoch J, et al. Combined use of cerebrospinal fluid and naloxone reduce risk of paraplegia in thoracoabdominal aneurysm repair. J Vasc Surg 1994;19:236–246.
81. Robertson C, Foltz R, Grossman R, Goodman C. Protection against experimental ischemic spinal cord injury. J Neurosurg 1986;64:633–642.

Paraanastomotic Aortic Aneurysms: A Continuing Surgical Challenge

Alan B. Lumsden, M.D., and Robert B. Smith III, M.D.

Paraanastomotic aneurysms (PAAs) of the aorta, although uncommon, continue to represent a formidable surgical challenge, despite advances in endovascular grafting. PAAs may follow bypass for occlusive or aneurysmal disease, may occur early or late, and may be classified as pseudoaneurysms or true aneurysms.

The incidence of PAAs may be underestimated because routine screening after aortic grafting is not the standard of care. Unlike groin pseudoaneurysms, proximal anastomotic pseudoaneurysms are less likely to be clincally detected because of their location within the retroperitoneum. Edwards and colleagues,[1] using life table analysis, demonstrated an incidence of PAA as high as 27% at 15 years after grafting. Detection of aortic PAAs is usually a result of increasing size, symptom development, or serendipity.

They have the same risk of rupture as primary aneurysms and the same dire consequences. Surgical repair is the optimal management before development of symptoms.

PAAs may be classified as true aneurysms of the residual aortic segment or pseudoaneurysms arising at the suture line. In our series at Emory University Hospital, true aneurysms (19%) were much less common than false aneurysms (81%).

Etiology

The cause of any anastomotic aneurysm is probably multifactorial.[2, 3] True aneurysms may represent an abnormality in collagen metabolism.[4, 5] True PAAs most commonly occur after bypass grafting for aneurysmal disease. The same connective tissue defect that contributed to the initial aneurysm can result in progressive dilation of a residual aortic segment.[1, 6, 7] True PAAs therefore result from inadequate resection of the diseased infrarenal aorta at the time of the initial operation. However, progressive dilation of an even shorter infrarenal segment, when combined with aneurysmal dilation of the pararenal and suprarenal aorta, can also lead to development of PAA degeneration, even after an adequate initial procedure.

False aneurysm formation due to suture line dehiscence may result from a combination of technical factors: poor choice of suture material (eg, silk, braided polyester), prosthesis dilation (ie, Dacron), type of anastomosis (ie, end to side), severity or progression of atherosclerosis (ie, multilevel disease), vessel-graft compliance mismatch, and infection (eg, periprosthetic, aortoenteric fistula [AEF]).[2, 3] Early PAA formation has been associated with a complicated postoperative course after the primary aortic procedure.[1] It was also linked in our experience to α_1-antitrypsin deficiency, recurrent PAA, and graft infection.[7]

Presentation

Most patients are totally asymptomatic, with their PAAs detected by chance, but symptoms can include abdominal pain and back pain. Physical examination may reveal a pulsatile mass in a patient who is otherwise asymptomatic, but frequently the findings are not diagnostic.[1, 6, 8] Most PAAs are detected late and are therefore large at the time of diagnosis; the average size was approximately 7 cm in our series.[7] The mean interval from the time of the primary aortic procedure to PAA diagnosis is 8 to 10 years. A femoral artery false aneurysm is an associated finding in approximately 25% of patients with PAAs and should be an indication to intensify surveillance.[1, 4, 8, 9] In contrast, approximately 15% of patients with a femoral pseudoaneurysm have associated PAA.[3]

Rupture of a PAA may manifest early or late during postoperative follow-up and is associated with a poor outcome.[9, 10] Two patients in our study complaining of abdominal and back pain had early contained rupture of false aneurysms after bypass grafting. The characteristic presentation of AEF is bleeding and abdominal or back pain in a patient with a history of bypass grafting of the abdominal aorta. This classic triad was found in all three of our patients with PAA and associated AEF.[7]

Imaging Studies

Patients who are symptomatic and who have femoral PAAs or a palpable abdominal mass should have imaging of the proximal anastomosis performed. Ultrasonography can be helpful diagnostically, and several academic centers have documented its high accuracy.[11, 12] However, this examination is operator dependent, and results vary between institutions.[11–14]

Computed tomograpy (CT) scanning demonstrates PAA size and extent of involvement, as well as synchronous disease processes in the abdomen.[12, 14, 15] In particular, CT scanning helps the surgeon to determine whether there is an adequate infrarenal aortic segment to permit infrarenal clamping. Frequently, however, the aorta and aneurysm are tortuous, making this determination difficult.

Aortography, the gold standard for defining the aneurysm and associated anatomy, facilitates planning of the operative approach and selection of the appropriate surgical procedure. It helps define the relationship of the renal arteries to the aneurysm.

In the future, magnetic resonance imaging and spiral CT scanning will have an increasing role in the diagnosis of PAA and may surpass standard angiography.[16] Proper preoperative evaluation of PAA patients before operative intervention is essential because of their frequently advanced age and multiple medical problems.

Treatment

Surgical Therapy

Elective surgical management of PAA lesions is the treatment of choice, because these lesions progressively increase in size and may rupture with time.[10] Morbidity and mortality rates are acceptable for asymptomatic patients undergoing elective repair, as reported in our series and by others.[6-8] For the good-risk patient, we advocate operative intervention for any PAA larger than 5 cm in diameter. Any suspicion of an infection lowers this threshold. Poor-risk patients or patients in whom the aneurysm involves the visceral segment may be monitored until the aneurysm is 6 cm; beyond that size, there must be a clear reason for avoiding intervention.

Operative repair mostly involves excising the diseased segment of the artery and graft and placement of an interposition prosthesis. End-to-side proximal anastomosis in patients with occlusive disease has been implicated as a causative factor for operative failure, but the importance of preserving the pelvic circulation must not be ignored.[8, 17, 18] A bifurcated graft can be used if iliofemoral aneurysmal disease or generalized graft fatigue is present. Operative management of PAA involving the renal and visceral vessels is more challenging, and a thoracoabdominal approach gives excellent proximal exposure and expedites repair.

Operative complications are common and increase in the urgent setting or when other aortic graft complications exist (eg, AEF, graft infection).[6, 9, 19, 20] The surgical mortality rate for these complicated reoperations is substantially higher than that associated with the initial aortic reconstruction (21% in our series of 29 patients).[7]

It is imperative to obtain operative cultures in every case, even if suspicion for a graft infection is minimal. The clinical judgment of an experienced vascular surgeon is crucial in the management of these frequently elderly and frail patients. Observation with ultrasonographic surveillance should be considered as an option for patients with small, asymptomatic PAAs or for high-risk patients with asymptomatic PAAs and who are poor operative candidates.

Endovascular Therapy

Transluminally placed endografts may have a role in the management of selected patients with PAAs. Those with PAAs that involve the visceral segment should be excluded for consideration, but those with focal pseudoaneurysms or those with normal segments of infrarenal aorta may be helped by such an approach.

Surveillance

Several reports show PAA to be an important problem, and each makes a plea for increased surveillance.[1, 6-8] However, the method and frequency of follow-up are still unclear, and limited short- and long-term information after bypass grafting of the abdominal aorta precludes informed recommendations. It is known that most PAAs occur late after aortic grafting (8 to 10 years) and that early PAA development is associated with a complicated postoperative course after the primary aortic procedure.[1, 6]

Ultrasonography and CT scanning appear to be the most effective diagnostic modalities, but each has advantages and disadvantages. Ultrasonography is inexpensive and quick, but the results obtained depend on the operator and institution. CT scanning is accurate and reproducible, but it is also expensive and time consuming. Ultrasonography may be the preferred study in this era of cost containment because of its substantially reduced cost ($300 versus $850 for CT in our center).

The data from our study and those from others lend support to the proposal for routine screening.[1, 6–8] Our follow-up policy in the past has been purely clinical, without routine radiographic surveillance. We now recommend an ultrasonographic examination at 5 years from the time of the original aortic prosthetic reconstruction and every 2 years thereafter. Patients at high risk for an early PAA should be followed more closely, with an ultrasonographic examination every 2 years. Risk factors for aneurysm formation, such as associated iliofemoral aneurysms or possible graft infection, require increased surveillance. The pattern of late presentation and increased incidence over time, as evidenced by life table analysis, argues for lifetime surveillance.[1, 6, 8] Early detection and elective operative repair of PAAs is essential to minimize morbidity and mortality.

References

1. Edwards JM, Teeffey FA, Zierler RE, Kohler TR. Intraabdominal paraanastomotic aneurysms after aortic bypass grafting. J Vasc Surg 1992;15:344–353.
2. Briggs RM, Jarstfer BS, Collins GJ. Anastomotic aneurysms. Am J Surg 1983;146:770–773.
3. Gaylis H, Dewar G. Anastomotic aneurysms: facts and fancy. Surg Annu 1990;22:317–340.
4. Deak SB, Ricotta JJ, Mariani TJ, et al. Abnormalities in the biosynthesis of type III procollagen in cultured skin fibroblasts from two patients with multiple aneurysms. Matrix 1991;12:92–100.
5. Tilson MD, Seashore MR. Fifty families with abdominal aortic aneurysms in two or more first order relatives. Am J Surg 1984;147:551–553.
6. Curl GR, Faggioli GL, Stella A, et al. Aneurysmal change at or above the proximal anastomosis after infrarenal grafting. J Vasc Surg 1992;16:855–860.
7. Allen RC, Schneider J, Longenecker L, et al. Paraanastomotic aneurysms of the abdominal aorta. J Vasc Surg 1993;18:424–432.
8. Gautier C, Borie H, Lagneau P. Aortic false aneurysms after prosthetic reconstruction of the infrarenal aorta. Ann Vasc Surg 1992;6:413–417.
9. Plate G, Hollier LA, O'Brien P, et al. Recurrent aneurysms and late vascular complications following repair of abdominal aortic aneurysms. Arch Surg 1985;120:590–594.
10. Sladen JG, Gerein AS, Miyagishima RT. Late rupture of prosthetic aortic grafts. Am J Surg 1987;153:453–458.
11. Gooding GA, Effeney DJ, Goldstone J. The aortofemoral graft: detection and identification of healing complications by ultrasonography. Surgery 1981;89:94–101.
12. Hilton S, Megibow AJ, Naidich DP, Bosniak MA. Computed tomography of the postoperative aorta. Radiology 1982;145:403–407.
13. Turnipseed WD, Acher CW, Detmer DE, et al. Digital subtraction angiography and B-mode ultrasonography for abdominal and peripheral aneurysms. Surgery 1982;92:619–626.
14. Mark A, Moss AA, Lusby R, Kaiser JA. CT evaluation of complications of abdominal aortic surgery. Radiology 1982;145:403–407.
15. Nevelsteen A, Suy R. Anastomotic false aneurysms of the abdominal aorta and iliac arteries [letter]. J Vasc Surg 1989;10:595.
16. Guinet C, Buy JN, Ghossain MA, et al. Aortic anastomotic pseudoaneurysms: US, CT, MR, and angiography. J Comput Assist Tomogr 1992;16:182–188.
17. Mikati A, Marache P, Watel A, et al. End-to-side aortoprosthetic anastomoses: long-term computed tomography assessment. Ann Vasc Surg 1990;4:584–591.
18. Melliere D, Labasttie J, Bequemin JP, et al. Proximal anastomosis in aortobifemoral bypass: end-to-end or end-to-side? J Cardiovasc Surg 1990;31:77–80.
19. Dennis JW, Littooy FN, Greisler HP, Baker WH. Anastomotic pseudoaneurysms: a continuing late complication of vascular reconstructive procedures. Arch Surg 1986;121:314–317.
20. Treiman GS, Weaver FA, Cossman DV, et al. Anastomotic false aneurysms of the abdominal aorta and the iliac arteries. J Vasc Surg 1988;8:268–273.

Alternative Approach for Management of Infected Aortic Grafts

Dhiraj M. Shah, M.D., R. Clement Darling III, M.D.,
Paul B. Kreienberg, M.D., Benjamin B. Chang, M.D.,
and Philip S. K. Paty, M.D.

Infection of an aortic graft is one of the most fearsome complications of vascular surgery. Despite tremendous improvement in the management of infected vascular grafts, the outcome of treatment for infected aortic grafts has been less than optimal. The standard of treatment for such infection usually entails complete removal of the prosthesis, debridement, and drainage, followed by revascularization of the lower limbs using an extraanatomic bypass. Although this treatment presumably represents the gold standard, the technique, whether performed simultaneously or in staged procedures, still results in significant morbidity and mortality. Literature reports, even from recent series, cite an average mortality rate of 21% and an amputation rate of 22%.[1-3]

Many centers have attempted to use alternative approaches, including graft removal and in situ reconstruction with autogenous or prosthetic materials or with allografts.[4-10] In some cases, when the entire graft is not involved, a conservative approach of partial graft excision is used along with anatomic bypasses outside the infectious process.[11] Inherent to the traditional and newer approaches to management is creation of an aortic stump, which may contain the infection and has the potential risk for subsequent rupture; placement of a bypass, prosthesis, or biologic tissue in the infected field, which maintains the potential for subsequent infection; or failure to remove the entire graft, which might have been involved in infection.

We have employed a technique that potentially avoids such problems. It involves in-line replacement of an aortic graft through clean plane by the retroperitoneal approach, followed by transperitoneal removal of the infected prosthesis and debridement, keeping the two fields separate from each other.[12] In this chapter, we present our experience with in-line aortic graft replacement and compare it with other methods of treatment in a concurrent series.

Patient Information and Treatment Options

Between 1987 and 1997, we performed 17 in-line graft replacements and compared the results with two other approaches: (1) the traditional technique of transabdominal removal of an infected aortic graft and extraanatomic bypass using axillobifemoral grafting[12] and (2) partial graft excision, with or without adjunctive bypass (as needed when the entire graft was not infected).[9] The patient information, including demographics, original surgery, clinical presentation, reoperative procedure, and results, was retrieved from our vascular registry and patient chart review.

A computed tomography (CT) scan or tagged leukocyte scan usually was obtained to document infection when a patient presented with signs and symptoms of graft infection. Arteriography was done to help formulate the management plan. In selected cases, patients with possible aortoenteric interactions were evaluated by gastrointestinal endoscopy. For some patients who presented with a sinus, sinograms were obtained.

Aortic in-line bypass was the procedure of choice and was considered for treating most aortic graft infections. A relative contraindication was the absence of adequate uninfected infrarenal aorta, a problem that can sometimes be circumvented by suprarenal aortic clamping and bypass, with or without renal and visceral revascularization.

When the infection was confined to one limb, we managed this graft with partial graft excision, debridement, drainage, and antibiotic therapy. One of the contraindications to the in-line bypass was CT evidence of extensive infection, soft tissue destruction, and fluid collection around the proximal aortic anastomosis. In such cases, we used traditional treatment of complete graft excision and axillobifemoral bypasses.

Surgical Technique

After induction of general endotracheal anesthesia with cardiovascular monitoring, patients were placed in a modified right lateral decubitus position. With the aid of a suction beanbag (Olympic Vac-Pac), patients were positioned with the left chest at about 45 to 60 degrees and the pelvis rotated 20 to 30 degrees relative to the plane of the table. The table break was positioned at the level of the iliac crest and flexed as necessary to open up the space between the rib cage and iliac crest.

The skin incision originated at the lateral edge of the rectus abdominous muscle, 5 cm below the umbilicus, and extended obliquely through the 10th intercostal space to or beyond the posterior axillary line. After division of the musculature, the peritoneum and left kidney were swept medially and cephalad. The aorta was approached above the level of the renal arteries, and dissection was carried out in a proximal to distal fashion. Such exposure allows for dissection of the aorta just below the renal arteries, without entering the infected field. When the original anastomosis bordered the left renal artery, the left crus was divided to permit access to the suprarenal aorta. With adequate length of the infrarenal aorta, two clamps may be placed approximately 1 cm apart below the renal arteries. Transection of the aorta, flush with the distal clamp, created a neck for the new anastomosis (Fig. 21–1). The distal aorta was oversewn with 3-0 polypropylene suture.

Extension of the infectious process to the level of the renal arteries mandates suprarenal clamping and renal reimplantation, polytetrafluoroethylene (PTFE) bypass, or both. Multiple Gram stains and bacterial cultures are obtained from the new site. If previous infected grafts were placed through the left flank, a right retroperitoneal in-line bypass was used when an uninfected infrarenal neck of aorta was available for crossclamping.

After the proximal anastomosis was completed, the graft limbs were tunneled through clean tissue planes to the appropriate level for distal anastomosis (Fig. 21–2). The left graft limb can be tunneled laterally under the inguinal

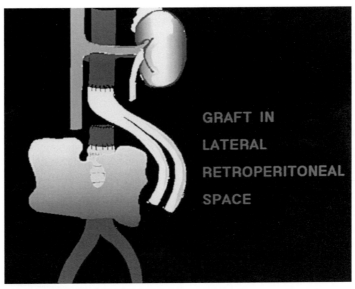

Figure 21-1. The diagram shows an in-line aortic graft replacement through a retroperitoneal approach in a clean field. Aortic root division was performed.

ligament into the sartorius sheath. Alternatively, the psoas fascia can be used as a path for the left graft limb. The right graft limb can be taken through the space of Retzius (ie, prevesical space). This graft limb is then passed medially under the inguinal ligament. If this space has been traversed by infection, the right limb can be passed retroperitoneally over the inferior vena cava and out through a counterincision made on the right side, just above the anterosuperior iliac spine. The graft limb is then routed laterally under the inguinal ligament.

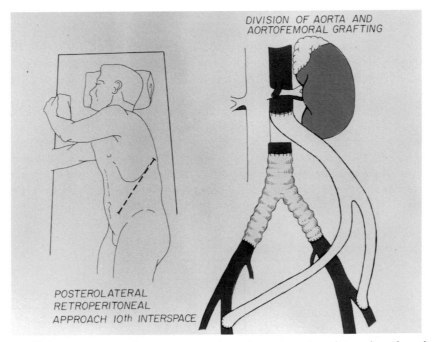

Figure 21-2. The diagram shows a new aortic graft anastomosis and tunneling through a noncontaminated area.

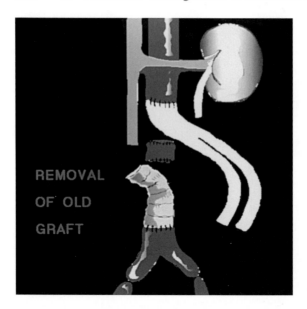

REMOVAL

OF OLD

GRAFT

Figure 21-3. An infected aortic graft is removed through a trans- peritoneal approach. The dia- gram shows graft removal after an in-line bypass is performed.

Distal anastomoses are carried out at uninfected sites. For infected aorto- femoral grafts, a lateral approach to the profunda femoris or superficial femoral artery avoids contact with the virulent field. Infected tube or aortoiliac grafts can be managed with bypassing to the common femoral or external iliac arteries.

On completion of the in-line bypass, the wounds are closed and dressed with a plastic barrier. The infected graft is then removed transabdominally with groin counterincisions as indicated (Fig. 21–3). Several weeks of appro- priate antibiotic therapy conclude the treatment. Patients are then monitored clinically with CT scans and tagged leukocyte scans at 6-month intervals.

Operative Results

Eleven men and 6 women, with an average age of 62 years (range, 47 to 73 years), received aortic in-line bypasses. Atherosclerotic risk factors are listed in Table 21–1. Time until presentation averaged 5.7 years (range, 5 months to 15 years).

Fifteen (88%) of the 17 original procedures were done through the transab- dominal route. The remaining two were done using a left retroperitoneal exposure (one aortobifemoral and one aortobiiliac). Clinical presentations (Table 21–2) varied, but 63% had some sort of groin involvement. Twenty-five percent of patients presented with gastrointestinal bleeding, though none of these patients' conditions was grossly unstable. At operation, eight patients

Table 21–1.
Demographics and Risk Factors

Risk Factor	Patients
Male/female	11/6
Heart disease	7 (44%)
Diabetes	4 (25%)
Hypertension	9 (56%)
Smoker	14 (87%)
Age	62 yr (range, 47–73)

Table 21–2.
Clinical Presentation

Clinical Presentation	Patients
Groin process, including sinus, mass, and infection	8 (47%)
Gastrointestinal bleeding	4 (25%)
Sepsis	1 (6%)
Graft occlusion	1 (6%)
Combination of above	3 (19%)
Total	17

had evidence of an aortoenteric fistula or erosion. Seven patients had mixed gram-positive and gram-negative infections, three had *Staphylococcus epidermidis* infections only, three had *Staphylococcus aureus* infections only, two had *S. epidermidis* and *S. aureus* infections, and one had only anaerobic infections.

All reoperative procedures (Table 21–3) entailed initial in-line revascularization, followed by same-day or staged removal of the infected graft. All patients with episodes of gastrointestinal bleeding had their aortoenteric processes dealt with at the time of graft removal. The 15 transabdominal cases were all treated through the left retroperitoneum, followed by transabdominal graft removal (eight at the same sitting, seven staged). Two cases required reimplantation of the left renal artery. A right retroperitoneal approach was employed in dealing with the other two cases done originally through the left flank. Both of the original operations, done for occlusive disease, left enough infrarenal aorta that in-line bypass could be performed through the right retroperitoneum.

There were no immediate postoperative deaths and no amputations. Two significant complications did occur: one duodenal tear and one case of necrotizing fasciitis. Both patients died; one death was related to sepsis 2 months after the operation, and the other resulted from myocardial infarction 5 months after surgery.

Follow-up averaged 36 months (range, 2 to 120 months) for the remaining 15 patients. Twelve (78%) are still alive, with no recurrent graft infection. Four (28%) patients developed isolated graft limb thromboses that required surgical intervention. One (7%) of these patients, who had severe multilevel disease and needed an infrainguinal bypass at the time of the in-line bypass, required

Table 21–3.
Reoperative Procedures

Procedure	Patients	
	Staged	*Combined*
Left retroperitoneal in-line aortobifemoral bypass and transabdominal graft removal	2 (12%)	8 (47%)
Left retroperitoneal in-line aortobifemoral bypass plus left renal artery reimplantation and transabdominal graft removal	2 (12%)	0
Left retroperitoneal in-line aortobifemoral bypass plus in situ femoral–posterior tibial bypass and transabdominal graft removal	1 (6%)	0
Left retroperitoneal in-line aortoiiliac (external iliacs) bypass and transabdominal graft removal	0	2 (12%)
Right retroperitoneal in-line aortobifemoral bypass and transabdominal graft removal	2 (12%)	0

an above-knee amputation at 3 months. At the time of these operations, infection was not clinically evident. All surveillance test results have been negative.

Extraanatomic Bypass and Complete Graft Removal

Twelve patients had extraanatomic bypasses coupled with complete graft removal. The mean age was 68 years (range, 45 to 80 years). These patients tended to present earlier than the in-line bypass group (average, 3.6 years). Clinical presentations varied. Five (42%) patients had a septic component. There were three (24%) perioperative deaths, all related to sepsis. Another patient died 4 months after surgery. The remaining eight patients did well, without any episodes of graft infection or limb loss.

Partial Graft Excision With or Without Revascularization

Nine patients who had partial graft excisions, with or without revascularization, had an average age of 66 years at the time of surgery. Seven (78%) presented with some type of groin infectious process, a pseudoaneurysm (four) or groin drainage (three). Five patients were managed with partial graft excision and bypass around the infected field; the other four patients were treated only with partial graft excision, and limbs remained viable through collateral blood supply. No perioperative deaths occurred. One patient died 7 months after surgery. The other eight patients did well, with no known episodes of reinfection or limb loss.

Achievements and Complications of Alternative Approaches

Intracavitary aortic bypass infections mandate total graft excision coupled with a revascularization procedure to the lower extremities. Management has traditionally consisted of graft removal and extraanatomic bypass. Such operations have been performed in combined or staged fashions with revascularization preceding or following graft removal.[1–3] Of all these variations, it appears that extraanatomic bypass followed by staged complete graft removal affords the best results. Reilly and colleagues[3] have the largest experience with this approach, reporting a 16% mortality rate and 23% amputation rate. Even with the implementation of the "best case scenario," the risk for aortic stump blowout still exists.

O'Hara and associates,[2] in reporting a large study, observed that aortic stump blowout accounted for 32% of the deaths of patients operated for aortoenteric fistulas. Creative techniques to secure the stump closure (ie, jejunal patch, omental patch, or prevertebral fascia flap) may lessen the risk of blowout but do not necessarily avoid it.[13, 14]

Vascular surgeons' concern about the significant complication rates provided the impetus to develop alternative strategies for managing infected aortic grafts. Such techniques combine removal of infected graft with in situ conduit replacement. Autogenous in situ reconstructions employ various conduits, such as native endarterectomized aortoiliac vessels, iliac or common femoral arteries, and superficial or deep veins from the lower extremities.[5, 6, 9] Clagett and coworkers[5] reported their experience with the creation of a neo-aortoiliac system from lower extremity deep and superficial veins. Hospital mortality and amputation rates of 10% support its efficacy, though conduit stenosis is of concern with greater saphenous vein reconstructions, and chronic limb edema may complicate deep vein harvests.

In situ bypass with prosthetic has gained popularity in certain centers. Key to embarking on such a procedure is assessment of the severity of graft infection. Jacobs and colleagues[7] demonstrated that in situ bypasses of severe aortic graft infections were prone to reinfection; for six patients, the reinfection rate was 100%, and the mortality rate was 83%. However, low virulent processes could be bypassed safely; among 12 patients, no reinfection or deaths occurred. These observations are echoed in the report of Bandyk,[4] who successfully treated 17 coagulase-negative staphylococcal graft infections (a low-virulence organism). The prosthetic in situ bypass affords good results when the operative field is not grossly contaminated. In highly contaminated cases, cadaveric allograft may be more resistant to reinfection.[6, 8, 9]

Although an in situ reconstruction avoids creation of an aortic stump and achieves good results in relatively less virulent infection, it is not as desirable in high-virulence situations. The retroperitoneal in-line PTFE bypass through clean tissue planes, followed by transabdominal graft removal, avoids creation of an aortic stump and traversing an infected field in all intracavitary and severe extracavitary aortic graft infections. We define severe extracavitary infections as high-virulence situations, cases in which the entire graft limb appears to be involved with infection, or any possible involvement of the intracavitary graft. No 30-day deaths, and only two (12%) early deaths speak to its safe performance. Moreover, of the 15 long-term survivors, only 1 (7%) required an amputation, and no episodes of reinfection have become evident.

Theoretically, certain conditions are to be satisfied for the performance of in-line bypass for infected aortic grafts. An adequate amount of the uninfected aorta should be present between the proximal infected suture line and renal arteries to allow for division and anastomosis in a clean field. In one instance, however, a proximal anastomotic infection that bordered the left renal artery was dealt with by suprarenal clamping and transection of the aorta above the left renal but below the right, followed by aortic anastomosis with left renal reimplantation. Another patient who had had a left nephrectomy and had an aortic graft infection extending to the right renal artery was treated initially with a transabdominal hepatorenal bypass, followed by retroperitoneal supra-renal aortic transection and bypass and then with transabdominal graft removal.

In-line bypass is contraindicated when the CT appearance of the infectious process suggests that it would not be possible to stay out of the abscess cavity when placing the new graft. The patient should be in relatively stable condition so that the clean part of the operation can be performed before tending to aortic bleeding when an aortoenteric fistula exists. Routing of the graft limbs usually does not pose a major problem, because careful planning allows graft placement through clean areas.

When the graft infection is localized and less virulent, some patients can receive conservative treatment with antimicrobial therapy, with or without partial graft removal and bypass when the collateral circulation is inadequate. This management strategy has proved successful in prospective series,[11] and our limited experience supports this concept. However, this therapeutic approach is not possible in cases of virulent and whole graft infection.

Conclusions

Retroperitoneal PTFE in-line aortic bypass for aortic graft infection has provided satisfactory early results, with no immediate mortality and morbidity. Follow-up of 10 years reveals no evidence of reinfection. When technically feasible, it is an optimal choice for dealing with severe aortic graft infections.

References

1. Curl GR, Ricotta JJ. Total prosthetic graft excision and extra-anatomic bypass. *In* Calligaro KD, Veith FJ (eds). Management of Infected Arterial Grafts. St. Louis: Quality Medical Publishing, 1994:82-94.
2. O'Hara PJ, Hertzer NR, Beven EG, et al. Surgical management of infected abdominal aortic grafts: review of a 25-year experience. J Vasc Surg 1986;37:25-31.
3. Reilly LM, Stoney RJ, Goldstone J, et al. Improved management of aortic graft infection: the influence of operation sequence and staging. J Vasc Surg 1987;5:421-431.
4. Bandyk DF, Bergamini TM, Kinney EV, et al. In situ replacement of vascular prostheses infected by bacterial biofilms. J Vasc Surg 1991;13:575-583.
5. Clagett GP, Bowers BL, Lopez-Viego MA, et al. Creation of a neo-aortoiliac system from lower extremity deep and superficial veins. Ann Surg 1993;218:239-249.
6. Ehrenfeld WK, Wilbur BG, Olcott CN IV, et al. Autogenous tissue reconstruction in the management of infected prosthetic grafts. Surgery 1979;85:82-92.
7. Jacobs MJ, Reul GJ, Gregoric I, et al. In situ replacement of extra-anatomic bypass for the treatment of infected abdominal aortic grafts. Eur J Vasc Surg 1991;5:83-86.
8. Kieffer E, Bahnini A, Koskas F, et al. In situ allograft replacement of infected infrarenal aortic prosthetic grafts: results in forty-three patients. J Vasc Surg 1993;17:349-356.
9. Seeger JM, Wheeler JR, Gregory RT, et al. Autogenous graft replacement of infected prosthetic grafts in the femoral position. Surgery 1983;93:39-45.
10. Walker WE, Cooley DA, Duncan JM, et al. The management of aortoduodenal fistula by in situ replacement of the infected abdominal aortic graft. Ann Surg 1987;205:727-732.
11. Calligaro KD, Veith FJ, Schwartz ML, et al. Selective preservation of infected prosthetic arterial grafts–analysis of a 20-year experience with 120 extracavitary-infected grafts. Ann Surg 1994;220:461-471.
12. Leather RP, Darling RC III, Chang BB, et al. Retroperitoneal in-line bypass for treatment of infected infrarenal aortic grafts. Surg Gynecol Obstet 1992;175:491-494.
13. Buchbinder D, Leather R, Shah D, et al. Pathologic interactions between prosthetic aortic grafts and the gastrointestinal tract. Am J Surg 1980;140:192-198.
14. Goldsmith HS, de los Santos R, Beattie EJ, et al. Experimental protection of vascular prosthesis by omentum. Arch Surg 1968;97:872-874.

Prevention and Treatment of Aortic Graft–Enteric Fistula

Steven M. Santilli, M.D., Ph.D., Eugene S. Lee, M.D., and Jerry Goldstone, M.D.

One of the late complications of aortic reconstruction surgery is development of a fistula between the aortic graft and the intestine. These secondary aortic graft–enteric fistulas, although rare, are the most lethal complication of aortic reconstruction. They are usually encountered under urgent or emergency conditions and are difficult to manage for even the most experienced vascular surgeon.

Aortic graft–enteric fistulas are classified as primary or secondary aortoenteric fistulas (AEFs). Primary AEFs are rare, occur in the absence of prior aortic surgery, and usually involve erosion of a large aortic aneurysm into the duodenum.

Secondary AEFs are caused by erosion of a vascular prosthesis or suture line into a segment of adjacent bowel. In 1953, Brock first described a case of AEF after aortic replacement with a homograft, and in 1956, Clayton reported the first AEF after the implantation of a synthetic graft. The first successful treatment of this condition was reported by McKenzie in 1958. During the past 35 years, sufficient data have accumulated to estimate the incidence, pathogenesis, clinical presentation, diagnosis, and management of this condition.[1–4]

Incidence

The incidence of AEF is difficult to determine from the literature because of the long interval between graft implantation and the onset of clinical manifestations, because the fistulas are rare, and because patients commonly are not treated by the same surgeons for the graft implantation and complications. In one series, the average time between graft implantation and treatment of AEF was 6.1 years.[5] AEFs develop in approximately one third of cases of aortic graft infections, and aortic graft infections are thought to occur in 1% to 2% of patients who undergo aortic graft placement. The estimated incidence of AEF occurring after primary prosthetic aortic graft implantation is 0.3% to 0.6%.[5–7] Primary AEFs are even less common, with only about 200 cases reported in the world's literature.

The authors acknowledge the assistance of Connie Lindberg in the preparation of the manuscript.

Pathophysiology

Infection and mechanical erosion of the graft into the bowel are the primary causes of AEF formation. Hematogenous seeding of a graft, although experimentally achievable, probably accounts for few aortic graft infections. Most infected grafts are caused by contamination at the time of implantation. Graft contamination may also occur during secondary vascular reconstructive procedures, usually reoperations in the groin for occluded graft limbs. Graft limb reoperations have contributed to subsequent aortic graft infections in 40% to 46% of cases.[7, 8]

Once initiated, the graft infection spreads along the graft to the graft-artery anastomosis, eventually leading to formation of a pseudoaneurysm. As the pseudoaneurysm enlarges, it becomes adherent to and erodes into the previously mobilized, scarred, and fixed duodenum, producing a fistula. Fistulas that occur between the aortic suture line and the bowel are classified as *anastomotic AEFs*, and they most frequently involve the third or fourth portions of the duodenum. Other enteric sites occasionally involved in fistula formation because of their proximity to the graft limbs include the cecum, sigmoid colon, and appendix. Another possible cause of anastomotic AEFs is the anteriorly pointed suture "whiskers" from the cut ends of sutures that erode into overlying bowel. Another type of AEF is the so-called *periprosthetic aortoenteric erosion*, which occurs when a graft lies in direct contact with and erodes into a loop of bowel distant from the suture lines. These fistulas appear to be primarily mechanically induced, although infection may also play an important role in their pathogenesis.[9, 10]

In one series,[5] secondary AEFs occurred with equal frequency after aortofemoral or aortoiliac grafts, but AEF formation after tube (aortic-aortic) grafts was rare. Primary indications for the initial aortic operations were equally divided between aneurysmal and occlusive disease, and end-to-end aortic anastomoses were found to be twice as common as end-to-side anastomoses. Additional factors contributing to the development of graft infection and fistula formation, including emergency aortic reconstruction and subsequent reoperations on an aortic graft, were present in 67% of cases in this series.[5]

Prevention

Prevention is directed toward eliminating factors associated with AEF development. Aortic graft infections may be prevented by minimizing the chance of graft contamination at the time of graft implantation by using strict sterile technique and by proper patient preparation before operation, including prophylactic antibiotics and avoidance of contact of the graft with the skin. Although not supported by solid clinical data, soaking coated polyester grafts in an antibiotic solution before implantation has been associated with a reduced incidence of graft infection.[11] Suture line fistulas resulting from anastomotic suture whisker erosion may be prevented by interposing aneurysm wall (if available) or retroperitoneal tissue between the suture line and the peritoneal contents. Another technique is to slide a collar graft over the anastomotic area.

Interpositioning retroperitoneal tissue between the graft and the peritoneal contents can prevent aortoenteric erosions. This is accomplished by appropriate tunneling of graft limbs and by closure of retroperitoneal tissue, including the aneurysm sac when present, over the aortic graft to isolate it from the anteriorly located abdominal contents. Close attention to these and all other aspects of the operative procedure helps prevent infection and AEF formation after aortic graft placement.

Clinical Presentation

Patients with AEF may present with symptoms varying from nonspecific complaints to sudden, exsanguinating hemorrhage and sepsis. AEF usually is a more unstable, more septic, and more deadly clinical entity than an aortic graft infection alone. The most frequent presenting symptoms and findings in one report were positive blood or wound cultures (78.3%), gastrointestinal bleeding (66.7%), fever (66.7%), fever and chills (60.6%), and malaise (34.4%). Hemodynamic instability was demonstrated in only 12% of patients with AEFs, though most had systemic signs of sepsis.[5] In another series, the clinical manifestations were more subtle in a significant number of patients.

The clinical presentation varies with the type of AEF or periprosthetic erosion. For example, MacBeth and coworkers[9] found gastrointestinal bleeding in 14 of 15 patients with anastomotic AEFs but in only 50% of patients with aortoenteric erosions.

Clinical suspicion is extremely important in the evaluation and treatment of patients with AEF, especially because the signs and symptoms can be vague. For patients with aortic grafts who are clinically septic or who have gastrointestinal bleeding, the clinical diagnosis should be graft infection until proven otherwise. A patient with sepsis is more likely to have a fistula than a perigraft infection alone, but a patient with gastrointestinal bleeding does not necessarily have a fistula, because septic stresses associated with a perigraft infection may result in gastrointestinal bleeding from peptic ulcer disease, gastritis, or other stress erosions in the bowel. Not all graft AEFs bleed; gastrointestinal bleeding can occur in the absence of AEF; and demonstration of another cause of gastrointestinal bleeding does not exclude the diagnosis of AEF. These ideas are confirmed by results of a series demonstrating that only 66.7% of patients with proven AEF had any gastrointestinal bleeding (48.5% of these patients had acute bleeding, 15% had chronic blood loss, and 6.1% had occult blood loss), but 11% of patients with infected aortic grafts bled in the absence of a fistula.[5]

Diagnosis

Any patient with gastrointestinal bleeding at any time after an aortic operation, especially surgery involving placement of a prosthetic graft, should have graft infection and AEF placed high on the list of differential diagnoses, and this diagnosis should not be discarded until there is proof excluding this pathologic process. Unfortunately, even in experienced centers, the preoperative diagnosis of AEF is made in only about one third of patients with this disorder.[5, 6, 10, 12]

The diagnosis of AEF requires a high level of intuitiveness, a thorough history, and a careful physical examination. The most reliable abdominal physical finding is a pulsatile abdominal mass, which points to the presence of a pseudoaneurysm, but this finding is rarely encountered. Assessment then requires one or more diagnostic studies, which may include esophagogastroduodenoscopy (EDG), computed tomography (CT), or magnetic resonance imaging (MRI) of the abdomen and pelvis and eventually may include arteriography.

EGD is the most important diagnostic test when gastrointestinal hemorrhage exists. The test can be performed in the intensive care unit while the patient is undergoing resuscitation and is being prepared for operation or in the operating room immediately before operation. EGD, performed by an experienced endoscopist with the surgeon in attendance, requires a thorough examination to the level of the distal duodenum. AEFs are typically found in the third and fourth portions of the duodenum but have no typical appearance. They can appear as ragged mucosa, as a red spot, or rarely, as graft material seen protruding through the bowel wall (which clearly establishes the diagnosis). The presence of a nonfistulous source of upper gastrointestinal bleeding (eg, peptic ulcer disease, gastritis) does not exclude AEF.

The EGD must be complete and include the fourth portion of the duodenum. In some cases, ongoing bleeding from an uncertain source in the third or fourth portion of the duodenum is the only abnormality found. The diagnosis of AEF is established when the fistula is seen or a bleeding site is identified in the distal duodenum with an entirely normal esophagus, stomach, and proximal duodenum. Using these criteria, one study found that EGD was abnormal in more than one-half the patients who had secondary AEF; however, graft material was seen in only two patients. The high false-negative rates of EGD in part result from the fact that endoscopy to the fourth portion of the duodenum has seldom been documented in reported series.[5]

A CT scan with intravenous contrast directly assesses the retroperitoneum, perigraft space, and the relationship between the duodenum or other bowel segments and the graft (Fig. 22–1). Normal CT findings do not exclude an AEF or graft infection. Findings that strongly suggest the diagnosis of an infection include perigraft fluid for more than 2 to 3 months and perigraft gas for more than 2 to 3 weeks after aortic surgery; an increase in perigraft soft tissue; pseudoaneurysm formation; loss of the continuous aneurysm wrap around the graft; thickening of the adjacent bowel wall; and prosthetic graft erosion into the lumen.[5, 6, 13, 14] Gas around a graft is more likely to be caused by AEF than a gas-forming organism. One series demonstrated that CT scans were abnormal in all cases of AEF but diagnostic in only 8 of 33 cases.[5]

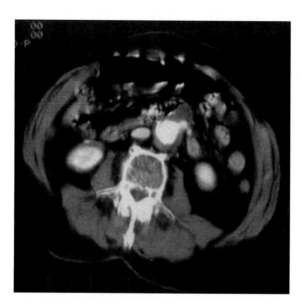

Figure 22–1. Computed tomography (CT) scan of a patient who had a Dacron aortofemoral graft placed 4 years earlier. He presented with upper gastrointestinal bleeding in the fourth portion of the duodenum. This CT scan demonstrates a pseudoaneurysm of the proximal graft anastomosis, which protrudes anteriorly and is adjacent to the duodenum. At laparotomy, he was found to have a pseudoaneurysm of the proximal anastomosis with erosion into the duodenum.

Magnetic Resonance Imaging

Since its first reported use in the diagnosis of prosthetic graft infection in 1985, there has been much interest in MRI for this purpose. The most useful feature of MRI is its ability to distinguish between fluid and surrounding tissue and thereby provide information about inflammatory reactions involving perigraft tissues. Neither CT nor ultrasonography are able to reliably distinguish between high-attenuation fluid and soft tissue without the additional invasive step of needle aspiration.

Perigraft tissue producing low signal intensity on T1- and T2-weighted images is considered to represent perigraft fibrosis or the wall of the native aorta wrapped around the graft. Perigraft fluid is seen as low to medium intensity on T1-weighted images and as high intensity on T2-weighted images. Inflammation in the surrounding tissue is characterized by nonhomogenously increased signal intensity and is a subtle clue to infection of an adjacent prosthesis such as retroperitoneal muscles adjacent to the graft (Fig. 22–2).

Olofsson and colleagues[15] prospectively compared the accuracy of MRI and CT in 18 of patients in whom retroperitoneal graft infections were confirmed or excluded by surgery. The presence and the extent of prosthetic graft infections were identified by MRI in 14 of 16 patients and correctly excluded in the other two. CT was accurate in only 5 of 12 patients and indeterminate or incorrect in the remaining six. Criteria for determining infection were fluid in the perigraft space and any concurrent inflammation seen in proximity to this fluid. CT and MRI were equally and completely accurate in confirming the absence of infection in the groin. When compared with the previously mentioned CT study by Low and associates,[14] it appears that the CT criteria used to assess the presence or absence of infection by Olofsson[15] were not nearly as inclusive, and this may explain the different results of the two studies.

In another prospective study of 24 patients with probable graft infections who eventually underwent surgery, there were 20 prosthetic graft infections documented at exploration. MRI correctly identified 17 of these. In the remaining three patients, prosthetic graft infection was diagnosed during sur-

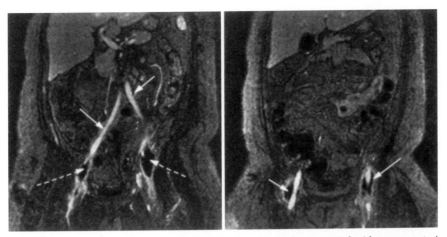

Figure 22–2. Magnetic resonance imaging (MRI) of a patient who presented with upper gastrointestinal bleeding with no identifiable source. This MRI documents a graft infection. The *solid arrows* show the limbs of the aortofemoral graft surrounded by perigraft inflammation. The *dashed arrows* demonstrate purulent material *(dark areas)* surrounding the limbs of the graft in the groins.

gery on the basis of lack of graft adherence to the perigraft fibrous capsule or overlying wrapped wall of native aorta. Four patients underwent exploration based on strong clinical indications; they were not found to have evidence of prosthetic graft infection, and MRI correctly excluded the diagnosis in all four cases. A specificity of 85% and a sensitivity of 100% were achieved. Corroborating the findings of previous CT studies, MRI documented that fluid normally should not be present around the graft 3 to 4 months after implantation.

Although accurate, MRI has limitations. It is unable to distinguish between gas and atherosclerotic calcifications, because both reveal a signal void seen as a black dot. Another limitation, although not unique to MRI, is its inability to detect AEF. Some patients are unable to tolerate the closed space and the lengthy scanning sessions needed to acquire adequate MRI data. The newer generation of "open" magnets may solve this problem. Despite these limitations, MRI is probably the most accurate of all direct imaging methods for determining the presence or absence of infection involving a retroperitoneal prosthetic arterial graft (Figs. 22–2 and 22–3).

Functional Imaging

Functional imaging studies using radioisotopes can detect inflammatory activity at the site of an arterial graft and its environment. Several isotopes and labels have been used for this purpose, including scans with gallium 67

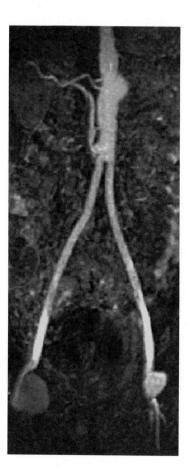

Figure 22–3. Magnetic resonance arteriogram of a patient with an aortoenteric fistula documents pseudoaneurysms at the proximal anastomosis and both distal anastomoses.

citrate, indium 111–labeled leukocytes, and indium 111–labeled immunoglobulin G.

Though arteriography is critical for planning a well thought out, carefully executed vascular reconstruction, it is not an important study for the diagnosis of AEF. In some series, arteriographic results were abnormal (usually a normal aortic lumen or an anastomotic false aneurysm) in 40% of cases but diagnostic in none[5] (Fig. 22–4). It is rare to find extravasation of dye into the intestinal lumen.[16] For purposes of the vascular reconstruction that is required to treat AEF, arteriography should visualize the entire abdominal aorta, the aortic graft, native vessels, and runoff into the lower extremities.

Most series reveal that institution of definitive treatment is usually delayed. In one report, the typical elapsed time between the onset of symptoms and definitive operative treatment was 84.8 days,[5] with most of the time delay occurring before referral for definitive treatment. Despite this relatively long delay before definitive treatment, relatively few patients required emergency treatment of their AEFs, and appropriate diagnostic studies were completed in most cases.[5] In septic or bleeding patients, EGD, CT or MRI, and arteriography can be accomplished within a few hours after admission, usually while the patient is being prepared for operation with fluid resuscitation and placement of appropriate invasive monitors.

Treatment

Preoperative Preparation

Surgical treatment should occur promptly after the diagnosis of AEF is strongly suspected or confirmed. Hematologic resuscitation with blood products should be guided by preoperative and ongoing laboratory evaluation. Although some patients have nutritional deficiencies because of their long illness, operations should not be delayed for nutritional replacement. All patients require broad-spectrum antibiotic coverage as soon as the diagnosis is suspected. Antibiotics should be effective against gram-positive (including *Staphylococcus epidermidis*, the most common organism responsible for vascular prosthetic graft infections),[2, 5, 6, 9, 12] gram-negative, and other enteric bacteria,

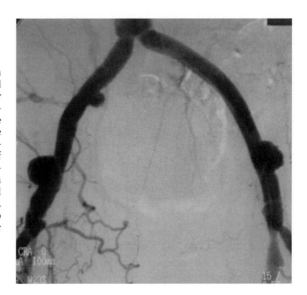

Figure 22–4. Arteriogram of a patient who had an aortofemoral bypass placed 20 years earlier and presented with lower gastrointestinal bleeding. The source was identified as proximal to the ileocecal valve. Arteriography revealed three pseudoaneurysms of the graft material not at the anastomotic sites. At operation, an aortoenteric fistula was identified between the small, proximal, right pseudoaneursm and two aortoenteric erosions at the larger pseudoaneurysms.

as well as any organism that has been cultured from draining wounds, aspirated perigraft fluid collections, or blood. Antibiotic coverage should remain quite broad until definitive intraoperative culture and sensitivity data are available, at which time antibiotic treatment can be tailored to the particular case.

Reconstructive Options

Autogenous tissue is the only material that can reliably be safely used when the vascular repair or reconstruction must traverse an infected field. Saphenous vein or endarterectomized superficial femoral artery are most often used as patches for repair of partial arterial wall defects (only with end-to-side anastomoses). Autogenous reconstruction can be performed by endarterectomizing previously bypassed native vessels or by autograft replacement of infected arteries with the saphenous vein (which can be fashioned into a large caliber by sewing segments together in a side-to-side or spiral manner), the superficial femoral vein, or a segment of endarterectomized superficial femoral artery.

Our preference is to use externally supported polytetrafluorethylene (PTFE) to construct an axillobifemoral revascularization of the lower extremities. We do not routinely perform arteriographic assessment of the axillary or subclavian arteries as donor vessels for axillobifemoral bypass; we instead rely on bilateral arm blood pressures to prevent placing the axillary anastomosis distal to a subclavian stenosis. Prosthetic materials should only be used outside of all infected fields, and a completely prosthetic revascularization is only possible when infected graft is confined to the aortic or aortoiliac position. If the femoral arteries are involved in the infectious process, the axillofemoral limb of the graft must be tunneled away from the infected field to the profunda femoris or middle to distal superficial femoral artery if it is patent.

An autogenous cross-femoral graft can then be constructed using the greater saphenous vein, superficial femoral vein, or endarterectomized, previously occluded, superficial femoral artery. These groin reconstructions can be extremely challenging and technically difficult, but long-term patency is better than when bilateral axillofemoral grafts are used.

Debate continues about the optimal method of treatment of AEF because of the continued publication of series with high mortality, amputation, and aortic stump disruption rates.[17-21] An operative plan should be chosen that is tailored to the patient's manifestations of fistula and infection and the existing vascular pathology. The goals of treatment are to prevent death due to hemorrhage and sepsis and then to prevent limb loss from ischemia.

Treatment Options

The traditional treatment plan for AEF consists of removal of the infected graft, repair of the fistula, and immediate extraanatomic bypass for revascularization of the lower extremities. One report challenged the traditional approach and recommended that the sequence be reversed, with extraanatomic bypass being performed first, followed by transabdominal removal of the infected graft and repair of the fistula. The time between lower extremity revascularization and infected graft excision may be immediate or staged, usually with 3 to 5 days between operations. A third treatment option, which has been proposed for selected patients, is in situ reconstruction with concomitant infected graft removal and repair of the enteric fistula.

The choice of operative therapy is primarily dictated by the clinical status of the patient. Treatment priorities are resuscitation of the unstable patient, control of bleeding, control of sepsis, and infected graft removal and revascularization of the lower extremities.

If the patient is actively bleeding and hemodynamically unstable, transabdominal control of the aorta must be accomplished first, followed by graft removal and fistula repair. Extremity revascularization then follows, using fresh sterile instruments and drapes. The staged treatment sequence usually is contraindicated in this circumstance, but controlling hemorrhage and repair of the fistula without graft excision sometimes can be a lifesaving initial operative procedure, with definitive care performed after stabilization of the patient.

Most patients present in a stable clinical state, eligible for an elective or semi-urgent procedure. The method of operative treatment (eg, traditional or reversed, staged or not staged) depends largely on the surgeon's preference. An AEF does not make the reversed staged approach unfeasible, because one third of patients with fistulas have no evidence of bleeding. Exsanguinating hemorrhage from the rupture of an aortic false aneurysm in the interval between extraanatomic bypass and removal of the infected aortic graft is rare.[5]

The overall mortality rates for the traditional approach to the treatment of AEF remain greater than 50%, with associated amputation rates of 8% to 10% and rates of aortic stump disruption averaging 21.6%.[17–21] These outcomes are based on small series that accumulate patients over long periods, and pooling these data does not provide a clear picture of the outcomes that can be achieved using a single consistent treatment plan. However, the data do suggest unacceptably high morbidity and mortality rates after the traditional one-stage approach to repair of AEF.

A contemporary series of patients with secondary AEF treated, whenever possible, with the reversed staged approach (ie, extraanatomic bypass [axillofemoral] first, followed several days later by infected graft excision and closure of the fistula) showed improved results. The perioperative death rate was 18.2%, the amputation rate and incidence of late deaths related to aortic graft infection were 9%, and the incidence of aortic stump disruption was 6%. Cumulative survival rates were 74.5% at 1 year, which stabilized and remained constant at 70% at 3 years (ie, this is essentially the cure rate). There were six failures of the extraanatomic bypass (two perioperatively, and four during late follow-up, an incidence of 18.2%), and one patient required a late amputation. The cumulative 4-year primary patency rate was 71%, and the secondary patency rate was 89.6%.[5]

Not all patients are candidates for the reversed staged procedure. A patient who presents with active bleeding that cannot be controlled or stabilized must be taken immediately to the operating room, the bleeding controlled, and the graft removed, followed by revascularization. Stable patients with active bleeding that stops can be considered for the reversed staged approach. The timing between extraanatomic bypass and infected graft removal depends on the clinical situation, but the interval should be kept as short as the patient's condition allows, usually 2 to 4 days. This short delay appears to confer some benefit in allowing the patient to recover physiologically from the first operation and thereby contribute to the lower morbidity and mortality rates associated with this technique.[5]

In situ reconstruction for secondary AEF has been reported in several small studies,[22–26] with only two studies using in situ prosthetic graft replacement exclusively.[24, 26] The most likely candidates are those with infection caused by low-virulence bacteria (eg, *S. epidermidis*) and no abscess around the graft. The reported morbidity and mortality rates were 30.4%, and the overall cure rate was 56.5%. This is a relatively new approach that requires further consideration and study. The advent of coated Dacron grafts with bonded antibiotics for slow, delayed release may make in situ graft replacement a more attractive option in the future.[5]

An approach introduced by Clagett and colleagues[27] employs superficial femoral veins as autogenous conduits for immediate revascularization of the lower extremities. The diameter and wall thickness make this an excellent aortic replacement, and its use has not been associated with significant lower extremity edema. Early results have been excellent, but most of the patients have had perigraft infection without accompanying AEF. Similar excellent results have been reported by Nevelsteen and coworkers from Belgium.[28]

An alternative approach by Kieffer and associates[29] uses preserved aortic homografts to replace infected prostheses. Originally introduced as a temporary bridge for eventual prosthetic in situ replacement, the results have been so good that very few of the homografts have had to be replaced, and it appears that this may be an effective long-term solution to the challenging problem of AEF.

Principles of Extraanatomic Bypass

Axillofemoral bypass is the most practical and reliable method for restoring circulation to the lower extremities in the presence of AEF. A 7- to 8-mm, externally reinforced PTFE graft has become our preference and the preference of several other groups for this purpose. The site of origin of the graft should be as far medial as possible on the inferior surface of the axillary artery. When AEF involves an aortoiliac graft, the groins are usually unaffected, and the femoral anastomosis is made to the common femoral artery. The absence of groin sepsis allows the cross-femoral limb to be synthetic. It should originate as close to the donor femoral anastomosis as possible. Use of an inverted C or gentle S configuration has not been shown to adversely affect long-term patency rates. Occasionally, the common iliac arteries can be sewn together to form an in situ autogenous femoral-femoral bypass.

When one or both femoral regions are involved with the infectious process, the reconstruction must be modified to avoid contamination of the axillofemoral graft. This is accomplished by routing the graft laterally out of the contaminated groin to the middle of the profunda femoris or superficial femoral artery (if patent). An autogenous cross-femoral graft constructed of saphenous vein, superficial femoral vein, or endarterectomized, previously occluded superficial femoral artery can then originate and terminate on the common femoral arteries, often using the anastomotic sites of the removed aortofemoral graft limbs. Whenever possible, retrograde perfusion of at least one iliac system should be maintained to ensure adequate pelvic circulation.

Principles of Aortic Graft–Enteric Fistula Repair and Infected Graft Removal

Graft removal and fistula repair are usually accomplished through a full-length midline incision. Proximal aortic control can be easily obtained at the supraceliac level when needed. Control of the distal graft limbs is followed by control of the fistula. This requires dissecting the graft from the adherent segment of the gastrointestinal tract. The bowel usually can be repaired primarily with a standard two-layer technique, but it must be done carefully to prevent subsequent breakdown and leakage. A large defect in the duodenum may require serosal patching and, in some cases, duodenal resection with an end-to-end anastomosis or a duodenojejunostomy. Placement of a feeding jejunostomy allows early postoperative enteral feeding while protecting the duodenal repair.

After vascular control and fistula repair, the infected aortic graft is completely removed and the segments are submitted for bacteriologic analysis. The most critical feature of aortic graft removal is the technique for handling the aortic stump, because the leading cause of perioperative death and late mortality from the treatment of AEF is dehiscence of the aortic stump. Most series report a low incidence of aortic stump disruption, but it has an associated mortality of 100%.[5, 17–21] Adequate debridement of the aortic stump is essential for a secure and durable closure. This occasionally necessitates relocating one or both renal arteries. Proximal portions of the debrided aortic wall should also be sent for culture, sensitivity analysis, and Gram's stain.

The aorta must be closed without tension using a double row of nonabsorbable, monofilament sutures: one row of horizontal mattress and the other of simple running sutures placed into healthy tissue. Temporary crossclamping of the suprarenal or supraceliac aorta is usually required to ensure adequate infrarenal aortic tissue to sew. Various methods of aortic stump reinforcement (eg, jejunal serosal patch, anterior spinal ligament patch, omental pedicle) may be helpful but have not yet proven beneficial in reducing the incidence of stump disruption and are no substitute for proper aortic debridement and closure. If the original aortic anastomosis was an end-to-side procedure, the same principles apply, unless maintenance of distal aortic perfusion is necessary. Retention of distal aortic perfusion usually requires the use of a patch to ensure an adequate aortic lumen.

Retroperitoneal tissue should be debrided and drainage considered in all cases with conspicuous pus. Infected femoral wounds should have excision of all necrotic and infected tissue, and the wounds should be packed open with antibiotic-soaked dressings. When an autogenous conduit is in the femoral area, noninfected subcutaneous tissue should be loosely approximated over the graft, with the remainder of the wound left open. In cases requiring extensive debridement, wound closure using rotated or free muscle flaps is frequently necessary to prevent drying and erosion of exposed vessels and to ensure wound healing.

Long-term Follow-up

Patients with positive proximal aortic wall cultures require appropriate imaging studies at regular intervals. CT or MRI scans of the abdomen are recommended to identify persistent infection in or about the aortic stump or the formation of a pseudoaneurysm. The appropriate duration of antibiotic therapy has yet to be determined, but it is recommended that therapy should be continued for at least 3 to 6 months.

Late infections may occur after treatment of AEF and usually involve prosthetic portions of the extraanatomic reconstruction used to revascularize the lower extremities. Most new graft infections occurred in the midportions of the axillofemoral graft, where a counterincision had been made to facilitate subcutaneous tunneling.[30] Abandoning the use of the counterincision in treating axillofemoral graft infections has significantly decreased the incidence of secondary graft infections.[5] The new graft infections occasionally have re-sulted in limb loss but have not been associated with death. For these reasons, patients should be reevaluated periodically for the remainder of their lives.

Conclusions

Secondary AEF is a rare and often lethal complication of prosthetic aortic reconstructions. It can manifest with a wide variety of symptoms. The diagnosis is definitively established in about one third of patients before operation. Treatment approaches include traditional repair, in which the graft is removed first and fistula repair by extraanatomic reconstruction immediately follows; reversed repair, which consists of extraanatomic bypass first, followed by infected graft removal and repair of the fistula; in situ repair, which consists of removal of the infected graft, repair of the fistula, and in situ vascular reconstruction using autologous material. We recommend the reversed staged approach, because it has significantly reduced the morbidity and mortality rates associated with this highly lethal condition.[5]

AEF remains a challenge for even the most experienced vascular surgeon, but successful treatment with long-term survival is possible in most cases. However, as with most devastating complications in vascular surgery, the most effective therapy is prevention.

References

1. Goldstone J, Effeney DJ. Prevention of arterial graft infections. *In* Bernhard VM, Towne JB (eds). Complications in Vascular Surgery. New York: Grune & Stratton; 1985:487.
2. Bergqvist D. Arterioenteric fistula. Acta Chir Scand 1987;153:81–86.
3. Connolly JE, Kwaan JHM, McCart PM, et al. Aortoenteric fistula. Ann Surg 1988;194:402.
4. O'Mara CS, Williams GM, Ernst CB. Secondary aortoenteric fistula: a 20-year experience. Am J Surg 1981;142:203.
5. Kuestner LM, Reilly LM, Jicha DL, et al. Secondary aortoenteric fistula: contemporary outcome with the use of extraanatomic bypass and infected graft excision. J Vasc Surg 1955;21:184.
6. Bunt TJ. Synthetic vascular graft infections. Secondary graft enteric erosions and graft enteric fistulas. Surgery 1983;94:1.
7. Reilly LM, Goldstone J, Ehrenfeld WK, et al. Gastrointestinal tract involvement by prosthetic graft infection: the significance of gastrointestinal hemorrhage. Ann Surg 1985;202:342.
8. Goldstone J, Moore WS. Infection in vascular prostheses: clinical manifestation and surgical management. Am J Surg 1974;128:228.
9. Macbeth GA, Rubin JR, McIntyre KE Jr, et al. The relevance of arterial wall microbiology to the treatment of prosthetic graft infections: graft infection vs. arterial infection. J Vasc Surg 1984;1:750.
10. Busuttil RW, Reese W, Baker JD, et al. Pathogenesis of aortoduodenal fistula. Experimental and clinical correlates. Surgery 1979;85:1–10.
11. Lachapelle K, Graham AM, Symes JF. Antibacterial activity, antibiotic retention, and infection resistance of a rifampin-impregnated gelatin-sealed Dacron graft. J Vasc Surg 1994;19:675–682.
12. Cooper A. The Lectures of Sir Astley Cooper on the Principles and Practice of Surgery with Additional Notes and Cases by Tyrell. 5th ed. Philadelphia: Haswell, Barrington, & Haswell, 1939.
13. Harris KA, Kozak R, Carrol SF, et al. Confirmation of infection of an aortic graft. J Cardiovasc Surg 1989;30:230.
14. Low RN, Wall SD, Jeffrey RB Jr, et al. Aortoenteric fistula and perigraft infection: evaluation with CT. Radiology 1990;175:157.
15. Olofsson P, Rabahie GN, Matsumoto K, et al. Histopathological characteristics of explanted human prosthetic arterial grafts: implications for the prevention and management of graft infections. Eur J Vasc Endovasc Surg 1995;9:143–151.
16. Kleinman LH, Towne JB, Bernhard VM. A diagnostic and therapeutic approach to aortoenteric fistulas: clinical experience with twenty patients. Surgery 1979;86:868.
17. O'Hara PJ, Hertzer NR, Beven EG, et al. surgical management of infected abdominal aortic grafts: review of a 25-year experience. J Vasc Surg 1986;3:725–731.
18. Plate G, Hollier LA, O'Brien P, et al. Recurrent aneurysms and late vascular complications following repair of abdominal aortic aneurysms. Arch Surg 1985;120:590–594.
19. Bergeron P, Espinoza H, Rudondy P, et al. Secondary aortoenteric fistulas: value of initial axillofemoral bypass. Ann Vasc Surg 1991;5:4–7.

20. Champion MC, Sullivan SN, Coles JC, et al. Aortoenteric fistulas. Incidence, presentation, recognition and management. Ann Surg 1982;195:314–317.
21. Trout HH III, Kozloff L, Giordano JM. Priority of revascularization in patients with graft enteric fistulas, infected arteries, or infected arterial prostheses. Ann Surg 1984;199:669–683.
22. Jacobs MJHM, Reul GJ, Gregoric I, et al. In-situ replacement and extra-anatomic bypass for the treatment of infected abdominal aortic grafts. Eur J Vasc Surg 1991;5:83–86.
23. Gozzetti G, Poggioli G, Spolaore R, et al. Aorto-enteric fistulae: spontaneous and after aortoiliac operations. J Cardiovasc Surg 1984;5:420–426.
24. Sorensen S, Lorentzen JE. Recurrent graft–enteric fistulae: case report. Eur J Vasc Surg 1989;3:583–585.
25. Vollmar JF, Kogel H. Aorto-enteric fistulas as postoperative complication. J Cardiovasc Surg 1987;28:479–484.
26. Walker WE, Cooley DA, Duncan JM, et al. The management of aortoduodenal fistula by in situ replacement of the infected abdominal aortic graft. Ann Surg 1986;205:727–732.
27. Clagett GP, Bowers BL, Lopez-Viejo MA, et al. Creation of a neo-aortoiliac system from lower extremity deep and superficial veins. Ann Surg 1993;281:239–249.
28. Nevelsteen A, LaCroix H, Suy R. Autogenous reconstruction with lower extremity deep veins: an alternative in the treatment of prosthetic infection after reconstructive surgery for aorto-iliac disease. J Vasc Surg 1995;22:129–134.
29. Kieffer E, Bahnini A, Koskas F, et al. In-situ allograft replacement of infected infrarenal aortic prosthetic grafts: results in forty-three patients. J Vasc Surg 1993;17:349–356.
30. Reilly LM, Goldstone J, Ehrenfeld WK, et al. Gastrointestinal tract involvement by prosthetic graft infection: the significance of gastrointestinal hemorrhage. Ann Surg 1985;202:342–348.

Treatment of Chylous Ascites After Abdominal Aortic Aneurysm Repair

Gabriel Carabello, M.D., and
William J. Quiñones-Baldrich, M.D.

Chylous ascites is the result of persistent extravasation of chyle into the peritoneal cavity. Spontaneous chylous ascites is most commonly associated with malignancy in adults and with congenital malformation of abdominal lymphatics in children.[19] Postoperative chylous ascites can occur after extensive retroperitoneal or mesenteric dissection, usually as a consequence of traumatic disruption of the lymphatic trunks or the cisterna chyli. Chylous ascites after abdominal aortic aneurysm (AAA) repair is one such example.

Although the incidence of chylous ascites is low, its manifestation is often dramatic and associated with significant morbidity. The leakage of large volumes of chyle into the peritoneal cavity can have grave mechanical, nutritional, and immunologic consequences. This chapter discusses the incidence, causes, clinical manifestations, diagnosis, and management of postoperative chylous ascites after AAA repair.

Anatomy of the Lymphatic Network

Lymphatic vessels drain interstitial fluid through a series of channels and lymph nodes to the venous system. Lymph from all parts of the body below the diaphragm, including the intestines, is directed toward lymph vessels and chains of lymph nodes that ascend around the great vessels of the retroperitoneum. Lymph below the diaphragm is eventually collected at the cisterna chyli, which is formed by the union of the paired lumbar lymphatic trunks with the intestinal lymphatic trunk. The cisterna chyli is the lower expanded end of the thoracic duct, located between the aorta and inferior vena cava and in front of the vertebral column at the L1-L2 level (Fig. 23–1).[7] It continues as the thoracic duct, passing through the aortic hiatus and entering the thorax, and it ascends the posterior mediastinum, running between the aorta and the azygous vein. In the mid-thorax, the thoracic duct inclines toward the left and terminates at the confluence of the left subclavian and left internal jugular veins.

The cisterna chyli can vary considerably in size, formation, and location. There may be no visible enlargement, and the lymphatic vessels may unite in highly variable patterns.[9] McVay[15] confirmed the unique variability of the abdominal lymphatic system, describing 16 distinctive anatomic variants of the lymphatic plexus of the abdomen and cisterna chyli (Fig. 23–2).

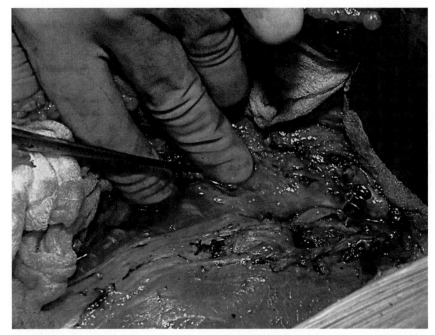

Figure 23-1. Cisterna chyli formed by the union of lumbar lymphatic channels in front of L1 to L2 vertebral bodies. The aorta has been mobilized in this dissection during exposure for anterior spinal fusion.

Physiology of Chyle

Chyle is rich in lymphocytes, chylomicrons, and proteins.[19] Chylomicrons are large-particle lipoproteins, 75 to 600 nm in diameter, that consist of 90% triglyceride and 10% phospholipid, cholesterol, and protein.[12] Chylomicrons are intimately associated with fat digestion and absorption, especially of long-chain fatty acids. The latter are absorbed into the intestinal lymphatics and eventually gain entrance into the venous system through the thoracic duct.[12] Medium-chain and short-chain fatty acids are water soluble and are absorbed directly into the portal venous system, bypassing the intestinal lymphatics.[12]

The biochemical properties of chyle have been well documented.[7, 17, 19, 25] It separates from the serum into a white creamy layer on standing that is odorless, sterile, and alkaline; has a specific gravity of more than 1.012; and is composed of more than 4% solids. The protein content is variable, approximating one half of the content of plasma. A predominance of lymphocytes is also characteristic. Fat content is higher than in any other fluid in the body, and fat globules may be seen under the microscope when stained with Sudan III. Other methods for demonstrating the fat content of the ascitic fluid are ether extraction or determination of blood triglyceride levels greater than 200 mg/dL.

The flow of chyle is variable. In the fasting state, lymph flow through the thoracic duct is less than 1 mL/min, but when the patient resumes an oral diet, lymph flow can exceed 225 mL/min.[27]

Incidence and Origin of Chylous Ascites

The incidence of chylous ascites is extremely low. A 20-year review from the Massachusetts General Hospital revealed an astonishingly low incidence

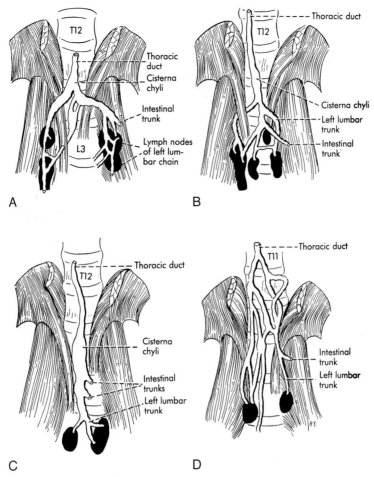

Figure 23–2. *A through D,* Four of 16 variants of the lymphatic plexus and cisterna chyli.

of 1 case in every 20,464 admissions, for a total of 24 adult cases. Of these, only one occurred postoperatively.[6] In 1986, Sarazin and Sauter[21] reviewed the world's literature and confirmed only 37 postoperative cases. The procedures involved with this complication included pancreaticoduodenectomy, vagotomy, celiac ganglionectomy, retroperitoneal node dissection, distal splenorenal shunting, mesocaval shunting, and radical nephrectomy. There have been only 28 reported cases of chylous ascites after abdominal aortic surgery.[1-6, 8, 10, 11, 13, 14, 16, 17, 20–24, 26, 27]

Although the incidence appears to be unequivocally low, evidence indicates the rate is increasing. In 1991, Quiñones-Baldrich and colleagues[27] reported six cases of chylous ascites occurring as a complication of aortic surgery during the 1970s, followed by seven cases during the 1980s and six cases in the early 1990s. However, since their report was published, another nine cases have been documented, bringing the total cases reported during the 1990s to 15. One plausible explanation for the increase is that more aortic procedures are being performed than in previous decades.

The mechanism by which chylous ascites forms after abdominal aortic surgery is unknown. One requirement is that a fistula must form between a lacerated cisterna chyli or a major abdominal lymphatic trunk and the peritoneal cavity. The condition may be further aggravated by interruption of lymphatic drainage from the abdomen as a result of prior trauma to the thoracic duct in the neck, obstruction by malignant lymph nodes, aneurysmal dilation, hyperplasia of the thoracic duct, or obstruction of the subclavian vein.[17] A transected lymphatic may not weep lymph during the operative procedure because of the low flow rate of lymph during the fasting state. However, on resumption of oral intake, chyle flow increases, and at this point, ascites may manifest. It is therefore prudent to ligate lymphatics during the course of dissection in the vicinity of the aorta. Similarly, closure of the retroperitoneum after aortic surgery may play an important role in preventing this complication.

Manifestations and Diagnosis

Patients with postoperative chylous ascites present in a characteristic manner. After recovery from their initial aortic reconstruction, most patients have abdominal distention, mild abdominal discomfort, and dyspnea (Fig. 23–3).[1-6] In a review of 22 cases by Pabst and coworkers,[17] the mean time from operation to the onset of abdominal distention was 18.4 days (range, 7 to 120 days), and only two patients developed symptoms later than 4 weeks postoperatively. The same investigators observed anorexia, weight loss or gain, weakness, nausea, vomiting, edema, and early satiety in their patients.

The diagnosis is relatively straightforward. In the review by Pabst and associates,[17] the presence of intraperitoneal fluid was documented by physical examination and confirmed by abdominal ultrasonography or computed tomographic scan. The recommended test to establish a definitive diagnosis is paracentesis.[17] In the 28 reported cases, paracentesis yielded the definitive diagnosis for 27 patients. The diagnosis for the remaining patient was made in the operating room while repairing a fascial dehiscence.[17] The hallmark of diagnosis is withdrawal of a milky, odorless fluid, along with the typical

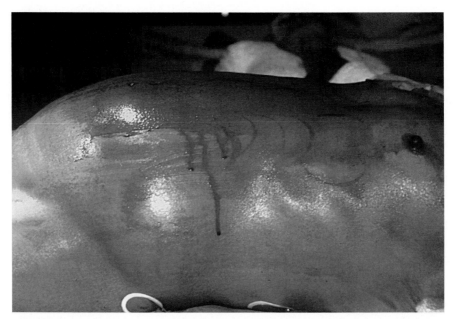

Figure 23–3. This patient presented 3 weeks after aortobirenal and mesenteric bypass with the typical abdominal appearance of distention and shifting dullness.

biochemical and analytical profile. Lymphoscintigraphy was used in isolated cases and was not required to establish the diagnosis in any of the 28 cases.

Management

Several regimens have been used to treat chylous ascites after aortic reconstructions. Management has included repeated therapeutic paracentesis; dietary control with a high-protein, low-fat, medium-chain triglyceride diet; total parenteral nutrition (TPN); diuretics; intravenous reinfusion of ascites; peritoneovenous shunting; and surgical closure of the leaking lymphatic vessel.[17]

Repeated therapeutic paracentesis was used in 13 of the 28 patients.[17, 18] It was not successful as a sole mode of therapy.[17] The success rate for resolution of the ascites when combined with a high-protein, low-fat, medium-chain triglyceride diet; diuretics; TPN; or some combination of these approaches has been approximately 50%.[17] Repeated paracentesis is not a benign procedure. Press and associates[19] reported that serious complications developed in 7 of 21 patients treated with this modality, including a case of peritonitis. The surgeon should be hesitant to proceed with this form of treatment in patients who have a recently placed vascular prosthesis, because graft infection may occur.

The use of high-protein, low-fat, medium-chain triglyceride diets has theoretical value. This regimen was popularized by Hashim to decrease the flow of lymph.[27] Medium-chain triglycerides are directly absorbed into the portal vein and not the intestinal lymphatics, as long-chain triglycerides are, and it is possible to predict a decrease in lymphatic flow, which would be beneficial in patients with chylous ascites. However, when this diet is used alone, it is not very successful.[17] Its use should probably be regarded as a complement to other treatment modalities.

The use of TPN as an adjunct to the overall treatment regimen is beneficial. TPN therapy provides nutrition; allows for bowel rest; diminishes the flow of lymph, which facilitates healing of transected lymphatics; and restores electrolyte balance in patients who are frequently immunodeficient, hypoalbuminemic, and cachectic. When TPN was used alone or in conjunction with diet or paracentesis, the chylous ascites resolved in 9 of 15 patients.[17]

The return of chyle to the body is an attractive and reasonable replacement therapy. Autotransfusion of chyle removed by paracentesis has been performed.[6] However, this procedure carries a significant risk of complications, and one case of sudden death has been reported.[27] Alternatively, chyle is returned to the body through peritoneovenous shunting. Of the 28 cases of chyloperitoneum forming after abdominal aortic surgery, five have been treated with peritoneovenous shunting.[17] Of these five patients, four had successful resolution of the chylous ascites, and one death occurred as a result of shunt sepsis.[17]

Operative exploration with direct ligation of the lymphatic fistula is highly effective. There have been five reported cases using this technique in 28 patients with chylous ascites occurring after abdominal aortic reconstruction, and the procedure was efficacious in all cases.[17] However, not all patients are candidates for reexploration, especially those who are debilitated, cachectic, and immunocompromised. We feel that this subset of patients may be better addressed with peritoneovenous shunting. If operative closure is planned, the patient should be fed cream the night before to help identify the leaking lymphatic fistula (Fig. 23–4).

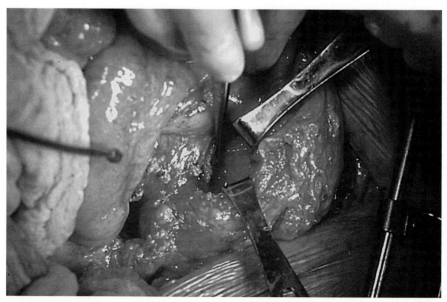

Figure 23–4. Operative findings in a patient with chylous ascites after aortic surgery. Notice the small pocket at the site of the chylous leak. Identification was made easier by feeding the patient cream the night before the operation. The leaking lymphatic vessel was suture ligated, and the patient had an uneventful recovery.

In our preferred management scheme for the treatment of chyloperitoneum after abdominal aortic surgery, the diagnosis of ascites is first confirmed by a combination of history, physical examination, and diagnostic imaging tests such as ultrasonography or computed tomography of the abdomen. Paracentesis is performed next to definitively diagnose the presence of chyle and to assist in therapy, especially if the patient is in respiratory distress. After chylous ascites has been unequivocally demonstrated, we proceed with a trial of conservative management, consisting of bowel rest and TPN, and we vigilantly look for resolution or progression. If the condition resolves, we administer a high-protein, low-fat, medium-chain triglyceride diet and monitor the patient for continued improvement. As the patient improves, she or he is advanced to a regular diet. If the patient fails to improve with conservative management, we proceed with surgical intervention in the form of reexploration with direct ligation of the lymphatic fistula or peritoneovenous shunting if the patient is too debilitated to withstand an operation.

References

1. Ablan CJ, Littooy FN, Freeark RJ. Postoperative chylous ascites: diagnosis and treatment. Arch Surg 1990;125:270–273.
2. Bahner DR Jr, Townsend R. Chylous ascites after ruptured abdominal aortic aneurysm. Contemp Surg 1990;36:37–39.
3. Boyd WD, Mcphail NV, Barber GC. Chylous ascites following abdominal aortic aneurysmectomy: surgical management with a peritoneovenous shunt. J Cardiovasc Surg 1989;30:627–629.
4. Bradham RR, Gregorie HB, Wilson R. Chylous ascites following resection of an abdominal aortic aneurysm. Am Surg 1970;36:238–240.
5. DeBartolo TF, Etzkorn JR. Conservative management of chylous ascites after abdominal aortic aneurysm repair. Mo Med 1976;73:611–613.
6. Fleisher HL, Oren JW, Sumner DS. Chylous ascites after abdominal aortic aneurysmectomy: successful management with a peritoneovenous shunt. J Vasc Surg 1987;6:403–407.
7. Garrett HE, Richardson JW, Howard HS, et al. Retroperitoneal lymphocele after abdominal aortic surgery. J Vasc Surg 1989;10:245–253.

8. Heyl A, Veen HF. Iatrogenic chylous ascites: operative or conservative approach? Neth J Surg 1989;41:5–7.

9. Hollinshead HW, Rosse C. The posterior abdominal wall and associated organs. *In* Hollinshead HW, Rosse C (eds). Textbook of Anatomy. Philadelphia: Harper & Row, 1985:677–711.

10. Jensen SR, Voegli DR, McDermott JC, et al. Lymphatic disruption following abdominal aortic surgery. Cardiovasc Intervent Radiol 1986;9:199–201.

11. Klippel AP, Hardy DA. Postoperative chylous ascites. Mo Med 1971;68:253–255.

12. Koltun WA, Pappas TN. Anatomy and physiology of the small intestine. *In* Greenfield LJ (ed). Surgery: Scientific Principles and Practices. Philadelphia: JB Lippincott, 1993:719–731.

13. Lopez-Enriquez E, Gonzales A, Johnson DC, et al. Chylothorax and chyloperitoneum: a case report. Bol Asoc Med P R 1979;71:54–58.

14. McKenna R, Stevick CA. Chylous ascites following aortic reconstruction. Vasc Surg 1983;17:143–149.

15. McVay CB. Thoracic cavity and its contents. *In* Anson BJ, McVay CB (eds). Surgical Anatomy. Philadelphia: WB Saunders, 1984:460–463.

16. Meinke AH III, Estes NC, Ernst CB. Chylous ascites following abdominal aortic aneurysmectomy: management with total parenteral hyperalimentation. Ann Surg 1979;190:631–633.

17. Pabst TS III, McIntyre KE Jr, Schilling JD, et al. Management of chyloperitoneum after abdominal aortic surgery. Am J Surg 1993;166:194–199.

18. Petrasek AJ, Ameli FM. Conservative management of chylous ascites complicating aortic surgery: a case report. Can J Surg 1996;39:499–501.

19. Press OW, Press NO, Kaufman SD. Evaluation and management of chylous ascites. Ann Intern Med 1982;96:358–364.

20. Sanger R, Wilmshurst CC, Clyne CA. Chylous ascites following aneurysm surgery. Eur J Vasc Surg 1991;5:689–692.

21. Sarazin WG, Sauter KE. Chylous ascites following resection of a ruptured abdominal aortic aneurysm. Treatment with a peritoneovenous shunt. Arch Surg 1986;121:246–247.

22. Savrin RA, High R. Chylous ascites after abdominal aortic surgery. Surgery 1986;98:246–247.

23. Schwein M, Dawes PD, Hatchuel D, et al. Postoperative chylous ascites after resection of an abdominal aortic aneurysm: a case report. S Afr J Surg 1987;25:39–41.

24. Stubbe LTFL, Terpstra JL. Chylous ascites after resection of an abdominal aortic aneurysm. Arch Chir Neerland 1979;31:111–113.

25. Vasko JS, Tapper RI. Surgical significance of chylous ascites. Arch Surg 1967;95:355.

26. Williamson C, Provan JL. Chylous ascites following aortic surgery. Br J Surg 1987;74:71–72.

27. Williams RA, Veto J, Quiñones-Baldrich WJ, et al. Chylous ascites following abdominal aortic surgery. Ann Vasc Surg 1991;5:247–252.

Management of Nonaortic Arterial Aneurysms

Treatment of Carotid Artery Aneurysms and Aortic Arch Vessel Aneurysms

Anil Hingorani, M.D., Marcel Scheinman, M.D., and Enrico Ascher, M.D.

Before World War II, syphilis was reported to be the most common cause of aneurysm formation.[1] Although atherosclerosis is now widely believed to be the main cause of carotid artery aneurysms (CAAs) or aortic arch vessel aneurysms (AAVAs), genetic, biochemical, and environmental factors have been sought and implicated in the development of these aneurysms.[2–12]

One of the most striking features of these aneurysms is the 14% to 50% association with concomitant aneurysms at other sites.[13–15] This consistent finding may suggest that systemic factors play a role in the cause of these aneurysms and that similar factors play a role in many types of aneurysms.

Therapy is directed toward prevention of embolic phenomena, avoiding rupture, and decompression of surrounding structures.[16] One of the most common complications of the repair of these aneurysms is neurologic deficit. Because aneurysms of the carotid artery and aortic arch vessels are rare disease processes, few large case series have been reported in the literature, and suggested treatments have varied. In an effort to help clarify these issues, we review some of the information concerning treatment of these aneurysms and the best reported outcomes from the larger series.

Extracranial Carotid Artery Aneurysms

History

The first account of surgical treatment of extracranial CAA was a carotid ligation performed by Ambroise Paré in 1552. The first attempted resection with restoration of the arterial flow was not performed until 1949.[1] The modern era of treatment of these aneurysms began with the first successful resection and end-to-end anastomosis, which was performed by Dimtza in 1952.[17] The first prosthetic graft replacement was performed in 1959 by Beall and associates.[18] They interposed a Dacron graft between the ends of the common and internal carotid arteries and used an internal shunt.

Presentation

Carotid aneurysms are defined by segments of the artery that are 150% of the internal carotid artery (ICA) diameter or 200% of the CCA diameter.[19] Because of the low incidence of these aneurysms, many vascular surgeons may go through their entire careers without encountering more than a handful of CAAs. CAAs make up only 0.4% to 4% of all aneurysms.[7, 20, 21] In a 7-year review of approximately 1000 carotid operations performed at the Mayo Clinic, only 19 cases of CAAs were identified.[22]

The most common site for these aneurysms is the common carotid bifurcation, followed by the ICA and CCA.[23] The most common causes, in decreasing frequency, are atherosclerosis, trauma, unknown origin, and fibromuscular disease.[2, 21] The presenting signs and symptoms, in decreasing frequency, are neck mass just below the angle of the mandible, hemiparesis, bruit, nerve compression, headache, and tinnitus.

Rarely, various surgeons have mistaken these lesions for an abscess protruding into the posterior pharynx and have tried to "incise and drain" these CAAs with disastrous results.[2, 24, 25] The differential diagnosis includes tortuosity of the carotid artery, carotid body tumors, enlarged cervical nodes, and brachial cleft cysts. Duplex ultrasonography can help to make the diagnosis, although magnetic resonance angiography (MRA) (Fig. 24–1), spiral computed tomography with intravenous contrast (Fig. 24–2), and standard angiography can also be useful in certain cases.(Fig. 24–3)

Treatment

Left untreated, the incidence of rupture is 10%, the rate of embolization is 50%, and the mortality rate is 71%.[8, 21] Because of this bleak outlook with conservative measures, operative repair is suggested when the diagnosis is made. The options for surgical treatment include resection with end-to-end anastomosis, bypass with vein or prosthetic material, and ligation with or without extracranial-intracranial (EC-IC) bypass. In the rare instance when ligation is necessary without EC-IC bypass, we suggest systemic anticoagulation for 5 to 7 days to decrease propagation of distal thrombus into the branches of the ICA.

Resection of the aneurysm and restoration of arterial flow has become the standard of treatment. In approximately 50% of these cases, redundancy of

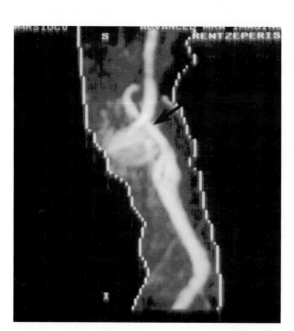

Figure 24–1. Magnetic resonance angiography of a carotid artery aneurysm *(arrow).*

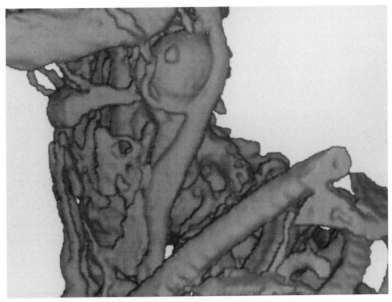

Figure 24-2. Three-dimensional computed tomography of a carotid artery aneurysm.

carotid artery allows resection and primary anastomosis.[16, 20] When this is not possible, an interposition graft is an option. The results of interposition of prosthetic or autogenous material have been equal, and either may be used.[26, 27]

When high exposure of the carotid is needed, the first step is to not become discouraged. The use of nasotracheal intubation, a headlight, and a self-retaining retractor can be helpful. Other options include division of the posterior belly of the digastric muscle, division of the styloid, mobilization of the parotid gland, subluxation of the mandible, mastoidectomy, and division of the styloid process or the stylomandibular ligament.[22]

One of the most important details in the repair of CAAs is to identify and

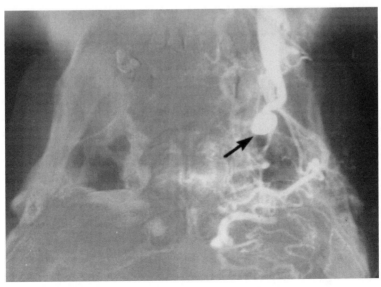

Figure 24-3. Standard angiogram of a carotid artery aneurysm.

preserve the adjacent cranial nerves. Often, there is an intense inflammatory reaction around these aneurysms that may involve the adjacent cranial nerves. Damage to these nerves can result in significant morbidity. However, careful dissection of the aneurysm with correct placement of self-retaining retractors in the subcutaneous tissues and the sternocleidomastoid muscle can avoid many of these injuries. Damage to these nerves tends to occur when repair of a larger aneurysm is attempted. Some surgeons have suggested not resecting these large aneurysms but instead performing an endoaneurysmorrhaphy to avoid injury to the adjacent cranial nerves.[22]

In our clinical practice, we have chosen to use of shunt when the ICA back pressure is less than 50 mm Hg.[28] We cite the literature suggesting a decreased rate of perioperative strokes with cerebral protection compared with using none.[2]

The role of endovascular techniques is a intriguing option. These procedures have been used in selected patients with high-risk situations or with very high aneurysms. One technique that has been used included obliteration of the aneurysm with detachable silicone balloons that were percutaneously inserted.[29] The role of stent grafts requires further documentation.

Results

The mortality rate for elective repair of CAA should be less than 5%.[22, 30, 31] Repair of CAA carried a mortality rate of 1.6% in one collected series of 66 patients and a rate of stroke of 4%.[32] Transient ischemia attacks occurred in 8.2% of patients during the perioperative period.[32] Cranial nerve injury occurs in 17% to 28% of patients.[21, 31] Long-term survival has been favorable, with a 10-year survival rate for CAA patients after repair of 80%. This is the same survival as for age- and sex-matched controls.

Innominate Artery Aneurysms

History

Many unsuccessful attempts were performed to repair innominate artery aneurysms (IAAs) until 1864, when Smyth operated on a patient who survived the operation and recovered from postoperative bouts of sepsis and hemorrhage.[33] After 11 years, the aneurysm recurred and bled, and the patient died. Triple ligation and excision was initially accomplished by Kimura in 1908.[34] These two approaches were associated with a high mortality rate of 54% to 78%, as reported for series collected from 1905 through 1946.[8, 35, 36]

Because one of the leading causes of death from this repair was the difficult exposure of the artery, several interesting techniques were developed to minimize the risk: introduction of agents to promote coagulation, such as gelatin insertion or the placement of a wire to pass electric current within the aneurysmal sac,[45] partial proximal or distal ligation,[35] creation of a fistula between the common carotid artery and jugular vein, and wrapping the aneurysm with cellophane to induce fibrosis in the periarterial layers.[36] However, these techniques often resulted in late rupture of the aneurysms.

In 1952, Kirby and Johnson[37] resected an IAA and reconstructed the vessel with an end-to-end anastomosis.[37] Two years later, Mahorner and Spencer[38] described the first bypass of an IAA with an end-to-side aortic homograft to the right common carotid artery. In 1957, DeBakey and Crawford[39] reported a revascularization using a bifurcated aortic homograft to the right common carotid and subclavian arteries. A Dacron graft was first used by Hejhal and colleagues[40] in 1965, and the first revascularization using a vein graft was performed by Schumacher and Wright in 1979.[36]

Presentation

IAAs are rare, with only three cases reported at the Massachusetts General Hospital over a 20-year period and 10 cases reported by Matas in a review of 1147 cases of aneurysms.[41–45] These aneurysms only account for 1 to 3% of all aneurysms.[42–45] The most common causes of IAAs are atherosclerosis, trauma, and infections.[31]

The most common presenting signs and symptoms are compression of the recurrent laryngeal, sympathetic, or brachial plexus nerves; mass; pain; bruit; transient ischemic attack; and dysphagia.[31, 55] The diagnosis can also be suggested in an asymptomatic patient by a superior mediastinal mass seen on chest radiography. The diagnosis can be confirmed with computed tomography with intravenous contrast, MRA, and angiography (Fig. 24–4).

Treatment

The preferred treatment is resection of the artery with restoration of the arterial flow. The standard approach is through a median sternotomy, with extension of the incision into the neck or right supraclavicular region, if needed. An 8- to 10-mm prosthetic graft is used to replace the aneurysmal artery. Aortic homografts, internal iliac or superficial femoral artery, or saphenous vein grafts may be used if the aneurysm is infected. Intraoperative electroencephalography monitoring or measurement of common carotid stump pressures should be used to assess cerebral protection during the procedure.[46, 47]

Results

With repair of an IAA, operative mortality ranges from 0% to 36%, with most larger series reporting mortality rates of less than 5%.[31] Operative morbidity ranges from 0% to 50%, with 5% to 16% of the patients suffering a

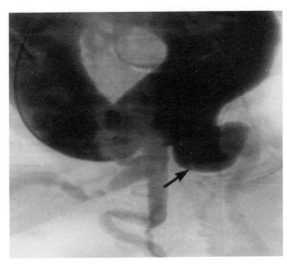

Figure 24–4. Standard angiogram of an innominate artery aneurysm *(arrow).*

cerebrovascular accident.[15, 60] Other major complications consist of transient ischemic attacks and peripheral nerve injury. Complications can be further avoided if a shunt is used when low back pressure is found.[36] Five-year survival after repair is 62.5% to 100%.[21, 31, 48]

Subclavian Artery Aneurysms

History

The first attempt to treat a subclavian artery aneurysm (SAA) was performed in 1818 in New York by Mott, who ligated the innominate artery for a traumatic SAA.[16, 49] However, the patient died after 26 days of sepsis and hemorrhage.

In 1864, the first successful treatment was performed in New Orleans by Smyth, who ligated the right common carotid and the innominate artery.[33] Halsted, in 1892, first successfully ligated and resected an SAA at the Johns Hopkins Hospital.[50] In 1913, Matas[51] described endoaneurysmorrhaphy as a new modality of repair for seven SAAs. Cellophane wrapping of SAA was first described in 1943, and arterial homografts, synthetic grafts, and replacement of segments of the aorta and great vessels became available in the 1950s.[52, 53] Bahnson has been credited with the first report of successful resection and graft replacement for SAA, which has become the standard of practice.[13, 14, 20, 54, 55] However, his two patients actually had IAAs treated by partial resection and lateral suture repair.

In 1993, May and colleagues from Australia reported the first transluminal placement of prosthetic graft stent device for treatment of an SAA.[56–58] We believe this technique will play a major role on the treatment of this type of disease in the near future.

Presentation

SAAs accounts for 1% to 4% of all aneurysms.[59] At the Mayo Clinic, one case was seen per year on average for more than 40 years.[31] Patients with SAAs may present with a pulsatile mass; chest, arm or shoulder pain; bruit, parasthesias, arm claudication, embolization, or rupture.[31, 60] Most of the aneurysms involve the right side.[13, 15, 31] Bilateral aneurysms are found in 5% to 12% of patients.[15, 60] A review of the literature on SAA found that the most common causes of were atherosclerosis, syphilis, and tuberculosis.[60]

Diagnosis can be made with duplex ultrasonography, computed tomography with intravenous contrast, MRA, and angiography (Fig. 24–5). Although in the past angiography was considered absolutely necessary before repair, there has been a trend to limit its use in favor of alternate modalities.

Treatment

Although ligation was the first form of treatment for SAAs, ligation can be followed by ischemia in one fourth of patients.[61–64] Because of this, the preferred technique has become resection of the aneurysm with restoration of arterial blood flow. The indications for surgery include an artery with twice the diameter of the uninvolved artery, embolization, or compressive symptoms.[65]

Intrathoracic SAAs are approached through a median sternotomy, with extension of the incision into the neck or supraclavicular region if necessary.[20]

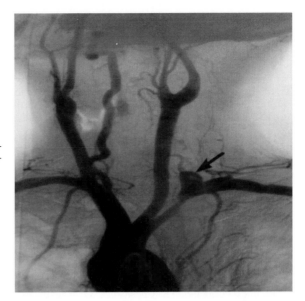

Figure 24–5. Standard angiogram of a subclavian artery aneurysm *(arrow)*.

The approach to repair a left intrathoracic aneurysm is through a left posterolateral thoracotomy. The supraclavicular approach is used for repair of the middle and distal segments of the subclavian artery. If thoracic outlet syndrome is diagnosed, the surgeon must resect the cervical rib or first rib to correct the underlying disorder. Replacement of the artery is performed with prosthetic material, although some have used the saphenous or hypogastric artery if the subclavian artery is small or infected. Cervical sympathectomy may be added as an adjunctive procedure if there is extensive microembolization with ulceration or gangrene.

Results

With the repair of SAA, the morbidity rate ranges from 7% to 21% and the 30-day mortality rate from 0% to 24%.[15, 31] The 5-year survival rate for these patients after surgical repair is 88%. This is the same as for controls if operative deaths are excluded.[14, 21, 31]

Conclusions

Aneurysms of the aortic arch vessels and the carotid artery are rare but can have devastating complications if left untreated. The various treatment options can be performed with very low complications. The morbidity and mortality of operative repair are substantially less than that of untreated cases, and elective repair of these aneurysms is warranted.

References

1. Kirby CK, Johnson J, Donald JG. Aneurysm of the common carotid artery. Ann Surg 1949;130:913.
2. Rittenhouse EA, Radke HM, Sumner DS. Carotid artery aneurysm. Arch Surg 1972;105:786.
3. Dehn TCB, Taylor GW. Extracranial carotid artery aneurysms. Ann R Coll Surg 1984;66:247.
4. Ekestrom S, Bergdahl L, Huttunen H. Extracranial carotid and vertebral artery aneurysms. Scan J Thorac Cardiovasc Surg 1983;17:135.
5. Mokri B, Piepgras DG, Sundt TM, et al. Extracranial internal carotid artery aneurysms. Mayo Clin Proc 1982;57:310.

6. Stewart MR, Moritz MW Smith RB, et al. The natural history of carotid fibromuscular dysplasia. J Vasc Surg 1986;3:305–310.
7. Welling RE, Taha A, Goel T, et al. Extracranial carotid artery aneurysms. Surgery 1983;93:319.
8. Winslow N. Extracranial aneurysm of the internal carotid artery. Arch Surg 1926;13:689.
9. Gandhi RH, Tilson MD. Arterial aneurysms: etiologic considerations. In Rutherford's Textbook of Vascular Surgery, 4th ed. Philadelphia: WB Saunders, 1995.
10. Tilson MD, Newman KM. Proteolytic mechanisms in the pathogenesis of aortic aneurysms. In Yao JST, Pearce WH (eds). Aneurysms—New Findings and Treatments. Norwalk, CT: Appleton & Lange, 1994:3–9.
11. Tilson MD, Ozvath KJ, Hirose H, Xia S. A genetic basis for autoimmune manifestations in the abdominal aortic aneurysms. (AAA) resides in the MHC class 2 locus DR B1. Ann N Y Acad Sci 1996;800:208–215.
12. Busuttil RW, Davidson RK, Foley KT, et al. Selective management of extracranial carotid arterial aneurysms. Am J Surg 1980;140:85–91.
13. Coselli JS, Crawford ES. Surgical treatment of aneurysms of the intra-thoracic segment of the subclavian artery. Chest 1987;91:704–708.
14. McCollum CH, DaGamma AD, Noon GP. Aneurysm of the subclavian artery. J Cardiovasc Surg (Torino) 1979;20:159.
15. Pairolero PC, Walls JT, Payne WS, et al. Subclavian-axillary artery aneurysms. Surgery 1981;90:757.
16. Thompson JE, Talkington CM. The surgery of carotid aneurysm. In Greenlaugh RM, Mannick JA (eds). The Cause and Management of Aneurysms. Philadelphia: WB Saunders, 1990.
17. Dimtza A. Aneurysm of the carotid arteries: report of two cases. Angiology 1956;7:218–227.
18. Beall AC, Crawford ES, Cooley DA, et al. Extracranial aneurysm of the carotid artery. Postgrad Med 1962;32:93–102.
19. DeJong KP, Zondervan PE, van Urk H. Extracranial carotid artery aneurysms. Eur J Vasc Surg 1989;3:557–562.
20. McCollum CH, Wheeler WG, Noon GP, DeBakey ME. Aneurysms of the extracranial carotid artery; twenty-one years' experience. Am J Surg 1979;137:196–200.
21. Zwolak RM, Whitehouse WM, Knade JE, et al. Atherosclerotic extracranial carotid artery aneurysms. J Vasc Surg 1984;72:946.
22. Sundt TM Jr, Pearson BW, Peipgras DG, et al. Surgical management of aneurysms of the distal extracranial internal carotid artery. J Neurosurg 1986;64:169.
23. Thompson JE, Talkington CM. The surgery of carotid aneurysms. In Greenlagh RM, Mannich JA (eds). The Cause and Management of Aneurysms. Philadelphia: WB Saunders, 1990.
24. Cunningham MJ, Reuger RG, Rothus WE. Extracranial carotid artery aneurysm: an unusual neck mass in a young adult. Ann Otol Rhinol Laryngol 1989;98:396–399.
25. Lane RJ, Wiesman RA. Carotid artery aneurysms: an otolaryngologic perspective. Laryngoscope 1980;90:987.
26. Busuttil RW, Davidson RK, Foley KT, et al. Selective management of extracranial carotid artery aneurysms. Am J Surg 1980;140:85–91.
27. Sundt TM Jr, Pearson BW, Peipgras DG, et al. Surgical management of aneurysms of the distal extracranial internal carotid artery. J Neurosurg 1986;64:169.
28. Ehrenfeld WK, Stoney RJ, Wylie E. Relation of carotid stump pressure to safety of carotid artery ligation. Surgery 1983;93:299–305.
29. Higashida RT, Hieshima GB, Halbach VV, et al. Cervical carotid artery aneurysms and pseudoaneurysms. Acta Radiol 1986;369:591.
30. Faggioli G, Freyrie A, Stella A, et al. Extracranial internal carotid aneurysms: results of a surgical series with long-term follow-up. J Vasc Surg 1996;23:587–595.
31. Bower TC, Pairolero PC, Hallet JW Jr, et al. Brachiocephalic aneurysm: the case for early recognition and repair. Ann Vasc Surg 1991;5:125–132.
32. Painter TA, Hertzer NR, Beven EG, et al. Extracranial carotid aneurysms: report of six cases and review of the literature. J Vasc Surg 1985;2:312–318.
33. Smyth AV. A case of successful ligature of the innominate artery. New Orleans Med Surg J 1869;22:464.
34. Greenough J. Operations on the innominate artery: report of a successful ligation. Arch Surg 1929;9:1484.
35. Sheen W. Original memoirs of ligation of the innominate artery, with report of a successful case. Ann Surg 1905;42:1.
36. Schumacher PD, Wright CB. Management of arteriosclerotic aneurysms of the innominate artery. Surgery 1979;85:489–495.
37. Kirby CK, Johnson J. Innominate artery aneurysm treated by resection and end-to-end anastomosis. Surgery 1953;33:562.
38. Mahorner H, Spencer R. Shunt grafts: a method of replacing segments of the aorta and large vessels without interrupting the circulation. Ann Surg 1954;139:439.
39. DeBakey ME, Crawford ES. Resection and homograft replacement of innominate and carotid arteries with use of shunt to maintain circulation. Surg Gynecol Obstet 1957;105:129–135.
40. Hejhal L, Firt P, Michal V, Hejnal J. Some interesting case reports in the field of reconstructive vascular surgery. J Cardiovasc Surg (Torino) 1965;6:409–415.

41. Brewster DC, Moncure AC, Darling RC, et al. Innominate artery lesions: problems encountered and lessons learned. J Vasc Surg 1985;2:99–112.
42. Prinotti C, Balzola F, Bruno G. Anerusima del tronco anonimo a partcolare avilupppo extratoracico. Minerva Med 1965;56:3662–3666.
43. Escande G, Dandjbakhch I, Christides C, et al. La cure chirurgicale des anaévrismes du tron artériel branchio-cephalique. Ann Chir Thorac Cardiovasc 1975;14:337.
44. Rundle F. Aneurysm of the innominate artery treated by surgery. Br J Surg 1971;25:172.
45. Matas R. Personal experience in vascular surgery: statistical synopsis. Ann Surg 1940;112:802.
46. Moore WS, Hall AD. Carotid artery back pressure: a test of cerebral tolerance to temporary carotid occlusion. Arch Surg 1940;112:802.
47. Hays RJ, Levinson SA, Wylie EJ. Intraoperative measurement of carotid back pressure as a guide to operative management for carotid endartectomy. Surgery 1972;72:953.
48. Stolf NAG, Bittencourt D, Verginelli G, Zerbini EJ. Surgical treatment of ruptured aneurysms of the innominate artery. Ann Thor Surg 1983;35:394–399.
49. Rhodes EL, Stanely JC, Hoffman GL, et al. Aneurysms of the extracranial carotid arteries. Arch Surg 1976;111:339.
50. Halsted WS. Ligation of the first portion of the left subclavian artery and excision of a subclavio-axillary aneurysm. Johns Hopkins Hosp Bull 1892;24:93.
51. Matas R. A summary of personal experience in the surgery of the subclavian arteries. Ann Surg 1940;112:802–806.
52. Muller GP. Subclavian aneurysm with report of a case. Ann Surg 1935;101:568.
53. Harrison PW, Chandy CA. A subclavian aneurysm cured by cellophane fibrosis. Ann Surg 1943;118:478.
54. Moloney GE. Excision of an aneurysm of the right subclavian artery: case history and discussion. Br J Surg 1955;43:94–96.
55. Thomas TV. Intrathoracic aneurysms of the innominate and subclavian arteries. J Thorac Cardiovasc Surg 1972;63:461–471.
56. May J, White G, Waugh R, et al. Transluminal placement of a prosthetic graft-stent device for treatment of subclavian artery aneurysm. J Vasc Surg 1993;18:1056–1059.
57. Marin ML, Veith FJ, Panetta TF, et al. Transluminally placed endovascular stented graft repair for arterial trauma. J Vasc Surg 1994;20:466–473.
58. Pastores SM, Marin ML, Veith FJ, et al. Endovascular stented graft repair of a pseudoaneurysm of the subclavian artery caused by percutaneous internal jugular vein cannulation: case report. Am J Crit Care 1995;4:472–475.
59. Dent TL, Lindenauer SM, Ernst CB, Fry WJ. Multiple arteriosclerotic arterial aneurysms. Arch Surg 1972;105:338–344.
60. Dougherty MJ, Calligaro KD, Savarese RP, DeLaurentis DA. Atherosclerotic aneurysm of the intrathoracic subclavian artery: a case report and review of the literature. J Vasc Surg 1995;21:521–529.
61. Pairolero PC, Walls JT, Payne WS, et al. Subclavian artery aneurysms. Surgery 1981;90:757–763.
62. Webb WR, Burford TH. Gangrene of the arm following use of the subclavian artery in a pulmonosystemic (Blalock) anastomosis. J Thorac Surg 1980;23:199–204.
63. Geiss D, Williams WG, Lindsay WK, Rowe RD. Upper extremity gangrene: a complication of subclavian artery division. Ann Thorac Surg 1980;30:487–489.
64. Folger GM, Shah KD. Subclavian steal in patients with Blalock-Taussig anastomosis. Circulation 1965;31:241–248.
65. Scher LA, Veith FJ, Haimovici H, et al. Staging of arterial complications of cervical rib: guidelines for surgical management. Surgery 1984;95:644–649.

Surgical Management of Aneurysms of Aberrant Subclavian Arteries

Edouard Kieffer, M.D.

Surgical management of aneurysms of aberrant subclavian arteries is often made difficult by their deep location in the posterior mediastinum. This chapter focuses on technical problems raised by these uncommon lesions, based on personal experience with 13 cases.[1, 2]

Embryology and Anatomy

Aberrant subclavian artery (ASA) is the most common anomaly of the aortic arch vessels.[3] It is found in approximately 0.5% of normal persons.

Although its embryologic origin remains a subject of debate, ASA probably results from an abnormal interruption of the fourth aortic arch, usually the right, which is destined to disappear. Normally, this interruption occurs between the origin of the subclavian artery and the dorsal aorta, with the anterior part of the arch becoming the innominate artery. In the case of an ASA, the interruption takes place between the origins of the common carotid and subclavian arteries. When the left fourth aortic arch persists, the ASA is on the right side. When the right fourth aortic arch persists, as is the case in 0.1% of individuals, the ASA is on the left. In the latter case, the left ligamentum arteriosum usually contributes to a complete vascular ring around the tracheoesophageal axis.

The ASA arises from the posteromedial aspect of the aortic arch, occasionally from an aortic diverticulum called Kommerell's diverticulum. Although the exact origin of Kommerell's diverticulum remains unknown, it is believed to be the remnant of the posterior segment of the fourth aortic arch. From there, the ASA courses obliquely cephalad and crosses the midline anterior to the spine and posterior to the esophagus to reach the supraclavicular fossa. After coursing through the scalene triangle, the ASA assumes the route of a normal subclavian artery.

An ASA is usually asymptomatic. It may occasionally cause esophageal compression and result in so-called dysphagia lusoria in children and adults.[1] Aneurysmal formation is the most common and serious complication of ASA in adults.[2] The aneurysm usually involves the origin of the artery from the descending thoracic aorta (Fig. 25–1), raising the question of its relationship to a preexisting Kommerell's diverticulum. An aneurysm, usually of the saccular type, rarely develops in the midportion of an ASA that has normal proximal and distal segments.

Because of intraluminal thrombus formation (see Fig. 25–1), such aneu-

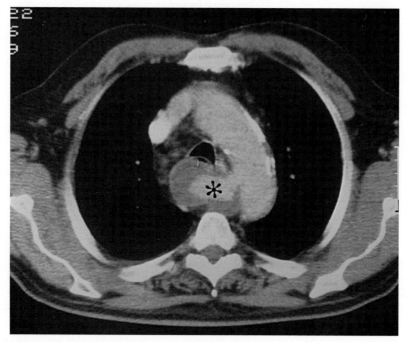

Figure 25–1. Computed tomography scan of an aneurysm of the proximal portion of an aberrant subclavian artery. Notice the large implantation on the proximal descending thoracic aorta and a significant mural thrombus.

rysms may be responsible for thromboembolic complications in the upper extremity or vertebrobasilar territory through the ipsilateral vertebral artery. They may compress the esophagus (Fig. 25–2), trachea, and venous system, resulting in dysphagia, dyspnea, and superior vena cava syndrome, respectively.

Rupture is the most serious complication. Although it is more common in large aneurysms, rupture has occurred in aneurysms not exceeding 4 cm in diameter.[4] Rupture usually occurs in the mediastinum or right pleural cavity, sometimes at a rate slow enough to permit diagnosis and surgical management. However, rupture into the esophagus results in massive hemorrhage and rapid death, sometimes preceded by small, sentinel hemorrhages.

Treatment

Indications for Surgery

Although their natural history is not fully known because of the scarcity of cases, aneurysms of ASA clearly threaten the patients' lives. They are presumed to be at least as morbid as aortic aneurysms, and indications for treatment are similar.[2] Surgery is indicated for patients with complicated or symptomatic aneurysms. Asymptomatic aneurysms in good-risk patients should probably be resected, regardless of their size. Poor-risk patients with small (<4 cm) aneurysms should probably be observed using spiral computed tomography (CT) scans with three-dimensional reconstruction at 6-month intervals. Surgery should be considered when the aneurysm is expanding or when its diameter reaches 4 cm.

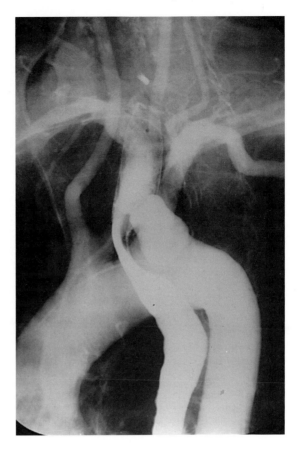

Figure 25–2. Combined esophagogram and aortogram show esophageal compression by an aneurysm of an aberrant subclavian artery. (From Berguer R, Kieffer E. Surgery of the arteries to the head. New York: Springer-Verlag, 1992.)

Principles of Surgical Treatment

The surgical treatment of ASA aneurysms aims to exclude the aneurysm while preserving blood flow to the distal subclavian artery.

Aneurysm Exclusion

Isolated distal exclusion (Fig. 25–3) may be justified in selected patients as a palliative procedure to eliminate the risk of distal embolization.[1] In most patients, however, proximal and distal exclusion is necessary to avoid or treat aneurysm expansion and rupture.

Although distal exclusion can be performed by ligating the artery distal to the aneurysm through a cervical incision on the side of the ASA, proximal exclusion is more demanding. Ligation of the ASA close to its origin is rarely feasible, because most aneurysms involve the origin of the ASA from the descending thoracic aorta. Lateral clamping of the descending thoracic aorta and suturing of the origin of the aneurysm (Fig. 25–4) is often difficult and hazardous because of the broad base of the aneurysm, the fragility of its wall, and the presence of intraluminal thrombus.

In most patients, proximal exclusion of the aneurysm entails intraaortic work, including patching of the orifice of the aneurysm[2, 5-7] (Fig. 25–5) or grafting of the portion of aorta that gives origin to the aneurysm[2, 8] (Fig. 25–6). These procedures may be achieved with crossclamping of the aorta (with or without distal aortic perfusion) or with circulatory arrest.[2, 5, 7] Provisions

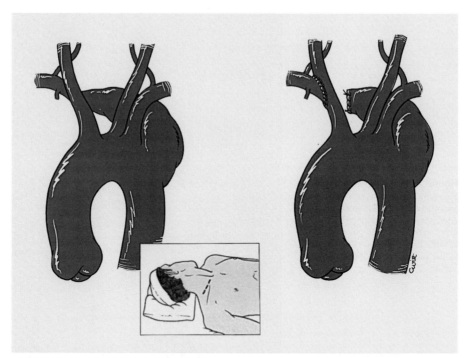

Figure 25–3. Diagram shows isolated distal exclusion of an aneurysm of an aberrant subclavian artery. Reestablishment of arterial continuity is achieved by transposition of the distal subclavian artery to the neighboring common carotid artery. The *inset* shows the incision line and positioning of the patient. (Kieffer E, Chemla E, Castier Y. Aneurysms of aberrant subclavian arteries: an approach to surgical management. Ann Vasc Surg [in press].)

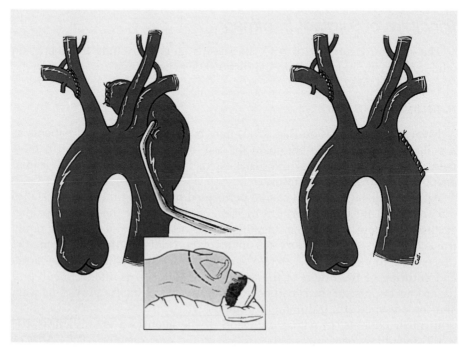

Figure 25–4. Diagram shows lateral clamping of the descending thoracic aorta and suturing of the origin of an aneurysm of an aberrant subclavian artery. The *inset* shows the incision line and positioning of the patient. (Kieffer E, Chemla E, Castier Y. Aneurysms of aberrant subclavian arteries: an approach to surgical management. Ann Vasc Surg [in press].)

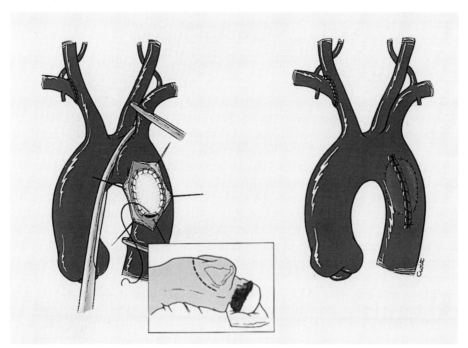

Figure 25–5. Diagram shows endoaortic patch closure of the origin of an aneurysm of an aberrant subclavian artery. The *inset* shows the incision line and positioning of the patient. (Kieffer E, Chemla E, Castier Y. Aneurysms of aberrant subclavian arteries: an approach to surgical management. Ann Vasc Surg [in press].)

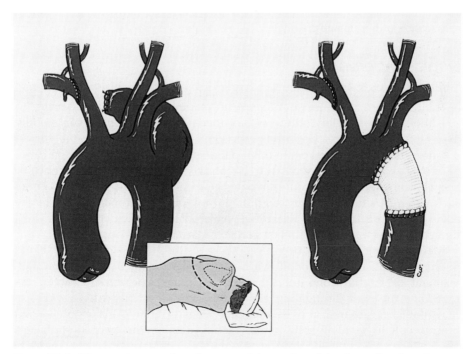

Figure 25–6. Diagram shows graft replacement of the portion of the descending thoracic aorta giving rise to an aneurysm of an aberrant subclavian artery. The *inset* shows the incision line and positioning of the patient. (Kieffer E, Chemla E, Castier Y. Aneurysms of aberrant subclavian arteries: an approach to surgical management. Ann Vasc Surg [in press].)

should be made for left heart bypass or cardiopulmonary bypass in the surgical management of patients with aneurysms of ASA.[2, 9, 10]

Distal Revascularization

Division of the ASA without restablishement of arterial continuity can lead to ischemic complications in the upper limb or the vertebrobasilar territory.[1,9,11] Although ligation alone may be safe in pediatric patients, the risk of early or late ischemic complications, with or without a subclavian steal syndrome, is higher for adults. As suggested by most reports, my colleagues and I feel that reconstruction of ASA is mandatory.

The simplest technique is transposition of the distal ASA to the neighboring common carotid artery, reconstituting an innominate artery.[1, 6, 10, 12] Carotid artery to subclavian artery bypass may be considered in patients with extensive atherosclerotic disease of the subclavian artery or contralateral carotid artery occlusion to avoid simultaneous clamping of the carotid and vertebral arteries.

Transposition of the ASA to the ascending aorta is feasible in patients operated through a median sternotomy[7] or thoracotomy on the side of the ASA.[13] Although it entails interposition of a prosthetic graft, it may be proposed when the common carotid artery is occluded, is severely diseased, or has a small diameter.

Revascularization of the distal ASA must be performed *before* the aneurysm is repaired.[2, 14] This is the most efficient way to avoid distal embolization during arterial manipulations. Aortic crossclamping may have to be done proximal to both subclavian arteries, possibly leading to serious ischemic complications in the vertebrobasilar territory. The only exception to this rule is in patients operated on using deep hypothermia and circulatory arrest,[2, 5, 7] although it may be convenient to take advantage of the cooling period to revascularize the distal ASA.

Surgical Approach

The choice of the surgical approach can determine the success of the operation. Treatment of an ASA aneurysm requires a thoracic approach.

Although thoracotomy on the side of the ASA has been used successfully in a few patients,[11] this approach was sometimes used because the correct diagnosis had not been made. In other patients, the treatment of the aneurysm had to be abandoned or followed by secondary contralateral thoracotomy, or reestablishment of arterial continuity was performed by a debatable procedure such as an in situ interposition graft.[2] In any case, proximal control of the aneurysm is difficult and hazardous or even impossible through such a limited approach, especially when aortic crossclamping is necessary.

Median sternotomy has been used successfully in a few patients.[15] It has the theroretical advantage of allowing exclusion of the aneurysm and reestablishment of arterial continuity through a single approach. However, approaching the ASA through a median sternotomy requires extensive dissection of the aortic arch and its branches, usually after division of the left brachiocephalic vein. Despite ample mobilization of the tracheoesophageal tract, which should be encircled by a wide umbilical tape or a Penrose drain, the ASA remains deep, especially at its origin on the descending thoracic aorta. In some cases, control of the aorta may be difficult,[8] hazardous, or even impossible without deep hypothermia and circulatory arrest.

In most patients, thoracotomy on the side of the aortic arch (ie, contralateral to the ASA) is the safest and easiest way to control the aorta and the origin of the ASA.[2, 9, 10, 12, 14] It allows crossclamping and reconstruction of the aorta when necessary. Its only drawback is that a complementary incision (ie, contralateral cervicotomy) is necessary to reconstruct the distal ASA.

Proposed Surgical Management

In most elective cases, we advise a two-step procedure, beginning with reconstruction of the distal ASA through an ipsilateral cervicotomy and followed by posterolateral thoracotomy on the side of the aneurysm and proximal exclusion of the aneurysm. Median sternotomy and cardiopulmonary bypass should be used in patients with ruptured aneurysms or when a combined cardiac procedure (ie, myocardial revascularization) is scheduled. In such cases, deep hypothermic circulatory arrest greatly simplifies the operative procedure.

References

1. Kieffer E, Bahnini A, Koskas F. Aberrant subclavian artery: surgical treatment in thirty-three adult patients. J Vasc Surg 1994;19:100–111.
2. Kieffer E, Chemla E, Castier Y. Aneurysms of aberrant subclavian arteries: an approach to surgical management. Ann Vasc Surg (in press).
3. Stewart JR, Kincaid OW, Edwards JE. An atlas of vascular rings and related malformations of the aortic arch system. Springfield, IL: Charles C Thomas, 1964: 52–75, 98–123.
4. Wagner T, Thiry S. Aneurysma der arteria lusoria: writteilung von vier fallen. Schweiz Med Wochenschr 1976;106:15–21.
5. Baillot RG, Beven RG, Cosgrove DM. Aneurysm of an aberrant right subclavian artery: repair using circulatory arrest. Cleve Clin Q 1984;51:173–175.
6. Cooley DA. Surgical treatment of aortic aneurysms. Philadelphia: WB Saunders, 1986:175–184.
7. Verkroost MW, Hamerlijnck RP, Vermeulen FE. Surgical management of aneurysms at the origin of an aberrant right subclavian artery. J Thorac Cardiovasc Surg 1994;107:1469–1471.
8. Hunter JA, Dye WS, Javid H, et al. Arteriosclerotic aneurysm of anomalous right subclavian artery. J Thorac Cardiovasc Surg 1970;59:754–758.
9. Esposito RA, Khalil I, Galloway AC, Spencer FC. Surgical treatment for aneurysm of aberrant subclavian artery based on a case report and a review of the literature. J Thorac Cardiovasc Surg 1988;95:888–891.
10. Brown DL, Chapman WC, Edwards WH, et al. Dysphagia lusoria: aberrant right subclavian artery with a Kommerell's diverticulum. Am Surg 1993;59:582–586.
11. Austin EH, Wolfe WG. Aneurysm of aberrant subclavian artery with a review of the literature. J Vasc Surg 1985;2:571–577.
12. Berguer R, Kieffer E. Surgery of the arteries to the head. New York: Springer-Verlag, 1992:190–197.
13. Kiernan PD, Dearani J, Byrne WD, et al. Aneurysm of an aberrant right subclavian artery: case report and review of the literature. Mayo Clin Proc 1993;68:468–474.
14. Harrison LH Jr, Batson RC, Hunter DR. Aberrant right subclavian artery aneurysm: an analysis of surgical options. Ann Thorac Surg 1994;57:1012–1014.
15. Jebara VA, Arnaud-Crozat E, Angel F, et al. Aberrant right subclavian artery aneurysm: report of a case and review of the literature. Ann Vasc Surg 1989;3:68–73.

Treatment of Visceral Artery Aneurysms

Alan B. Lumsden, M.D., and Robert B. Smith III, M.D.

Splenic Artery Aneurysms

Splenic artery aneurysm (SAA) is the most common type of visceral artery aneurysm. The incidence varies from 1.6% in an unselected autopsy population[1] to 7.1% in autopsies performed on patients who died of cirrhotic portal hypertension.[2] However, a much higher incidence of 10.4% was reported by Bedford and Lodge,[3] who specifically looked for SAAs in 250 autopsies carried out on patients who were older than 60 years of age when they died. In clinical situations, SAAs are being increasingly recognized with the use of visceral angiography, Doppler ultrasonography, and computed tomography (CT).

Etiology

The first report of SAA was made in 1770 by Beaussier,[4] who recounted an anatomic dissection that he had performed 10 years earlier. Before 1952, only 204 cases had been recorded.[5] The precise mechanism of aneurysmal dilation of the splenic artery is unknown, but views have not changed markedly since the proposals published by Trimble and Hill in 1942.[6] They identified two factors: preliminary weakness of the arterial wall and a concomitant rise in blood pressure. Fibromuscular dysplasia is a recognized etiologic factor that is readily demonstrated by angiography.

Stanley and Fry[2] demonstrated internal elastic lamina disruption and diminution of elastic fibers in the SAAs of multiparous women. They suggested that preexisting fibrodysplasia associated with repeated pregnancies that increased intravascular volume and portal congestion may promote aneurysmal dilatation. The hormonal effects of pregnancy, particularly those of relaxin, may further weaken the arterial wall. This set of conditions also affects patients with liver disease and portal hypertension with splenomegaly, for whom the reported incidence of SAA is as high as 20%.[2, 7] Patients with systemic hypertension have an increased incidence of SAA. Atherosclerotic changes seen in some excised specimens, however, are most likely secondary events, because they are not uniformly present in all lesions.[2]

We reported management of 44 SAAs at Emory University Hospital.[8] In contrast to studies that report most patients with SAA as being older than 60 years,[9, 10] our patients' average age was 48 years at diagnosis. This difference probably reflected the large proportion of patients with portal hypertension (70% of our patients), which may have accelerated pathogenesis. There is a particular interest in portal hypertension and liver transplantation at our institution, which serves as a referral center for such patients. These patients tend to be in a younger age group than the elderly patients who are cited in other reports. Possibly for the same reasons, the marked preponderance of multiparous women described in other studies[9, 10] was not present in our series.

The splenic artery is the visceral vessel that is also most likely to develop pseudoaneurysms.[11] These lesions are caused by disruption of the vessel wall as a result of the direct action of elastase and other digestive enzymes released by the inflamed pancreas[12] or caused by penetrating or blunt trauma.[13] In contrast to true aneurysms, pseudoaneurysms, particularly those caused by pancreatitis, may be extremely fragile[14] and are more likely to be a source of bleeding. These lesions therefore tend to be symptomatic and have readily distinguishable etiologic factors. The finding of a "cyst within a cyst" on CT suggests a pseudoaneurysm within a pseudocyst,[15] but as in true SAAs, the most valuable investigative modality remains visceral angiography. In view of the expected difficulties with the operative approach, transcatheter embolization is the treatment of choice for pseudoaneurysms.

Symptoms and Signs

Symptoms and clinical findings for SAAs are rare. Most of our patients were asymptomatic.[16] The aneurysms were discovered incidentally in the course of managing associated conditions, which in our patients were primarily the manifestations of portal hypertension. Chronic, vague epigastric and left hypochondrial pain may be reported.[17] Development of acute left upper quadrant pain indicates that rupture may have occurred, especially when signs of hypovolemia exist. Two patients in our series who were not previously diagnosed presented in this manner and received emergency treatment. Their aneurysms had ruptured.

No reliable physical signs indicate the presence of an SAA. Bruits are thought to arise from turbulent aortic flow, and a palpable mass in the left upper quadrant is more likely to be an enlarged spleen. An SAA may occasionally be suspected with the appearance of calcification in a corresponding area on an abdominal roentgenogram. However, calcified aneurysms were demonstrated in only four patients, which may reflect the preponderance of portal hypertension in this series that prompted diagnosis. All four patients with calcified SAAs had no other identifiable vascular causes, and most of the reported aneurysms in the literature were initially detected as calcified ring shadows on abdominal radiographs.

Imaging

Although Doppler ultrasonography is a noninvasive investigation with minimal risk to the patient, visualization of the splenic artery remains essentially operator dependent. CT easily delineates most SAAs. Angiography is required as a preoperative planning tool and for evaluating embolization. Magnetic resonance (MR) angiography and spiral CT angiography may further assist clinicians in the diagnosis and more accurate assessment of SAAs.

Risk of Rupture

Interest in SAA is based on concern about rupture, a risk now recognized to have been overestimated in early reports that cited rates up to a 10%.[17, 18]

More contemporary series suggest rates are closer to 2%.[19] Nevertheless, rupture does occur, and certain high-risk groups can be identified. Surgery has been the traditional method of treatment, but percutaneous embolization has gained popularity.

Although there are no absolute determinants of impending rupture, several factors guide the decision to treat patients with SAAs (Table 26–1). Sudden left upper quadrant pain usually indicates rupture has occurred, and any patient in this situation should undergo emergency surgery, particularly when signs of hypovolemia are evident. About 25% to 30% of these patients may spontaneously stabilize, albeit temporarily.[5, 15] Sudden circulatory collapse and death usually ensue within 48 hours in untreated cases. These are the recognized features of the double-rupture phenomenon, in which initial aneurysmal bleeding tamponades in the lesser sac, followed by inevitable rupture into the general peritoneal cavity.

Reports of ruptured SAAs after liver transplantation are appearing with increasing frequency.[20, 21] Ayalon[20] recommends ligating the splenic artery in all patients undergoing orthotopic liver transplantation who have documented SAAs. He suggests that the drop in portal pressure after transplantation may be associated with an increase in splenic arterial flow that may rupture an existing SAA.[20] At our institution, SAAs encountered during liver transplantation are treated during the same procedure.

Treatment

There is a general consensus that women anticipating pregnancy and patients with symptomatic aneurysms should be promptly treated. Although this is widely recommended, the indications for treating aneurysms that are larger than 2 cm are less definite.[10, 17, 19] With the use of various investigative modalities, SAAs are being diagnosed with increasing frequency. Although most lesions are small, asymptomatic and nonenlarging aneurysms larger than 2 cm are detected. The mean SAA diameter in patients who have been monitored is less than 2 cm. Trastek and colleagues[10] described 19 patients who were observed for a maximum of 19 years (mean, 7.4 years) and who had a mean SAA diameter of 1.4 cm. Only one aneurysm increased in size, but none of the patients experienced any difficulties related to the aneurysms.[10]

Prospective studies are needed to help determine the natural history of SAAs larger than 2 cm. The acquired data may allow readjustment of the "threshold" diameter for active treatment of a disease that has a greater than 0.5% operative mortality rate.[22] Our practice is to treat patients with asymptomatic SAAs larger than 3 cm or smaller aneurysms in higher-risk groups.

Preservation of the spleen should be a consideration, although this may

Table 26–1.
Treatment Guidelines for Splenic Artery Aneurysms

Size of Aneurysm	Age of Patient	Comorbidity	Management
<2 cm	<40 yr	None	Treat
<2 cm	>60 yr	No risk factors for rupture	Observe
2–4 cm	<70 yr	Yes	Observe; assess every 6 mo with CT
>4 cm	All ages	If not prohibitive	Treat

prove impossible in treating distal and intrasplenic aneurysms. Unfortunately, 70% of SAAs in patients with portal hypertension are in this category, and one half of these aneurysms are the multiple variety.[2, 23] The recommended procedure for more proximal aneurysms is exclusion of the lesion with proximal and distal ligation of the splenic artery. Opening the aneurysm to oversew feeding vessels from within the lesion may be necessary. Distal ligation is mandatory to prevent backfilling of the aneurysm from the abundantly supplied spleen. Excision of the aneurysm is the operation of choice for middle-third lesions.

Successful ligation of an SAA with endoscopic methods has been reported.[24] We recommended laparoscopic ligation in young pregnant women, in whom alternative modes of treatment may be more hazardous. Alternatives to surgical treatment of SAA have evolved within the realms of interventional radiography. Percutaneous embolization with Gianturco coils and Gelfoam sponges has been reported with favorable results.[25–27] One patient in our series with severe Parkinson's disease received this treatment but died of unrelated causes 1 year later. No long-term follow-up studies of patients treated by embolization are available.

Conclusions

We agree that observant treatment is a reasonable option for patients with aneurysms smaller than 3.0 cm. Long-term follow-up studies are needed to determine the reliability of incorporating Doppler ultrasonography, MR angiography, and spiral CT angiography in the observant treatment program for these patients. Prospective studies are also needed to assess the efficacy of embolization and the incidence of bleeding or rebleeding. More active treatment is reserved for patients whose aneurysms have ruptured or are at a high risk for rupture. Patients in the latter category include pregnant women and those anticipating pregnancy, patients with symptomatic or expanding aneurysms, and liver transplant candidates who have SAAs.

The diagnosis of SAA is not necessarily an indication for surgery. Controversy remains about adhering to the recommendation that all SAAs larger than 2 cm in diameter should be treated. As experience is gained, this criterion is being less strictly adhered to. Pseudoaneurysms, particularly those of traumatic origin, should be treated, preferably by percutaneous embolic means.

Hepatic Artery Aneurysms

Wilson first described a hepatic artery aneurysm (HAA) in 1809 as a lesion the "size and shape of a heart involving the left hepatic artery."[28] Since then, only about 400 cases have been reported. HAAs are the second most common visceral artery aneurysm, comprising 20% of splanchnic artery aneurysms. The natural history of HAAs typically is enlargement, rupture, and life-threatening hemorrhage.[29] Heightened clinical suspicion with conclusive diagnosis and effective treatment are imperative in the successful management of patients with these aneurysms. We have reported the largest series of hepatic artery aneurysms in the literature.[30]

Incidence and Etiology

The true incidence of HAAs cannot be ascertained, but HAAs are being encountered with increasing frequency, a development that may result from a combination of augmented referral patterns, enhanced clinical awareness, improved imaging techniques, and a possible shift in cause. Traditionally, atherosclerosis has been the most common cause of HAAs, although reservations remain about whether it is the primary process.[31] Atherosclerotic aneurysms comprised most early HAAs in our series, but an increased number of HAAs discovered in the latter years resulted from trauma or were of iatrogenic origin (50% of aneurysms in the past 6 years). Mycotic lesions were probably the single most common cause of HAAs at the start of the century but gradually diminished in incidence and became rare by the late 1970s (Fig. 26–1).[32] There was only one mycotic aneurysm in our series, but there is concern that these aneurysms, particularly in association with endocarditis, may reappear with increasing frequency because of the rise in intravenous substance abuse and the prevalence of immunocompromised patients.

A 2:1 male to female preponderance is observed for HAAs, probably reflecting the atherosclerotic origin in most cases.[31–37] Pseudoaneurysms typically affect younger, male individuals, reflecting a traumatic cause.

Risk of Rupture

There is controversy regarding the incidence of aneurysmal rupture, with values ranging from 20%[31] to 80%.[33, 34] The risk of rupture probably has been overestimated, because reported data is weighted toward symptomatic and ruptured aneurysms. HAAs may also come to attention because of erosion into the biliary tree, erosion into the portal veins with development of portal hypertension and its sequelae, or rupture into the retroperitoneum or peritoneal cavity.[29] Quincke's classic triad of jaundice, biliary colic, and gastrointestinal bleeding suggests hemobilia and occurs in one third of patients.[35] Bleeding

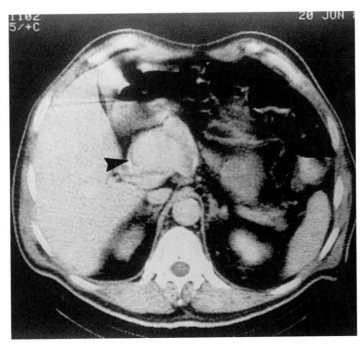

Figure 26–1. A massive, mycotic intrahepatic pseudoaneurysm in a patient with bacterial endocarditis and embolic infarction of the spleen. (From Lumsden AB, Mattar SG, Allen RC, et al. Hepatic artery aneurysms: the management of 22 patients. J Surg Res 1996;60:345–350.)

into the abdominal cavity is a catastrophic event, with a mortality rate of 82%.[34]

Symptoms and Signs

Symptoms and signs, when present, are varied, and a high level of suspicion is required. The most common symptom is vague, right-sided or epigastric abdominal pain, as demonstrated in 41% of our patients. It is unclear, however, how pain correlates with the state of the aneurysm and whether it heralds impending rupture. Nevertheless, it serves the purpose of directing diagnostic efforts toward underlying abnormalities.

Plain abdominal radiographs or upper gastrointestinal contrast studies may suggest an underlying HAA when a rim of calcification in the right hypochondrium or a smooth filling defect in the duodenum is demonstrated. Ultrasonography and contrast-enhanced CT scanning can provide the diagnosis in most cases (Fig. 26–2A and B).[38] MRI has been applied to good effect in the diagnosis of HAAs.[39] Color duplex ultrasonography has also been used effectively to determine blood flow in some aneurysms (Fig. 26–2C) and can demonstrate arterialization of the portal system when a fistula is present.[36] It is also useful for monitoring intrahepatic aneurysms that have been embolized to ensure their continued occlusion.[40]

The standard preoperative investigation in HAAs is selective angiography (Fig. 26–2D). This modality defines the location of the lesion and its collateral pathways. If the gastroduodenal artery is not visualized, a superior mesenteric artery or left gastric artery injection should be performed. This procedure is valuable in planning surgical strategies for proximal aneurysms. It is likely,

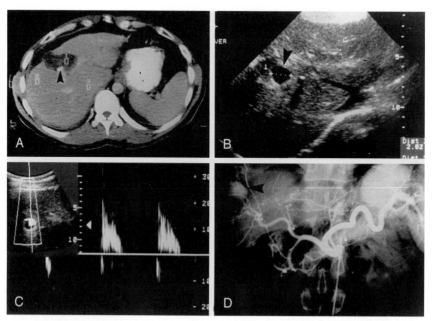

Figure 26–2. An intrahepatic pseudoaneurysm, diagnosed several months after a right upper quadrant gunshot wound. *A,* Computed tomography demonstrates the contrast-filled lumen, surrounded by organizing liver tissue. *B,* Gray-scale ultrasonography depicts the 2-cm aneurysm lumen, and Doppler interrogation confirms the arterial flow characteristics. *C,* Celiac arteriography. *D,* The pseudonaneurysm arises from a branch of the right hepatic artery. (From Lumsden AB, Mattar SG, Allen RC, et al. Hepatic artery aneurysms: the management of 22 patients. J Surg Res 1996;60:345–350.)

however, that spiral CT angiography and MR angiography will become the studies of choice in the future.

Treatment

Unless severe comorbidities disqualify the patient, all HAAs larger than 1 cm in diameter should be treated. Treatment options are largely determined by the anatomic location of the aneurysm (Table 26–2). Extrahepatic aneurysms warrant surgical treatment, except in high-risk patients and in those with saccular aneurysms. Common HAAs, such as an aneurysm proximal to a patent gastroduodenal artery, may be ligated and excised, because the liver continues to receive arterial blood through collaterals such as the pancreaticoduodenal and gastroduodenal arteries. However, the response of liver parenchyma to hepatic artery ligation is unpredictable. Countryman and coworkers[29] suggest temporary clamping of the hepatic artery with inspection of the liver for any change in color before definite ligation. Intraoperative Doppler ultrasonography performed before and after clamping can help predict subsequent compromise. Dougherty and associates[33] recommend vascular reconstruction at all times in good-risk patients.[33] One patient in our series unexpectedly sustained an area of central liver necrosis after ligation of a proximal aneurysm. It is our policy, if easily performed, to reconstruct with reversed saphenous vein grafts.

Extrahepatic aneurysms involving the hepatic artery propria usually require vascular reconstruction. Simple ligation of the hepatic artery propria at sites beyond the gastroduodenal artery frequently results in significant liver ischemia. The preferred conduit in these procedures is the reversed autogenous saphenous vein graft.

Until the advent of transcatheter embolization, most intrahepatic HAAs inevitably warranted resection along with relevant liver tissue. These hepatic resection procedures caused considerable morbidity and, in our series, resulted in the formation of one postlobectomy abscess. Interventional radiologists have contributed to the treatment of HAAs, and successful percutaneous embolization was first reported in 1977. Since then, several reports have supported the use of this technique.[27, 41, 42] An advantage of selective arterial embolization is its precision in limiting hepatic devascularization. It is of particular value in cases of posttraumatic pseudoaneurysms and, because of

Table 26–2.
The Recommended Therapy of Hepatic Artery Aneurysms According to Site

Site	Treatment
Intrahepatic artery	Embolization
Hepatic artery proper	
Good-risk candidate	Surgery
Poor-risk candidate	Observation for <2 cm diameter; surgery for >2 cm diameter
Saccular aneurysm	Embolization
Common hepatic artery	
Good-risk candidate	Aneurysmectomy
Poor-risk candidate with patent gastroduodenal artery	Embolization
Hepatic arterioportal fistula	Embolization
Intrahepatic	Surgery, intraaneurysmal oversewing
Extrahepatic	of venous communicants

its lower morbidity, represents an attractive option in treating all high-risk patients.[43]

Percutaneous embolization has become the preferred method of treating intrahepatic aneurysms. This development, however, is not without its complications, as exemplified by one of our patients in whom embolization failed because of migration of the embolic material. This case illustrates the need for follow-up documentation of aneurysmal occlusion. The natural history of embolized aneurysms is unknown, and there is potential for recanalization and repeat aneurysmal formation. In our series, three patients (42% of embolized patients) developed early recanalization but were re-embolized without difficulty to achieve total aneurysmal occlusion.

This experience emphasizes that follow-up imaging of the aneurysm is necessary after embolization. If the aneurysm has been effectively imaged by color-flow duplex ultrasonography, it is the modality of choice for follow-up; otherwise, repeat angiography is necessary. Embolization occasionally may be used preoperatively to reduce surgical blood loss.[37]

Conclusions

HAA is a life-threatening lesion. Although several diagnostic modalities, such as MR angiography and spiral CT, may be helpful in particular situations, selective angiography remains the gold standard.

Surgery is the preferred treatment for extrahepatic lesions. Therapeutic embolization has achieved a recognized role in the treatment of HAAs and has been safe and effective for most patients who received it. In our series, close cooperation between surgeons and radiologists about the diagnostic and therapeutic aspects of management resulted in favorable outcomes.

Renal Artery Aneurysms

The exact incidence of renal artery aneurysms is estimated to be 0.09% to 0.7% after angiographic studies performed for renal and nonrenal disease.[44, 45] The incidence rises to 2.5% among patients evaluated for hypertension and up to 9.2% among patients with fibromuscular disease involving the renal artery.[46] Complications appear to be uncommon but include renovascular hypertension; renal infarction from embolization, dissection, or thrombosis; and arteriovenous fistula formation.[45]

Etiology and Incidence

The causes are numerous, but fibromuscular disease[47] and congenital conditions are the most common. Aneurysms have also been reported in transplanted kidneys.[48] Post-stenotic dilations, false aneurysms, aneurysms resulting from renal artery dissections,[49] mycotic and inflammatory aneurysms, and arteritis-induced aneurysms[50] have also been described.[51] The role of atherosclerosis is controversial and in many cases may be a secondary phenomenon.[52] Frequently, classic atherosclerotic changes are found within the aneurysm despite a paucity of atherosclerosis in adjacent arteries. Nevertheless, the only predisposing factor identified in most cases was atherosclerosis.

Stanley[45] suggested that these aneurysms be classified into four types: true macroaneurysms, aneurysmal dissections, fusiform microaneurysmal dilations, and microaneurysms resulting from arteritis. The first two categories represent aneurysms amenable to surgical intervention and are the types treated in this report.

Renal artery aneurysms are slightly more common in women than men and more frequently affect the right than the left renal artery, an observation reported previously[27] and confirmed in this report. This sex and site predilection reflects the increased frequency of fibromuscular disease in women and its occurrence in the right renal artery.[27] Most renal artery aneurysms are saccular, have an average diameter of 1.3 cm,[47] and develop at the primary or secondary renal artery bifurcations. More than 90% of macroaneurysms are extraparenchymal.

Hypertension may cause and be caused by renal artery aneurysms; it is associated with up to 70% to 80% of cases.[27, 53] Preexisting hypertension in patients with congenital defects of the internal elastic lamina and media may predispose to aneurysm formation. The mechanism of hypertension induction by renal artery aneurysms may be occult stenoses, arterial compression, parenchymal embolization, branch vessel compromise, or arteriovenous fistula.[54] Detection of an aneurysm with significant hypertension is generally regarded as an indication for repair, even in the absence of demonstrable stenosis. However, without lateralizing renins, successful repair may occur in the absence of significant improvement in hypertension.[53, 55]

Risk of Rupture

The fear of aneurysm rupture has driven surgeons to early repair. However, the true risk of rupture of renal artery aneurysms has been overestimated. Early reports cited rupture rates up to 24%[56, 57] and claimed that rupture was most likely to develop in aneurysms larger than 2 cm. Larger series have refuted these ideas; in 28 patients followed for a mean of 36 months, rupture did not occur.[45] Tham monitored 69 patients for a mean of 4.3 years without ruptures developing in any of them; however, only three patients had aneurysms larger than 2.5 cm.[58]

A disproportionate number (>19) of ruptures have occurred during pregnancy.[59] Most occur in the third trimester, although not associated with labor, and have a 70% maternal mortality rate and almost 100% fetal mortality rate. Increased intraabdominal pressure, the hyperdynamic state of pregnancy, and altered wall tension because of increased estrogen and progesterone levels may all contribute to the risk of rupture. Preexisting defects and fragmentation of the internal elastic lamina may render the renal artery susceptible to aneurysmal changes. Accumulation of ground substance with a loss of elastic tissue and smooth muscle cells is characteristic. Such preexisting defects may predispose the renal artery to aneurysmal changes in the altered hemodynamic and hormonal environment of pregnancy. Most renal artery aneurysms occurring in pregnancy are situated within the left kidney; those in nonpregnant patients are more common on the right. Because of the increased rupture risk and high morbidity and mortality, it is widely held that aneurysms detected in women planning pregnancy should be repaired prophylactically.

Treatment

Management options include observation, transcatheter occlusion, and surgical intervention. Indications for intervention include an aneurysm size larger than 2.5 cm, renovascular hypertension with lateralizing renins, symptomatic aneurysms, documented expansion, renal embolization, and young women anticipating pregnancy (Table 26–3).

Therapeutic arterial embolization with a variety of agents has been described in the management of renal artery aneurysms.[50, 60] This approach may be particularly useful in patients with saccular aneurysms, small bleeding aneurysms in patients with arteritis, and in high-risk patients. Transcatheter embolization may be the treatment of choice for intraparenchymal lesions. Surgeons have considerable experience in transcatheter occlusion of a variety of visceral artery aneurysms.[27] Although direct experience with embolization of renal artery aneurysms remains limited, in the specific situations described and in the absence of significant renal artery stenosis or concomitant disease warranting surgical intervention, embolization should be strongly considered as primary therapy.

Aneurysmectomy and arteriorrhaphy with or without patch angioplasty is the simplest method of aneurysm resection with reconstitution of the renal artery. It is most easily applied to saccular aneurysms with a narrow neck on the parent artery. Ligation and bypass is appropriately applied to fusiform aneurysms. Opening the aneurysm with oversewing of feeding vessels from within the sac is optimal to preclude progressive enlargement of a ligated aneurysm. This technique may also be applied to closure of an arteriovenous fistula from within the aneurysm sac.

When multiple aneurysms are associated with an abnormal renal artery (eg, fibromuscular disease, dissection) or intraparenchymal involvement is evident, in vivo repair with hypothermic perfusion is desirable.[61, 62] This technique provides optimal visualization for evaluating the extent of disease by permitting mobilization onto the abdominal wall, ensuring a blood-free field, allowing complex microsurgical repairs, and protecting against renal ischemia. The kidney may be replanted back into the renal fossa or autotransplanted into the iliac fossa. In average-size patients, adequate mobilization can be achieved while leaving the ureter intact. Obese patients may require ureteric transection, with the procedure performed on the bench.

If an observant approach is selected, lifelong follow-up is necessary. Contrast-enhanced CT scanning is the imaging modality of choice. The patient should be instructed that flank pain or hematuria requires immediate evaluation. Blood pressure should be monitored, and development of hypertension requires arteriography.

Superior Mesenteric Artery Aneurysms

Superior mesenteric artery (SMA) aneurysms are rare aneurysms but a particular challenge when encountered. They frequently are caused by fungal infection and often involve the SMA close to the aorta. The presenting features are usually pain and an epigastric mass, often with coexisting subacute bacterial endocarditis or other infectious sources.

Table 26–3.
Indications for Surgical Repair of Renal Artery Aneurysms

Aneurysm >2.5 cm in diameter
Renovascular hypertension with lateralizing renins
Symptomatic aneurysms
Aneurysms in women planning pregnancy
Aneurysm with distal embolization

Treatment is mandatory and usually requires oversewing the SMA at the aorta and bypass grafting with reversed saphenous vein from the infrarenal aorta to more distal SMA or one of its branches. Morbidity and mortality rates are high.

Celiac Aneurysms

Celiac aneurysms are the least common visceral aneurysms. Usually caused by atherosclerosis, they represent a risk of rupture that is difficult to define because of their rarity. They should be repaired in low-risk patients and in any patient if they are larger than 3 cm, enlarging, or symptomatic.

Bypass from the aorta to a distal cuff of celiac artery is optimal. Ligation is reasonable when grafting is technically difficult. When the operation is undertaken in a cirrhotic patient, the hepatic artery must be revascularized.

Miscellaneous Visceral Artery Aneurysms

Pseudoaneurysms of the left gastric, pancreaticoduodenal, gastroduodenal, and colic arteries have been described and are usually complications of pancreatitis or prior surgical intervention. Surgical repair is a challenge, and we primarily choose transcatheter embolization. Because of recanalization after embolization of visceral artery aneurysms, we perform follow-up angiography and re-embolization when indicated.[27]

References

1. Sheps SG, Spittel JA, Fairbairn JF, Edwards JE. Aneurysms of the splenic artery with special reference to bland aneurysms. Proc Staff Meet Mayo Clin 1958;33:381–390.
2. Stanley JC, Fry WJ. Pathogenesis and clinical significance of splenic artery aneurysms. Surgery 1974;76:898–909.
3. Bedford PD, Lodge B. Aneurysms of the splenic artery. Gut 1960;1:312–320.
4. Beaussier M. Sur un aneurismie de l'artere splenique: dont les parois se sont ossifies. J Med Clin Pharmacol (Paris) 1770;32:157.
5. Owens JC, Coffey RJ. Aneurysm of the splenic artery, including a report of 6 additional cases. Int Abstr Surg 1953;97:313–35.
6. Trimble WK, Hill JH. Congestive splenomegaly (Banti's disease) due to portal stenosis without hepatic cirrhosis; aneurysms of the splenic artery. Arch Pathol 1942;34:423.
7. Boijsen E, Efsing HO. Aneurysm of the splenic artery. Acta Radiol 1969;8:29–41.
8. Mattar SG, Lumsden AB. The management of splenic artery aneurysms: experience with 23 cases. Am J Surg 1995;169:580–584.
9. DeVries JE, Schattenkerk ME, Malt RA. Complications of splenic artery aneurysm other than intraperitoneal rupture. Surgery 1982;91:200–204.
10. Trastek VF, Pairolero PC, Joyce JW, et al. Splenic artery aneurysms. Surgery 1982;91:694–699.
11. Gadacz TR, Trunkey D, Kieffer RT. Visceral vessel erosion associated with pancreatitis. Arch Surg 1978;113:1438–1440.
12. Mandel SR, Jaques PF, Mauro MA, Sanofsky S. Non-operative management of peripancreatic arterial aneurysms. Ann Surg 1987;205:126–128.
13. Sculley RE, Galbadini JJ, McNeely BU. Case records of the Massachusetts General Hospital. N Engl J Med 1981;304:1533–1538.
14. Gangahar DM, Carveth SW, Reese HE. True aneurysms of the pancreatico-duodenal artery: a case report and review of the literature. J Vasc Surg 1985;2:741–742.
15. Lumsden AB, Riley JD, Skandalakis JE. Splenic artery aneurysms. *In* Skandalakis JE, Gray SW (eds). Problems in general surgery—the spleen. Philadelphia: JB Lippincott, 1990:113–121.
16. Derchi LE, Biggi E, Cicio GR, et al. Aneurysms of the splenic artery: noninvasive diagnosis by pulsed Doppler sonography. J Ultrasound Med 1984;3:41–44.
17. Busuttil RW, Brin BJ. The diagnosis and management of visceral artery aneurysms. Surgery 1980;88:619–625.
18. Spittel JA, Fairbairn JF, Kincaid OW, Remine WH. Aneurysm of the splenic artery. JAMA 1961;175:452–456.
19. Stanley JC, Wakefield TW, Graham LM, et al. Clinical importance and management of splanchnic artery aneurysms. J Vasc Surg 1986;3:836–840.

20. Ayalon A, Wiesner RH, Perkins JD, et al. Splenic artery aneurysms in liver transplant patients. Transplantation 1988;45:386–389.

21. Brems JJ, Hiatt JR, Klein AS. Splenic artery aneurysm rupture following orthotopic liver transplantation. Transplantation 1988;45:1136–1137.

22. Stanley JC, Messina LM, Zelenok GB. Splanchnic and renal artery aneurysms. *In* Moore WS (ed). Vascular Surgery: a Comprehensive Review. Philadelphia: WB Saunders, 1991:335–349.

23. Puttini M, Aseni P, Brambilla G, Belli L. Splenic artery aneurysms in portal hypertension. J Cardiovasc Surg 1982;23:490–493.

24. Hashizume M, Ohta M, Ueno K, et al. Laparoscopic ligation of splenic artery aneurysm. Surgery 1993;113:352–354.

25. Tarazov PG, Polysalov VN, Ryzhkov VK. Transcatheter treatment of splenic artery aneurysms. J Cardiovasc Surg 1991;31:128–131.

26. Reidy JF, Rowe PH, Ellis FG. Splenic artery aneurysm embolization—the preferred technique to surgery. Clin Radiol 1990;41:281–282.

27. Salam TA, Lumsden AB, Martin LG, Smith RB. Nonoperative management of visceral aneurysms and pseudoaneurysms. Am J Surg 1992;164:215–219.

28. Guida PM, Moore SW. Aneurysms of the hepatic artery: report of five cases with a brief review of the previously reported cases. Surgery 1966;60:299.

29. Countryman D, Norwood S, Register D, et al. Hepatic artery aneurysm: report of an unusual case and review of the literature. Am Surg 1983;49:51.

30. Lumsden AB, Mattar SG, Allen RC, Bacha EA. Hepatic artery aneurysms: the management of 22 patients. J Surg Res 1996;60:345–350.

31. Stanley JC, Messina LM, Zelenock GB. Splanchnic and renal artery aneurysms. *In* Moore WS (ed). Vascular Surgery: a Comprehensive Review, 4th ed. Philadelphia: WB Saunders, 1993:435.

32. Stanley JC, Zelenock GB. Splanchnic artery aneurysms. *In* Rutherford RB (ed). Vascular Surgery, 3rd ed. Philadelphia: WB Saunders, 1989:969.

33. Dougherty MJ, Gloviczi P, Cherry KJ, et al. Hepatic artery aneurysms: evaluation and current management. Int Angiol 1993;12:178.

34. Rogers MD, Thompson JE, Garrett WV, et al. Mesenteric vascular problems: a 26-year experience. Ann Surg 1982;195:554.

35. Stouffer JT, Weinman MD, Bynum TE. Hemobilia in a patient with multiple artery aneurysms: a case report and review of the literature. Am J Gastroenterol 1989;84:59.

36. Lumsden AB, Allen RC, Sreeram S, et al. Hepatic arterioportal fistulae. Am Surg 1993;5:722.

37. Skudder PA. Visceral artery aneurysms. *In* Persson AV, Skudder PA (eds). Visceral Vascular Surgery. New York: Marcel Dekker, 1987:145.

38. Kibbler CC, Cohen DL, Cruicshank JK, et al. Use of CAT scanning in the diagnosis and management of hepatic artery aneurysm. Gut 1985;26:752.

39. Zalcman M, Matos C, Gansbeke DV, et al. Hepatic artery aneurysm: CT and MR features. Gastrointest Radiol 1987;12:203.

40. Warshauer DM, Keefe B, Mauro MA. Intrahepatic hepatic artery aneurysm: computed tomography and color-flow Doppler ultrasound findings. Gastrointest Radiol 1991;16:175.

41. Goldblatt M, Goldin AR, Schaff MI. Percutaneous embolization for the management of hepatic artery aneurysms. Gastroenterology 1977;73:1142.

42. Baker KS, Tisnado J, Cho SR, Beachley MC. Splanchnic artery aneurysms and pseudoaneurysms: transcatheter embolization. Radiology 1987;163:135.

43. Schmidt B, Bhatt GM, Abo MN. Management of post-traumatic vascular malformations by catheter embolization. Am J Surg 1980;140:332.

44. Edsman G. Angiography and suprarenal angiography. Acta Radiol 1965;155:104–116.

45. Stanley JC, Rhodes EL, Gewertz BL, et al. Renal artery aneurysms: significance of macroaneurysms exclusive of dissections and fibrodysplastic mural dilations. Arch Surg 1975;110:1327–333.

46. Stanley JC, Gerwertz BL, Bove EL, et al. Arterial fibrodysplasia: histopathologic character and current etiologic concepts. Arch Surg 1975;110:561–566.

47. Castenada-Zuniga W, Zollikofer C, Vadlez-Davila O, et al. Giant aneurysms of the renal arteries: an unusual manifestation of fibromuscular dysplasia. Radiology 1979;133:327–330.

48. Fleshner NE, Johnston KW. Repair of an autotransplant renal artery aneurysm: case report and literature review. J Urol 1992;148:389–391.

49. Scully RE, Mark EJ, McNeely WF, McNeely BU. Case records of the Massachusetts General Hospital: weekly clinicopathological exercises—case 9-1990: a 39-year-old man with hypertension, a renal-artery aneurysm and eosinophiluria. N Engl J Med 1990;322:612–622.

50. Smith DL, Wernick R. Spontaneous rupture of a renal artery aneurysm in polyarteritis nodosa: critical review of the literature and report of a case. Am J Med 1989;87:464–467.

51. Goldman MH, Tilney NL, Vineyard GC, et al. A twenty year survey of arterial complication of renal transplantation. Surg Gynecol Obstet 1975;141:758–760.

52. Hubert JP Jr, Pairolero PC, Kazmier FJ. Solitary renal artery aneurysm. Surgery 1980;88:557–561.

53. Youkey JR, Collins GJ Jr, Orecchia PM, et al. Saccular renal artery aneurysm as a cause of hypertension. Surgery 1985;97:498–501.

54. Pliskin MJ, Dresner ML, Hassell LH, et al. A giant renal artery aneurysm diagnosed postpartum. J Urol 1990;144:1459–1461.

55. Cummings KB, Lecky JW, Kaufman JJ. Renal artery aneurysms and hypertension. J Urol 1973;109:144–148.

56. Harrow BR, Sloane JA. Aneurysm of renal artery: report of five cases. J Urol 1959;81:35–41.
57. Ippolito JJ, LeVeen HH. Treatment of renal artery aneurysms. J Urol 1960;83:10–16.
58. Tham G, Ekelund L, Herrlin K, et al. Renal artery aneurysms: natural history and prognosis. Ann Surg 1983;197:348–352.
59. Richardson AJ, Liddington M, Jaskowski A, et al. Pregnancy in a renal transplant recipient complicated by rupture of a transplant renal artery aneurysm. Br J Surg 1990;77:228–229.
60. Saltiel AA, Matalon TAS, Patel SK. Embolization of a giant renal arterial aneurysm. J Urol 1990;144:1227–1228.
61. Kent KC, Salvatierra O, Reilly LM, et al. Evolving strategies for the repair of complex renovascular lesions. Ann Surg 1987;206:272–278.
62. Dubernard JM, Martin X, Gelet A, Mongin D. Aneurysms of the renal artery: surgical management with special reference to extracorporeal surgery and autotransplantation. Eur Urol 1985;11:26–30.

The Isolated Hypogastric Artery Aneurysm

Louis M. Messina, M.D., Linda Reilly, M.D., and Ronald J. Stoney, M.D.

Atherosclerotic aneurysms of the hypogastric artery are uncommon, and they are rare in the absence of infrarenal aortic or associated common iliac aneurysms.[1] A 1967 review by Silver and associates[2] found three isolated hypogastric aneurysms in 671 patients with abdominal aortic aneurysms. In the 20th century, 56 cases of isolated hypogastric aneurysms have been reported in the English literature.[1–37] Although most of the aneurysms have been characterized as atherosclerotic, some have been associated with infection, trauma, or pregnancy.[14] Hypogastric aneurysms are aneurysms of the true pelvis, unlike aneurysms of the common iliac artery, which are located at the pelvic brim. This chapter reviews the clinical presentation, diagnostic evaluation, and treatment of hypogastric artery aneurysms.

Diagnosis

Diagnosis of isolated aneurysms of the hypogastric artery by routine physical examination is difficult because of their rarity and their location within the pelvis.[15–17] Nonetheless, most patients become symptomatic because of complications caused by the aneurysm, compression, or erosion into adjacent structures, such as the bladder, ureter,[18–25] and rectum.[26–28] Symptoms in these circumstances are caused by urinary obstruction or constipation. Nerve compression most frequently involves the sciatic nerve, although a femoral neuropathy and an obturator neuropathy have also been reported.[33–37] Among 33 isolated atherosclerotic aneurysms of the hypogastric artery occurring in 32 patients, only two were considered to be asymptomatic, but one half of the aneurysms ruptured.[29–32]

Physical examination may be helpful when the physician is alert to the possibility of an aneurysm. Rectal examination can identify the presence and size of hypogastric aneurysms, because they are usually adjacent to the rectum and not palpable by abdominal examination.[26–28] The suspicion of an isolated internal iliac artery aneurysm mandates computed tomographic (CT) scanning for definitive diagnosis[15–17] (Fig. 27–1). This imaging technology is useful when applied to these aneurysms within the pelvis and, when combined with aortography, can clearly define the configuration, anatomy, and coexistent structures. Three-dimensional helical CT imaging provides a graphic representation of these aneurysms (Fig. 27–2).

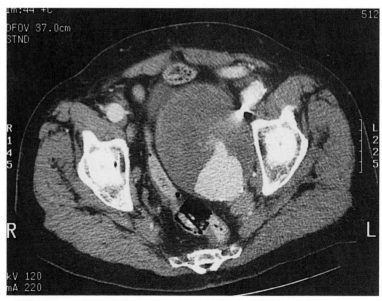

Figure 27–1. Computed tomography scan of the pelvis shows a large, right intestine iliac aneurysm.

Treatment

Surgical treatment must be tailored to the clinical manifestation and anatomy of the isolated internal iliac aneurysm itself.[6–13] Exposure may be difficult because of its location within the pelvis. The neck of the internal iliac artery, as it originates from a common iliac bifurcation, is easily exposed for proximal control. The distal ramification of the aneurysm may preclude external mobilization and clamp control, and in these circumstances, the aneurysm may be opened and the outflow vessels managed from within the aneurysm sac by endoaneurysmorrhaphy. It may be safer because the inflammation and fibrotic response surrounding the aneurysm may involve the ureter, bladder, or rectum and can complicate exposure and lead to organ damage if mobilized excessively.

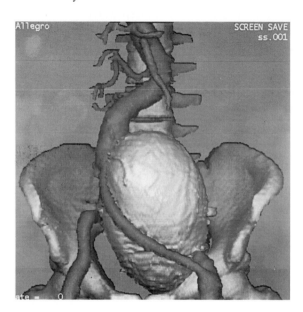

Figure 27–2. Helical computed tomography with three-dimensional reconstruction graphically demonstrates a right internal iliac aneurysm.

Unilateral ligation of an internal iliac aneurysm is well tolerated, provided contralateral iliac artery flow is adequate. If ligation of bilateral internal iliac aneurysms is undertaken, gluteal claudication and left colon ischemia are possible sequelae, particularly if the inferior mesenteric artery perfusion is inadequate. Interposition grafting in the internal iliac artery is possible but is rarely considered because all but one of the cases reported have involved a unilateral aneurysm. This contrasts with the pattern seen when hypogastric aneurysms occur in conjunction with aortic and common iliac artery aneurysmal disease. Under these circumstances, hypogastric aneurysms tend to be bilateral. Endovascular exclusion using coils or stents are options that may be quite effective and safe in controlling isolated hypogastric aneurysm.

A case at our hospital illustrates the application of these new treatment modalities and the inherent difficulties in diagnosis because of the location of these aneurysms deep in the pelvis. The workup of patient referred for repair of a pararenal aneurysm failed to identify a distal right internal iliac aneurysm. At operation, the lack of common iliac aneurysmal disease prompted a tube replacement of the pararenal and infrarenal aorta. No additional pelvic aneurysms were identified. Later, this patient had a pelvic CT (Fig. 27–3) performed for abdominal pain, and the right internal iliac artery aneurysm was identified. An aortogram (Fig. 27–4) identified an isolated aneurysm 3 cm in its transverse diameter, which occurred 5 cm beyond the origin of the right internal iliac artery. Using selective right catheterization, this aneurysm was occluded effectively with two Gianturco coils (Fig. 27–5). The contralateral internal iliac artery was normal, and the patient's graft repair was intact. The patient has remained asymptomatic for 18 months.

Conclusions

Heightened clinical suspicion is required to diagnose isolated hypogastric artery aneurysms. Most patients develop symptoms related to compression or obstruction of adjacent structures or rupture. Surgical management consists of endoaneurysmorrhaphy and preservation of external iliac artery flow.

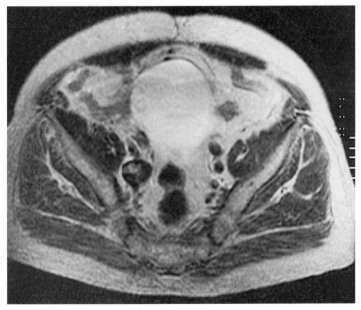

Figure 27–3. Computed tomography scan shows a moderate-size, right internal iliac aneurysm.

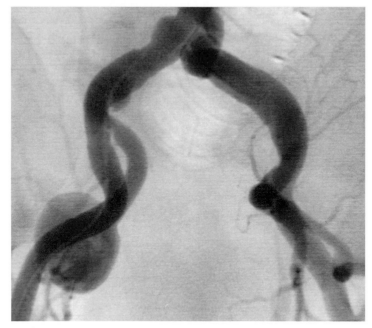

Figure 27–4. The aortogram shows an isolated distal right internal iliac aneurysm.

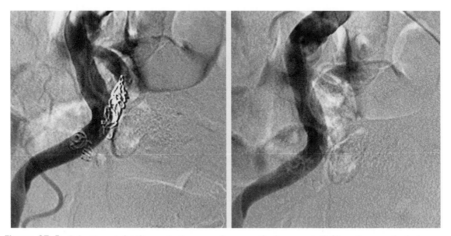

Figure 27–5. Selective right iliac arteriogram shows coil placement *(left)* and an occluded aneurysm *(right)*.

References

1. Krupski WC, Bass A, Rosenberg GD, et al. The elusive isolated hypogastric artery aneurysm: novel presentations. J Vasc Surg 1989;10:557–562.
2. Silver D, Anderson EE, Porter JM. Isolated hypogastric artery aneurysm: review and report of three cases. Arch Surg 1967;95:308–312.
3. Perdue GP, Mitternthal MJ, Smith RB, Salam AA. Aneurysms of the internal iliac artery. Surgery 1982;93:243–246.
4. McCready RA, Pairolero PC, Gilmore JC, et al. Isolated iliac artery aneurysms. Surgery 1983;93:688–693.
5. Richardson JW, Greenfield LJ. Natural history and management of iliac aneurysms. J Vasc Surg 1988;8:165–171.
6. Gilifillan I, Fell G, King B, French J. Unusual isolated iliac artery aneurysm. Br J Surg 1986;73:375.
7. Drisi-Kacemi A. Isolated internal iliac aneurysm: report of one case and review of the literature. J Cardiovasc Surg (Torino) 1988;29:68–69.
8. Markowitz AM, Norman JC. Aneurysms of the iliac artery. Ann Surg 1961;154:777–787.
9. Frank IN, Thompson HT, Rob C, Schwartz SI. Aneurysm of the internal iliac artery. Arch Surg 1961;83:956–958.
10. Short DW. Aneurysms of the internal iliac artery. Br J Surg 1966;53:17–19.
11. Kasulke RJ, Clifford A, Nichols K, Silver D. Isolated atherosclerotic aneurysms of the internal iliac artery. Arch Surg 1982;117:73–77.
12. Brin BJ, Bustatill RW. Isolated hypogastric artery aneurysms. Arch Surg 1982;117:1329–1333.
13. Fothergill WC, Donagal D. Aneurysm of the internal iliac artery. J Obstet Gynecol 1914;26:32–35.
14. MacLaren A. Aneurysm of the internal iliac artery following a severe instrumental delivery: operation and partial cure. Ann Surg 1913;117:73–77.
15. Lineaweaver WC, Slore F, Alexander RH. Computed tomographic diagnosis of acute aortoiliac catastrophes. Arch Surg 1982;117:1095–1097.
16. Marcus R, Edell SL. Sonographic evaluation of iliac artery aneurysms. Am J Surg 1980;140:667–670.
17. Samuelsson L, Albrechtsson U. Ruptured aneurysm of the internal iliac artery. J Comput Assist Tomogr 1982;6:842–844.
18. Goodwin WE, Shumacker HB. Aneurysm of the hypogastric artery producing urinary tract obstruction: report of a case. J Urol 1947;57:839–844.
19. Anderson EE, Silver D. Aneurysm of hypogastric artery presenting with bladder neck obstruction. Urology 1979;13:646–649.
20. Nelson RP. Isolated internal iliac artery aneurysms and their urological manifestation. J Urol 1980;124:300–303.
21. Safran R, Sklenicka R, Kay H. Iliac artery aneurysm: a common cause of ureteral obstruction. J Urol 1975;113:605–609.
22. Smith HW, Campbell EW, Dagher FJ. Bilateral ureteral obstruction secondary to hypogastric artery aneurysm: a case report. J Urol 1977;117:796–797.
23. Marino R, Mooppan UMM, Sein TA, et al. Urological manifestations of isolated iliac artery aneurysms. J Urol 1987;137:232–234.
24. Redman JF, Campbell GS. Ureteral obstruction secondary to iliac artery aneurysm. Urology 1975;6:212–214.
25. Kaynan A, Rosenberg JB, Szuchmacher P. Ureteral obstruction secondary to iliac artery aneurysms. Mt Sinai J Med 1978;45:334–337.
26. Victor DW, Werdick GM, Proudfoot RW. Internal iliac artery aneurysm presenting as severe constipation. J Ky Med Assoc 1987;85:310–312.
27. Victor DW, Halverson JB, Butcher HR. Internal iliac artery aneurysm: unusual cause of lower abdominal and pelvic symptoms. Mo Med 1979;78:424–426.
28. Jackman RJ, McQuarrie HB, Edwards JE. Fatal rectal hemorrhage caused by aneurysm of the internal lilac artery: report of case. Proc Staff Meet Mayo Clinic 1948;23:305–308.
29. Perry MO, Leventhal M. Ruptured hypogastric artery aneurysms. Am J Surg 1968:115:828–829.
30. Palmer PE. Massive retroperitoneal hemorrhage with unusual presentation. JAMA 1974;227:1422.
31. Datta MC, Henson FG, Vaughan ED, Nolan SF. Leaking left hypogastric artery aneurysm causing bilateral ureteric obstruction. Urology 1979;13:646–649.
32. Wirthlin LS, Warshaw AL. Ruptured aneurysms of the hypogastric artery. Surgery 1973;73:629–633.
33. Chapman EM, Shaw RS, Kubick CS. Sciatic pain from arteriosclerotic aneurysm of pelvic arteries. N Engl J Med 1964;271:1410–1411.
34. Soimakallio S, Oksala I. Sciatic pain from an aneurysm of the internal iliac artery. Ann Chir Gynaecol 1982;71:172–174.
35. Dang MT, Janati A, Higgins DC, et al. Radicular compression syndrome caused by ruptured iliac artery aneurysm: case report and review of the literature. Electromyogr Clin Neuropysiol 1987;27:447–449.
36. Waldman I, Broun AI. Femoral neuropathy secondary to iliac artery aneurysm. South Med J 1977;70:1243–1244.
37. Crews DA, Dohlman LE. Obturator neuropathy after multiple genitourinary procedures. Urology 1987;24:504–505.

Treatment of Sciatic Artery Aneurysms

Gordon L. Hyde, M.D., and Chester C. Yavorski, M.D.

Sciatic artery aneurysm is a rare but clinically relevant vascular problem. It develops in a persistent sciatic artery (PSA), a congenital anomalous condition in which the early fetal circulation in the lower extremity persists. PSA was first described by Green in 1832,[11] and 172 cases have been reported in the world literature.[7, 14, 22, 25] On the basis of angiographic studies, the incidence of PSA has been estimated to be 0.01% to 0.05%.[5, 7, 14, 20] The condition can affect male and female patients from 6 months to 89 years of age (mean, 54 years). PSAs are prone to aneurysmal dilation and as such may rupture, develop thrombosis, embolize distally, or compress the sciatic nerve. This chapter discusses the embryology and anatomy of PSAs and the pathophysiology, diagnosis, and treatment of sciatic artery aneurysms.

Embryology and Anatomy

During development of the embryo, the sciatic artery matures as the main axial artery and provides the primary blood supply to the lower limb bud. It passes dorsally along the developing mesenchymal skeletal structures and runs distally to the sole of the foot. As the embryo grows and develops, portions of this axial artery regress as the femoral artery develops. The common and superficial femoral arteries, as extensions of the external iliac artery, supersede and replace the sciatic artery and its branches to the mid-thigh.[16] The superficial femoral artery joins the popliteal artery and continues distally as the posterior tibial artery. The sciatic artery eventually persists as the popliteal, anterior tibial, and peroneal arteries. Interruption of this normal process or failure of the sciatic artery to involute results in atresia of the superficial femoral artery and persistence of the sciatic artery (Fig. 28–1).

The PSA is anatomically a continuation of the internal iliac artery.[16] After giving rise to the superior gluteal and internal pudendal arteries in the pelvis, the sciatic artery courses through the greater sciatic foramen below the piriformis muscle, where it then enters the thigh.[30] In the thigh, the PSA runs beneath the gluteus maximus along the posterior aspect of the adductor magnus, finally passing into the popliteal fossa, where it continues as the popliteal artery. The sciatic artery frequently is found within the posterior medial sheath of the sciatic nerve,[30] although it may accompany the posterior cutaneous nerve or lie within or adjacent to the sheath of the sciatic nerve.[3] When the artery is found within the sheath of the sciatic nerve, the nerve is usually splayed out over the artery. This splaying becomes more pronounced with aneurysmal dilation, creating a potential hazard to the nerve when the aneurysm is resected.[4] This anatomic relationship explains why patients

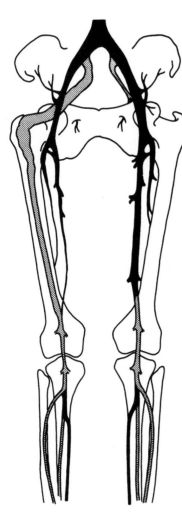

Figure 28–1. Schematic drawing of a persistent sciatic artery to the right leg and a normal pattern to left leg. Normal popliteal, peroneal, and anterior tibial arteries are derivatives of the sciatic system. *Dotted area*, primitive sciatic artery and its derivatives; *solid area*, external iliac artery and its derivatives. (Adapted from Steele G Jr, Sanders RJ, Riley J, Lindenbaum B. Pulsatile buttock masses: gluteal and persistent sciatic artery aneurysms. Surgery 1977;82:201–204.)

frequently appear with sciatica, pain in the leg or foot, or both. Most commonly, aneurysmal dilation occurs at the level of the greater trochanter, just under the gluteus maximus muscle, although it may extend far down the posterior thigh.[4]

A clinically convenient definition of the two forms, complete and incomplete, in which the PSA can exist was first proposed by Bower and colleagues[4] in 1977. This simple classification system provides a useful way of interpreting the pathologic features and of planning surgical intervention for patients with PSAs. A PSA is considered *complete* when it is the main supply to the extremity and changes little in its course to the popliteal artery. This configuration occurs in 71% of all cases reported in the world literature. The superficial femoral artery may be normal or entirely absent in these cases.[1] However, in 55% of the cases, the superficial femoral artery is hypoplastic or aplastic and provides flow to the lower limb through collateral vessels, which usually end just above the knee.[14] The PSA is considered *incomplete*[9] if its continuity is interrupted or its connection to the internal iliac or popliteal arteries is by small collateral vessels.[17, 19]

From an anatomic perspective, the sciatic artery aneurysm may be easily approached through a posterolateral buttock curvilinear incision, splitting the gluteus maximus muscle in the direction of its fibers.[17] If proximal control

Table 28–1.
Location of Sciatic Artery Aneurysms in 172 Cases of Persistent Sciatic Arteries

Location	Patients (N = 172)	Percent of Total
Right side	33	40.7
Left side	32	39.5
Bilateral	8	9.9
Unknown	8	9.9
Total	81	47.1

cannot be achieved through this incision, an anterior lower abdominal retroperitoneal approach may be made to control the internal iliac artery.[9]

Pathophysiology

Although a PSA may exist as a normally functioning vessel, early atheromatous degeneration and aneurysm formation are common. Aneurysms were detected in 81 (47.1%) of the 172 reported cases of PSA. The PSA may occur on either side (40.7%, right side; 39.5%, left side); and 9.9% of PSAs are bilateral (Table 28–1).

The cause of aneurysm formation is unclear, but the literature has suggested congenital and acquired mechanisms.[16] Some investigators attribute the aneurysms to a congenitally abnormal vessel wall with reduced elastic elements.[2, 16] Others believe that the aneurysms occur because the PSA is exposed to frequent trauma as the result of its location in a relatively exposed position of the buttock region and close to the sharp edges of the bony pelvic structures.[12, 16] Hypertension, infection, and atherosclerosis may also play a role.[27] We believe that the cause of PSA is probably a combination of congenital and acquired factors.

Diagnosis

The symptoms described by the patients discussed in the 172 reported cases of persistent sciatic arteries are outlined in Table 28–2. Patients most often report symptoms of acute ischemia (32%); however, sciatic artery aneurysms may be suggested by a buttock mass (26.2%). This mass may or may

Table 28–2.
Symptoms of 172 Patients With Persistent Sciatic Arteries

Symptom Status	Patients (N = 172)	Percent of Total
Symptomatic	103	59.9
Ischemia	55	32.0
Acute	24	13.9
Chronic	31	18.0
Gluteal mass	45	26.2
Painful	17	9.8
Painless	10	5.8
Pulsatile	24	13.9
Gluteal pain	6	3.5
Asymptomatic	65	37.8
Unknown	4	2.3

not be painful, but it is pulsatile in more than one half of the cases. When patients report symptoms of a buttock mass, the clinician should suspect a sciatic artery aneurysm and should always palpate the buttock to exclude this condition. The uncommon but pathognomonic finding of an absent femoral pulse with strong popliteal and distal pulses suggests a PSA.[10]

A suspected sciatic artery aneurysm may be confirmed diagnostically with Doppler ultrasonography[4] by following the course of the sciatic nerve down the posterior thigh.[5] Computed tomography or magnetic resonance imaging also can be used.[25, 31, 32]

Angiography is valuable in confirming the diagnosis of sciatic artery aneurysm, determining that the aneurysm is related to a PSA, defining the vascular anatomy of the distal extremity, and planning the appropriate surgical intervention. Without the angiogram, surgical exploration could have disastrous results.[20] Angiographically, the internal iliac artery courses laterally at the level of the femoral head and is recognized as a PSA. When a PSA is found, an aneurysm is present in 47% of the sciatic arteries visualized.

If oblique views are obtained, the sciatic artery aneurysm is usually located at the level of the greater trochanter, below which the persistent sciatic artery with its ectatic and irregular walls can be visualized.[16] The sciatic artery often appears dilated and runs a very tortuous course; this finding gives rise to the term *arteriomegaly*.[28] The superficial femoral artery may appear hypoplastic and in its normal position, although it gently tapers to an end above the knee without direct communication to the popliteal artery. This hypoplastic vessel may be mistaken for a normal-sized, superficial femoral artery that is occluded at the adductor canal. An unusually small superficial femoral artery that is not continuous with the popliteal artery suggests the possibility of a PSA.[17]

It may be difficult to visualize the popliteal and tibial vessels with arteriography. In the presence of a PSA, routine arteriography may suggest that the runoff vessels are occluded. Poor visualization of the runoff vessels may occur for two reasons. First, the sciatic artery is usually large, tortuous, and slow flowing, with poor distribution of contrast in the runoff vessels. Second, arteriography may fail to opacify the sciatic artery if the catheter is not proximal to the origin of the internal iliac artery. When a sciatic artery aneurysm or a PSA is suspected, selective internal iliac artery injection of contrast with delayed timing should be performed to demonstrate the distal runoff and collateral flow. If this cannot be accomplished, exploration of distal vessels should be performed before the limb of a patient with ischemia resulting from a sciatic artery aneurysm is amputated.

When a sciatic artery aneurysm is diagnosed, the contralateral extremity should be examined carefully for the presence of a similar aneurysm, because 10% of all cases are bilateral. The differential diagnosis must also include gluteal artery aneurysms and hypogastric artery aneurysms, which require only ligation or endovascular thrombosis.[6, 21, 23] Because gluteal artery aneurysms and hypogastric artery aneurysms are usually clinically indistinguishable from sciatic artery aneurysms, arteriography is necessary for a definitive diagnosis.

Treatment

Throughout the literature, the reported treatment of sciatic artery aneurysms has varied markedly according to available techniques and ingenuity. In early cases, misdiagnosis of sciatic artery aneurysm as a gluteal abscess or buttock tumor led to unsuccessful results. Historically, sciatic artery aneurysms were treated by injection of ferric chloride. Initially, ferric chloride injection appeared to be successful, but this technique subsequently failed and was quickly abandoned.[24] More aggressive approaches, such as ligation of the sciatic artery aneurysm, have proved successful when the femoral arterial system was developed sufficiently to maintain viability of the leg.[17, 20, 30] However, when patients have a complete PSA without adequate collateralization in the hypoplastic femoral arterial system, ligation of the sciatic artery aneurysm must be followed by some form of bypass if disastrous results are to be avoided.[4, 19, 26, 30] The ischemia caused by a thromboembolic event can be worsened by ligation of the sciatic artery aneurysm. In selected cases, intraarterial thrombolytic therapy may be useful before definitive surgical revascularization.[5]

Excision of the sciatic artery aneurysm with end-to-end interposition grafting has been successful.[4, 13, 18] However, this technique has several disadvantages. The intimate relationship between the sciatic nerve and the sciatic artery aneurysm causes the nerve to be attenuated and stretched out over the surface of the aneurysm. Attempts at excision or mass ligation can cause injury to the sciatic nerve.[30] McLellan and Morettin[20] point out that the remaining anomalous sciatic artery is prone to further atheromatous degeneration and that ideal therapy requires complete exclusion. Moreover, blood flow is compromised when the patient sits on the graft.[20]

Endoaneurysmorrhaphy with end-to-end sciatic artery anastomosis has been successful and probably avoids nerve injury.[30] However, this technique does not address the problems of continued atheromatous degeneration and of compromised blood flow when the patient sits.

The current approach is proximal and distal ligation of the aneurysm in an area less adherent to the nerve and simultaneous femoropopliteal bypass graft.[1, 7, 8, 14, 17, 19, 32] This approach successfully fulfills all of the goals of surgical therapy, including ablation of the aneurysm, restoration of satisfactory arterial blood flow to the lower extremity, and prevention of future complications from the diseased sciatic artery.[17] However, an ileopopliteal graft may be a necessary bypass procedure in patients who have hypoplastic superficial femoral arteries.

With the emergence of minimally invasive surgery and endovascular procedures, another successful alternative includes femoropopliteal bypass grafting followed by percutaneous endovascular occlusion of the sciatic artery aneurysm.[1] Angiographic embolization with or without femoropopliteal bypass grafting has been successfully performed in selected cases.[15, 25] These endovascular techniques are appealing alternatives to ligation with femoropopliteal bypass because they reduce the chance for sciatic nerve injury while successfully satisfying the goals of surgical therapy. With continued advancements in endovascular techniques and improvements in the instrumentation used in these techniques, the need for surgical ligation or ablation of the sciatic artery aneurysm will be a matter of historical interest.

References

1. Becquemin JP, Gaston A, Coubret P, et al. Aneurysm of persistent sciatic artery: report of a case treated by endovascular occlusion and femoropopliteal bypass. Surgery 1985;98:605.
2. Benevenia J, Zimmerman MG, O'Neil M, et al. Aneurysm of a congenitally persistent sciatic artery presenting as a soft-tissue mass of the buttock: a case report. J Bone Joint Surg Am 1995;77:1724.
3. Blair CB, Nandy K. Persistence of the axis artery of the lower limb. Anat Rec 1965;152:161.

4. Bower EB, Smullens SN, Parke WW. Clinical aspects of persistent sciatic artery: report of two cases and review of the literature. Surgery 1977;81:588.

5. Brantley SK, Rigdon EE, Raju S. Persistent sciatic artery: embryology, pathology, and treatment. J Vasc Surg 1993;18:242.

6. Brin BJ, Busuttil RW. Isolated hypogastric artery aneurysms. Arch Surg 1982;117:1329.

7. Calleja F, Garcia Jimenez MA, Roman M, et al. Operative management of a persistent sciatic artery aneurysm. Cardiovasc Surg 1994;2:281.

8. Chleboun JO, Teasdale JE. A pulsatile gluteal mass due to sciatic artery aneurysm. Aust N Z J Surg 1995;65:907.

9. Clark FA Jr, Beazley RM. Sciatic artery aneurysm: a case report including operative approach and review of the literature. Am Surg 1976;42:13.

10. Cowie TN, McKellar NJ, McLean N, et al. Unilateral congenital absence of the external iliac and femoral arteries. Br J Radiol 1960;33:520.

11. Green PH. On a new variety of the femoral artery. Lancet 1832;1:730.

12. Hessling KH, Szkandera J, Theron L. Pulsatile gluteal mass revealed as a false aneurysm of a persistent sciatic artery. S Afr Med J 1988;73:245.

13. Hutchinson JE 3d, Cordice JW Jr, McAllister FF. The surgical management of an aneurysm of a primitive persistent sciatic artery. Ann Surg 1968;167:277.

14. Ikezawa T, Naiki K, Moriura S, et al. Aneurysm of bilateral persistent sciatic arteries with ischemic complications: case report and review of the world literature. J Vasc Surg 1994;20:96.

15. Loh FK. Embolization of a sciatic artery aneurysm an alternative to surgery: a case report. Angiology 1985;36:472.

16. Mandell VS, Jaques PF, Delany DJ, et al. Persistent sciatic artery: clinical, embryologic, and angiographic features. AJR Am J Roentgenol 1985;144:245.

17. Martin KW, Hyde GL, McCready RA, et al. Sciatic artery aneurysms: report of three cases and review of the literature. J Vasc Surg 1986;4:365.

18. Martinez LO, Jude J, Becker D. Bilateral persistent sciatic artery: a case report. Angiology 1968;19:541.

19. Mayschak DT, Flye MW. Treatment of the persistent sciatic artery. Ann Surg 1984;199:69.

20. McLellan GL, Morettin LB. Persistent sciatic artery: clinical, surgical, and angiographic aspects. Arch Surg 1982;117:817.

21. Rinaldi I, Fitzer PM, Whitley DF, et al. Aneurysm of the inferior gluteal artery causing sciatic pain: case report. J Neurosurg 1976;44:100.

22. Saey JP, Fastrez J. Acute ischemia of the lower limb and sciatic artery aneurysm. Cardiovasc Surg 1994;2:271.

23. Schorn B, Reitmeier F, Falk V, et al. True aneurysm of the superior gluteal artery: case report and review of the literature. J Vasc Surg 1995;21:851.

24. Shutze WP, Garrett WV, Smith BL. Persistent sciatic artery: collective review and management. Ann Vasc Surg 1993;7:303.

25. Sogaro F, Amroch D, Galeazzi E, et al. Non-surgical treatment of aneurysms of bilateral persistent sciatic artery. Eur J Vasc Endovasc Surg 1996;12:503.

26. Steele G Jr, Sanders RJ, Riley J, et al. Pulsatile buttock masses: gluteal and persistent sciatic artery aneurysms. Surgery 1977;82:201.

27. Taylor DA, Fiore AS. Arteriography of a persistent primitive left sciatic artery with aneurysm: a case report. Radiology 1966;87:718.

28. Thomas ML, Blakeney CG, Browse NL. Arteriomegaly of persistent sciatic arteries. Radiology 1978;128:55.

29. Vimla NS, Khanna SK, Lamba GS. Bilateral persistent sciatic artery with bilateral aneurysms: case report and review of the literature. Can J Surg 1981;24:535.

30. Williams LR, Flanigan DP, O'Connor RJ, et al. Persistent sciatic artery: clinical aspects and operative management. Am J Surg 1983;145:687.

31. Wilms G, Storme L, Vandaele L, et al. CT demonstration of aneurysm of a persistent sciatic artery. J Comput Assist Tomogr 1986;10:524.

32. Wolf YG, Gibbs BF, Guzzetta VJ, et al. Surgical treatment of aneurysm of the persistent sciatic artery. J Vasc Surg 1993;17:218.

Treatment of Infected False Aneurysm of the Femoral Artery

Frank T. Padberg Jr., M.D.

Active local infection and anatomic location are the critical distinguishing features of a false aneurysm of the femoral artery. The severity of adverse complications from peripheral aneurysms is amplified by the presence of infection, and the infection usually becomes the overriding consideration in management. The probability of tissue ischemia is directly related to anatomic location. Adverse factors associated with infected femoral artery pseudoaneurysm are summarized in Table 29–1 and include hemorrhage, compression injury of contiguous structures, ischemic limb loss, and life-threatening sepsis.

Arterial wall infection may originate locally or from a remote source such as endocarditis. According to one literature review,[1] the femoral artery (38%) and the aorta (31%) are the most common sites for arterial wall infection, accounting for more than two thirds of those reported. Septic emboli that emanate from a central source may involve any arterial distribution, including those to the extremities, the cerebra, and the viscera.[1, 20] Septic emboli may also emanate from a peripheral source and have an appropriately localized distribution.[9] The femoral site and a traumatic cause are the most common features, but a false aneurysm occurring after needle or catheter puncture may develop in any accessible extremity artery (ie, femoral, radial, brachial, axillary, and subclavian). Infection can complicate a pseudoaneurysm resulting from use of unsanitary needles and can develop when an otherwise uncomplicated false aneurysm is not recognized early in its course.

The infectious agents tend to represent common pathogens. Staphylococcal species predominate in femoral pseudoaneurysms, accounting for 16 (88%) of 18 cases in our report.[9] Of these, 19% were methicillin resistant. Brown and colleagues[1] reported a marked increase in the frequency of staphylococcal

Table 29–1.
Complications Associated With Infected Peripheral Aneurysm

Expansion and/or Rupture
Free hemorrhage
Contained aneurysm
Retroperitoneal extension
Occlusion or Thrombosis
Embolization, thrombotic
Embolization, septic
Ischemic limb loss
Systemic Sepsis
Originating locally with systemic manifestations
Originating centrally with peripheral manifestations

infections and associated this microbiologic profile with the increase in cases caused by trauma. *Staphylococcus aureus* in experimental graft infection is associated with tissue lysis and hemorrhage.[5] In the population of injectable drug abusers, human immunodeficiency virus (HIV) infection is also common. Recognition of this factor probably will increase as diagnostic and treatment methods improve.

Salmonella species have been associated with primary arterial wall infection of the aorta. By reviewing serial computed tomographic (CT) scans, several investigators have demonstrated that bacterial arteritis with this organism begins in a normal-diameter artery; the natural history of this infection unfolds during 2 to 5 weeks, during which the diameter enlarges and forms an unstable aneurysm.[6, 13]

Normally, the arterial wall is resistant to infection, but after its integrity is compromised, inflammation and necrosis potentiate intramural destruction. As an uncommon clinical event with a diffuse anatomic distribution and devastating consequences (see Table 29–1), arterial wall infections have been the subject of many small case series.[1, 6, 13]

Clinical nomenclature remains somewhat confusing because the terminology is not uniformly applied. Fortunately, the misleading term *mycotic aneurysm* has become less popular.[1, 19] Coined by Osler to describe a fulminating aortic wall infection originating in an infected aortic valve, the term mycotic aneurysm has been used by surgeons to describe almost any arterial infection, whether or not there is a fungal component. The terms *bacterial arteritis* and *infected pseudoaneurysm* have been employed to differentiate primary infections of the arterial wall from those occurring after local trauma.

Experience with the management of infected femoral false aneurysm has guided development of the management plan described in this chapter.

Significance of the False Aneurysm

Although exsanguinating hemorrhage is a real threat, free rupture through the skin is uncommon.[19] Usually, breakdown of the arterial wall produces extravasation and surrounding tissue necrosis from direct compression. Rapid expansion and the inflammatory response combine to exacerbate the damage. Expansion or contained rupture may also extend proximally above the inguinal ligament.

Symptomatic involvement of surrounding anatomic structures may be the first symptom of an enlarging aneurysm. Local compression may take the form of nerve injury, usually involving the femoral nerve that passes close to the femoral arterial bifurcation.[9] The vein may be compressed or thrombosed, resulting in symptoms of venous obstruction. Dermis, muscle, adipose tissue, and lymphatics may also be damaged.

Although bleeding and expansion are usually the major emergent issues, thrombotic events are also important management concerns. Significant limb ischemia is uncommon when the infected aneurysm is diagnosed; however, because the method of management may risk acute ischemia, preoperative consideration of this problem is important. Thrombosis of the superficial femoral artery may occur before surgical repair of the aneurysm, and the capacity for development of collateral blood flow should be assessed. Septic arterial embolization (Fig. 29–1) may originate in the aneurysm, a prosthetic graft, or heart valve. Localization to a single extremity suggests a peripheral source.

Sepsis and bacteremia from local injury have become more common, and

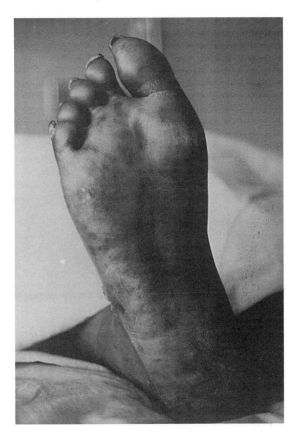

Figure 29–1. Multiple embolic petechiae are diffusely distributed on the plantar surface of this foot.

the frequency of involvement from a central source such as an infected cardiac valve has declined.[1] Bacteremia may seed true aneurysms, but this is probably less common than once assumed.[6] Extravasation of pressurized arterial blood leads to acute expansion, which is responsible for the severity of the complications associated with infected pseudoaneurysms. With infection of the arterial wall, tissue lysis and weakening occur, leading to rupture. Identification of physical findings of local injection trauma and an accurate history may be crucial to clarify the source.[8, 9]

Clinical Features and Assessment

An infected pseudoaneurysm of the femoral artery produces significant findings and symptoms. However, the diagnosis is not always obvious, even to the experienced vascular specialist. A painful mass in the groin was the only finding consistently observed in all our patients.[9] Without appropriate imaging studies, the tender groin mass might have been treated as a local infection. Although an infected arterial aneurysm may be the first manifestation of a systemic focus of bacteremia, suspicion of endocarditis is likely to focus the physician's initial attention elsewhere. A transthoracic or transesophageal echocardiogram is useful in assessing the valve. Because arterial wall infection is not a common clinical problem, delayed recognition is common. The delay in diagnosis averaged 17 days in our experience.[9]

The infected aneurysm expands rapidly and compresses surrounding tissues, producing localized swelling and pain. The mass often is not readily appreciated to be pulsatile or expansile. Bruit, however, is a common finding.

Surrounding erythema, edema, and localized cellulitis are accompanied by fever and leukocytosis. Preoperative examination of the distal circulation is important, because arterial thromboembolism implies occlusion and distal infection.

Both distal pulse examination and Doppler assessment of the ankle systolic pressure are essential preoperative observations. The rapidly expanding, infected pseudoaneurysm often produces local nerve injury by direct compression, and the resulting deficits are likely to produce sustained pain and functional disability long after the arterial problem is controlled. Careful documentation of sensory and motor functions is important because they are often not a priority for the initial examiner.

The temptation to perform incision and drainage of a tender mass in the groin should be avoided if the lesion may be an infected aneurysm. Suspicion of a purulent collection should prompt appropriate imaging studies. The absence of a pulsatile component to the mass is not sufficient to exclude an underlying pseudoaneurysm. A history of local needle or catheter entry by the physician, the patient, or another individual also should prompt further diagnostic investigation. Addicts with needle trauma are by nature wary of hospitals, delay visits for medical care, and still attempt to conceal their habit after seeking medical care. However, careful clinical examination and questioning may identify a site of injection or characteristic scars.[8]

Duplex ultrasonography is useful in diagnosing uncomplicated pseudoaneurysms. Arterial and venous thromboses are also readily identified by the experienced sonographer. However, local discomfort and hip flexion from the advanced lesion may preclude accurate placement of the probe. Moreover, accurate examinations are not always readily available on an emergent basis. Although direct compression therapy has had increasing success in management of the fresh, uncomplicated, catheter-induced pseudoaneurysm, compression therapy is unlikely to succeed with the infected aneurysm, because the arterial wall is diffusely damaged, the mass is usually too tender to permit compression, and the local infection is not controlled by this method.

The anatomic extent of the aneurysm, the hematoma, and the surrounding inflammatory mass is well defined by CT. A hematoma that infiltrates the surrounding structures is a common finding. Although essential for the evaluation of occult intraabdominal arterial infection, CT is not required for management of a femoral pseudoaneurysm. CT is particularly useful when the aneurysm extends above the inguinal ligament into the pelvis (Fig. 29–2). The rapid acquisition and high resolution of CT scanners have improved their utility.

Magnetic resonance imaging may be equally satisfactory. Magnetic resonance arteriography offers the potential advantage of static tissue imaging with concomitant characterization of arterial flow.

Arteriography is important because it defines the extent of the aneurysm and the arterial anatomy (Fig. 29–3). Unexpected findings, such as isolated involvement of the profunda femoris or a small branch artery, may permit more limited surgical therapy.[8, 9] The infected false aneurysm expands early in its course, and the intraluminal thrombus is often limited in extent, unlike the thick, laminated thrombus typically seen in the sac of a true aneurysm.

The extent of the arterial wall infection can be determined only by direct surgical visualization. Preexisting arterial occlusive disease is uncommon in the youthful population using illicit drugs, but thrombotic events occur with some frequency in those with infected pseudoaneurysms (Figs. 29–1 and 29–4). Embolization is ominous and implies an increased likelihood of limb

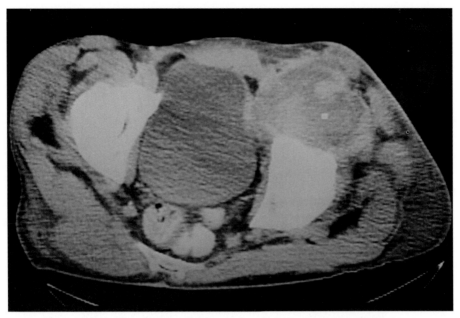

Figure 29–2. Computed tomographic examination demonstrates a large pseudoaneurysm *(small white square)* at the level of the acetabulum and femoral head. The aneurysm extends above the inguinal ligament into the pelvis.

loss.[8, 9] In the case of bacteremia with seeding from a remote source, additional aneurysmal sites and septic aneurysms may be unmasked by a thorough arteriographic survey.[20]

Treatment

Debridement and Ligation

Adequate debridement and complete excision of the infected arterial wall and surrounding necrotic tissue is essential to the successful management of the infected aneurysm. This can be accomplished only by obtaining control of all arterial flow contributing to the aneurysm. Arterial integrity is poor in the infected aneurysm, and premature entry into the lumen may occur during dissection. Proximal control of arterial inflow is secured before dissection of the aneurysm. If the infection extends into the pelvis, an oblique lower abdominal incision is required for proximal control and adequate debridement.

The superficial or profunda femoris arteries may be dissected next, but a careful approach is important because their preservation may be essential to limb survival. A Fogarty catheter with a syringe and three-way stopcock is prepared before aneurysm dissection because control of the patent profunda femoris or superficial femoral arteries are usually secured from within the opened aneurysm sac. This approach reduces blood loss and injury to the profunda femoris and superficial femoral arteries, veins, and nerves. Small arteries feeding the aneurysm may be ligated from within the sac or externally during the dissection.

After control of bleeding has been obtained and the aneurysm opened, debridement commences. At this time, the profunda femoris or superficial femoral arteries may also be dissected and controlling tapes applied. All

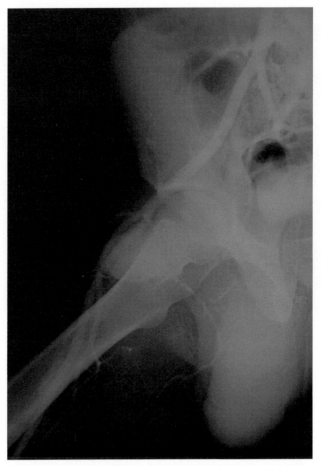

Figure 29–3. This arteriogram demonstrates a femoral pseudoaneurysm, which is superimposed on the femur. The hip is externally rotated, a position that relieves the tension exerted by the musculotendinous structures surrounding the expanding aneurysm.

necrotic debris surrounding the aneurysmal mass is excised to healthy tissue, determined by observation of adequate bleeding from the exposed surfaces. Abnormal arterial wall must be completely excised during the debridement to avoid postoperative hemorrhage. Involved muscle and tendon are easily recognized and excised as needed. Nerve that is clearly nonviable should be excised, but if there is any doubt, it can be left for subsequent debridement.

Adequate resection of involved skin is also required. Because the operative field is grossly infected, skin closure is deferred to facilitate frequent local wound care.

Careful definition of patent or occluded major veins is an important part of this process. The prime target of the addict, the vein, is frequently thrombosed or destroyed in the area of the aneurysm. Secure ligation and marking of the artery is essential to subsequent wound care outside of the operating suite. It has been our practice to doubly ligate the artery using a distinctive suture such as blue Prolene, which can easily be identified in the wound during daily dressing changes. Disappearance of the Prolene suture into the granulating tissue bed is a useful prognostic sign and indicates healing of healthy arterial wall. Lymphatic channels may remain open after debridement, producing large volumes of clear, serous drainage; careful observation of the open wound often permits direct ligation of persistent lymphatic leaks.

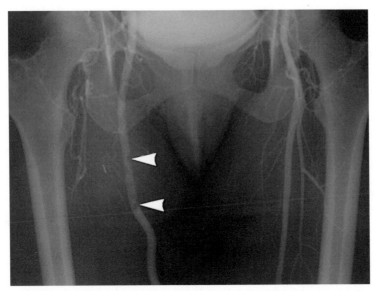

Figure 29–4. This arteriogram demonstrates multiple septic foci within the lumen of a polytetra-fluoroethylene bypass *(arrowheads)*. Septic embolization, caused by *Staphylococcus aureus* infection, was heralded by embolization to the foot. (From Padberg FT Jr, Hobson RW II, Lee BC, et al. Femoral pseudoaneurysm from drugs of abuse: ligation or reconstruction? J Vasc Surg 1992;15:642–648.)

The most effective treatment for the infected femoral aneurysm is simple ligation when limb viability can be ensured. Arterial reconstruction has been complicated by multiple repeat operations and a higher rate of amputation.[9] Detection of an audible Doppler signal at the ankle has proven satisfactory for determination of limb viability. When this signal has been present, the limbs have survived with neuromuscular function unchanged from the preoperative state.[9] A reduced likelihood of amputation correlated with ligation of only a single artery.[14]

Inadequate debridement may require reoperation for hemorrhage after arterial ligation. Similar to the procedure for aortic infections, complete excision of all diseased and infected tissue is the key to a successful operation.[1, 6, 9, 15] Just as infection of the aneurysm wall led to tissue breakdown, bleeding, and expansion, the ligated arterial wall must be capable of secure healing. Tissue necrosis rather than pressure is the probable culprit when postoperative bleeding problems occur.

Results of this management plan were satisfactory, with little complaint of persistent claudication.[9] Although some surgeons have advocated routine reconstruction for claudication,[10] this has not been required in our experience.[9] The mean ankle-brachial index in limbs that underwent arterial ligation was 0.63. Neurologic dysfunction was the major debilitating factor in the postoperative interval; it was unrelated to the form of management.

Vascular Reconstruction

When adequate circulation to the limb is doubtful, a wide array of challenging procedures may be employed to correct the problem. Autogenous tissue repair is desirable in the presence of infection but is not always available. In our report, the profunda femoris artery was reimplanted more distally onto an intact superficial femoral artery in one limb. Reddy and coworkers[14] advocated saphenous vein reconstruction and reported satisfactory results when this conduit was available. Rotational muscle flaps have been successful in the management of prosthetic graft infection, but they are less likely to succeed with the extent of local infection associated with this problem and the frequency of infections with organisms such as *S. aureus*.[9, 12] One attempt to employ a temporary prosthetic graft in the aneurysm bed was also plagued by recurrent infection.

Despite an increased incidence of graft infection, prosthetic bypass procedures through clean tissue planes probably remain a common method of revascularization. Because expansion of the infected aneurysm produces considerable local tissue reaction, tunnels passing near the common femoral artery are usually undesirable. The contralateral femoral artery has been avoided (and the femoral-femoral bypass) because of the risk of bilateral limb involvement. The remaining options include axillary to distal profunda bypass through a lateral thigh incision, axillary to popliteal bypass through a lateral incision, and iliofemoral bypass through the obturator foramen. Experience with each of these techniques has not shown one to be preferable to another.

Axillary-based procedures are performed through a standard infraclavicular incision to expose the proximal axillary artery. The dissection is carried as far medially as possible for proximal control and precise anastomosis; division of the pectoralis minor carries minimal morbidity and significantly enhances the exposure. With careful dissection, the axillary nerve trunks are easily excluded from the operative field, and the axillary vein is retracted. Caution is exercised in manipulation of the artery because the axillosubclavian arteries are particularly fragile. An S-shaped bevel facilitates a short parallel course for the prosthesis, with an end-to-side anastomosis. The graft is laid parallel to the distal course of the artery to provide flexibility and reduce strain on the anastomosis with motion of the shoulder.[18] The tunnel is made behind the pectoral musculature and descends along the anterior axillary line.

The lateral approaches for popliteal and profunda exposure are not everyday procedures, but they are readily accomplished by the experienced vascular surgeon.[7, 16, 18] For a profunda femoris anastomosis, the tunnel can often be made without a third counterincision. Because the inflammatory mass is so extensive in the groin, the tunnel may place the graft at risk; these grafts may be successfully placed lateral to the anterior superior spine, although this is less desirable than the standard site. Exposure of the distal profunda is similar to that of the superficial femoral, except that the sartorius muscle is reflected medially and the profunda femoris is found deep to the underlying fascia.[16] For more distal outflow, a third incision is usually required to complete the tunnel. The popliteal artery is easily exposed using a lateral thigh incision. The deep fascia may be incised laterally or posteriorly; the common peroneal nerve is identified first, and the popliteal artery is located in the anterior portion of the popliteal space. The resulting course of the graft is shorter and avoids an unnatural curve across the anterior thigh. Grafts 6 or 8 mm in diameter and made of polytetrafluoroethylene or Dacron have been successfully used; although there is no objective evidence to support its use, a graft reinforced with rings is preferred. Improved patency of axillofemoral grafts has made this option more attractive.[2, 18]

Grafts traversing the obturator foramen may originate from the common, external, or internal iliac artery.[11] An oblique incision, 2 to 4 cm proximal and parallel to the inguinal ligament, is made for the exposure. The peritoneum is reflected anteriorly and superiorly to expose the iliac bifurcation. The obturator membrane is identified by following the obturator artery and nerve, which exit the foramen in the anterior and lateral corner. The membrane is dense, and it is difficult to palpate instruments passed to it from either side; it cannot be easily penetrated by blunt instruments and should be incised anteromedially to the obturator artery and nerve. The distal incision is made in the medial, distal thigh, and the superficial femoral or popliteal artery is exposed and encircled. A tunneler is passed proximally to the obturator membrane from a plane below the adductor longus muscle. After the proximal anastomosis is completed, the graft is brought through the tunnel and the distal anastomosis performed.

Arteriography is often performed to evaluate the technical result. The artery distal to the anastomosis is insonated by Doppler to evaluate the arterial signal before and after construction of the new graft. The contribution from graft flow is assessed intraoperatively by Doppler insonation of the outflow artery to verify augmentation of arterial flow by the new graft during temporary occlusion of the graft.

Adjunctive pharmacologic measures remain unproved for these specific graft configurations, but aspirin has been shown to be of value for sustaining infrainguinal grafts.[4] Dextran infusion may be of value for enhancing initial patency, and warfarin sodium (Coumadin) also may prove to be of value.[3, 17] The use of aspirin and warfarin is the subject of an ongoing prospective, randomized, cooperative trial supported by the Veterans Administration.

Continued duplex surveillance may detect early intimal hyperplasia and can diagnose clinically asymptomatic graft occlusion. Delayed infectious complications are common and require similar ingenuity for their solution. Prosthetic grafts are at significant risk for secondary infection.[9] These patients are chronically colonized with staphylococci and may have increased susceptibility for bacterial infections by concomitant viral infections, such as HIV. New infected pseudoaneurysms may occur at the distal anastomosis, and the risk of bleeding remains high. Intraluminal infectious seeding of the prosthesis may lead to septic embolization; the risk of limb loss in this situation is high, and the options for further revascularization are limited. Although the subcutaneous course of the axillary-based graft is theoretically at risk from attempted self-cannulation for drug injection, we have not been able to document the occurrence of this complication.

Conclusions

Treatment of the infected femoral artery aneurysm is complicated by local tissue necrosis, delay in diagnosis, and the threat of limb ischemia. Adequate and complete debridement of the surrounding tissues and the involved arterial wall are critical to the success of any course of management. Femoral arterial ligation is well tolerated and leads to improved results when an audible Doppler signal is detected at the ankle. Revascularization usually requires a prosthetic extraanatomic approach and is complicated by frequent reoperative events and a higher rate of limb loss.

References

1. Brown SL, Busuttil RW, Baker JD, et al. Bacteriologic and surgical determinants of survival in patients with mycotic aneurysm. J Vasc Surg 1984;1:541–547.
2. El-Massry S, Saad E, Sauvage LR, et al. Axillofemoral bypass with externally supported knitted Dacron grafts: a follow-up through twelve years. J Vasc Surg 1993;17:107–115.
3. Flinn WJ, Rohrer MJ, Yao JST, et al. Improved long term patency of infrainguinal PTFE grafts. J Vasc Surg 1988;7:785–789.

4. Goodnight SM, Could BH, McAnulty JH, Taylor LH. Antiplatelet therapy: part 2. West J Med 1993;158:506–514.

5. Malone JM, Moore WS, Campagna G, et al. Bacteremic infectability of vascular grafts: the influence of pseudointimal integrity and duration of graft infection. Surgery 1975;78:211.

6. Oz MC, Brener BJ, Buda JA, et al. A ten-year experience with bacterial aortitis. J Vasc Surg 1989;10:439–449.

7. Padberg FT Jr. A lateral approach to the popliteal artery. Ann Vasc Surg 1988;3:397–401.

8. Padberg FT Jr. Infected femoral artery false aneurysm associated with drug abuse. *In* Ernst C, Stanley J (eds). Current Therapy in Vascular Surgery, 3rd ed. St. Louis: Mosby–Year Book, 1995:319–321.

9. Padberg FT Jr, Hobson RW II, Lee BC, et al. Femoral pseudoaneurysm from drugs of abuse: ligation or reconstruction? J Vasc Surg 1992;15:642–648.

10. Patel KR, Semel L, Clauss RH. Routine revascularization with resection of infected femoral pseudoaneurysm from substance abuse. J Vasc Surg 1988;8:321–328.

11. Pearce WH, Ricco JB, Yao JST, et al. Modified technique of obturator bypass in failed or infected grafts. Ann Surg 1983;197:344–347.

12. Perler BA, Vander Kolk CA, Manson PM, Williams GM. Rotational muscle flaps to treat localized prosthetic graft infection: long-term follow-up. J Vasc Surg 1993;18:358–365.

13. Reddy DJ, Shephard AD, Evans JR, et al. Management of infected aortoiliac aneurysms. Arch Surg 1991;126:873–879.

14. Reddy DJ, Smith RF, Elliot JP, et al. Infected false aneurysm in drug addicts: evolution of selective vascular reconstruction. J Vasc Surg 1986;3:718–724.

15. Reilly LM, Stoney RJ, Goldstone J, Ehrenfeld WK. Improved management of aortic graft infection: influence of operation sequence and staging. J Vasc Surg 1987;5:421–431.

16. Rutherford RB. Atlas of Vascular Surgery: Basic Techniques and Exposures. Philadelphia: WB Saunders, 1993:112–131.

17. Rutherford RB, Jones DH, Bergentz SE, et al. Efficacy of dextran 40 in preventing early postoperative thrombosis following lower extremity bypass. J Vasc Surg 1985;1:765–773.

18. Taylor LM Jr, Moneta GL, McConnell DB, et al. Axillofemoral grafting with externally supported polytetrafluoroethylene. Arch Surg 1994;129:588–595.

19. Yellin AE. Ruptured mycotic aneurysm. Arch Surg 1977;112:981–986.

20. Yeager RA, Hobson RW, Padberg FT, et al. Vascular complications related to drug abuse. J Trauma 1987;27:305–308.

Popliteal Artery Aneurysms

Marc E. Mitchell, M.D., and Jeffrey P. Carpenter, M.D.

Popliteal artery aneurysms, although the most common of the peripheral arterial aneurysms, occur infrequently, with a reported incidence of less than four cases in 100,000 in hospitalized patients.[9] They are found almost exclusively in men and are usually diagnosed during the sixth or seventh decade of life.[2, 5, 13, 14, 16, 19]

The popliteal artery is considered to be aneurysmal when its diameter is larger than 2 cm or greater than 150% the diameter of the normal adjacent popliteal artery.[7] Most popliteal aneurysms are fusiform and may involve the distal superficial femoral artery as well as the popliteal artery. Saccular aneurysms are less common but tend to have larger diameters and involve shorter segments of the popliteal artery. Atherosclerosis is thought to cause popliteal aneurysms in more then 90% of patients.[13, 19] Symptoms or complications are evident at the time of initial presentation of up to 79% of patients in surgical series.[16]

Popliteal aneurysms are unique in that they have a higher rate of thromboembolic complications and a lower risk of rupture than arterial aneurysms in other locations. Because the incidence of limb-threatening ischemia and limb loss rises dramatically with aneurysm thrombosis,[1–3, 5, 10, 12, 15, 17–19] most surgeons advocate surgical repair in symptom-free patients before complications develop. Thrombosis, distal embolization, rupture, and compression of adjacent structures are the clinical manifestations commonly produced by popliteal aneurysms. The incidence of bilateral popliteal aneurysms is high, ranging from 24% to 68% (Table 30–1). Popliteal aneurysms are frequently associated with aneurysmal disease elsewhere in the arterial circulation, particularly the

Table 30–1.
Frequency of Bilateral and Extrapopliteal Aneurysms in Patients With Popliteal Artery Aneurysms

Author	Patients	Popliteal Aneurysms (n)	Bilateral Aneurysms (%)	Extrapopliteal Aneurysms (%)	Aortic Aneurysms (%)
Anton et al.[1]	110	160	45	39	32
Carpenter et al.[2]	33	54	62	61	58
Evans et al.[4]	36	56	54		36
Reilly et al.[12]	159	244	53		21
Roggo et al.[13]	167	252	51	51	
Shortell et al.[14]	39	51	24		39
Szilagyi et al.[15]	62	87	40		45
Varga et al.[16]	137	200	54		33
Vermilion et al.[17]	87	147	68	55	42
Whitehouse et al.[18]	61	88	44		62
Wychulis et al.[19]	152	233	53	45	38

aorta. Extrapopliteal aneurysms are more common in patients with bilateral popliteal aneurysms, with an incidence as high as 78%.[18] Approximately 1% of patients with aortic aneurysms also have popliteal aneurysms.[18] Aortic, femoral, and iliac artery aneurysms must be searched for in any patient presenting with a popliteal artery aneurysm.

Clinical Presentation

Between 48% and 79% of patients requiring operation for popliteal artery aneurysms are symptomatic at the time of initial presentation (Table 30–2). The most common presenting symptoms include lower extremity ischemia, compression of adjacent structures, and rupture. Rupture of a popliteal aneurysm is rare, occurring in fewer than 7% of patients. When rupture does occur, life-threatening hemorrhage is unusual, but limb-threatening ischemia is common, with 50% to 75% of patients requiring amputation.[4, 17] Compression of adjacent neurologic and venous structures may give rise to pain in the popliteal fossa, diffuse leg pain, or swelling of the lower extremity. These symptoms affect in 5% to 13% of patients and are much more likely to occur if the aneurysm is large.[2, 17, 19]

Lower extremity ischemia from thrombosis of the aneurysm or distal embolization of aneurysm contents is the most common presenting symptom of popliteal artery aneurysms. Ischemia can be severe and acute, as in the case of thrombosis of the aneurysm along with the runoff vessels, or it may manifest as claudication resulting from chronic thrombosis of the aneurysm or distal embolization to segments of runoff vessels. Thrombosis occurs in as many as 55% of patients. Although many patients with acute aneurysm thrombosis present emergently with limb-threatening ischemia, aneurysm thrombosis is just as likely to produce less severe symptoms of claudication.[1, 2, 4, 13–18] Ischemia resulting from distal embolization of aneurysm contents is common, with up to 25% of patients demonstrating evidence of emboli.[4, 13, 17] Embolization can result in chronic occlusion of runoff vessels, adversely affecting graft patency and limb salvage after vascular reconstruction.

Most popliteal aneurysms are between 3 and 4 cm in diameter at the time of diagnosis,[3, 13, 18] but aneurysms as large as 15 cm have been reported.[19] Larger aneurysms are more likely to cause symptoms than smaller aneurysms; a diameter of approximately 3 cm is the point of demarcation.[2, 18] We have found that patent aneurysms tend to be smaller than thrombosed aneurysms, 2.7 cm compared with 3.4 cm.[2] However, size is not as important in the evaluation of popliteal aneurysms as it is in the evaluation of aneurysms in other locations, because the major risk of complications from popliteal aneurysms comes from thromboembolism, not rupture. Even small aneurysms can produce symptoms, including limb-threatening ischemia caused by thrombosis or distal embolization.

Diagnosis and Clinical Evaluation

The diagnosis of popliteal artery aneurysm is based on careful physical examination in conjunction with imaging studies of the popliteal artery. Most asymptomatic popliteal aneurysms are discovered as a prominent popliteal pulse or a pulsatile mass in the popliteal space found on physical examination.

Duplex ultrasonography has become the imaging study of choice for evaluation of popliteal aneurysms. It is useful in the evaluation of symptomatic and asymptomatic patients. Ultrasonography can differentiate a popliteal

Table 30-2.
Presenting Symptoms of Patients With Popliteal Artery Aneurysms

Author	Popliteal Aneurysms (n)	Symptomatic (%)	Thrombosed (%)	Emboli (%)	Ruptured (%)	Claudication (%)	LTI (%)
Anton et al.[1]	160	52	44			41	11
Carpenter et al.[2]	54	61	39	7	0	9	44
Evans et al.[4]	56	70	36	25	7	53	16
Reilly et al.[12]	244	54	36	13		30	41
Roggo et al.[13]	252	75	46	23	2	4	55
Shortell et al.[14]	51	71	55	8		35	22
Szilagyi et al.[15]	87	57				29	28
Varga et al.[16]	200	79			6	30	37
Vermilion et al.[17]	147	67	45	23	3	30	28
Whitehouse et al.[18]	88	55	24	6	0	14	28
Wychulis et al.[19]	233	48	28	10	3		12

LTI, limb-threatening ischemia.

aneurysm from other masses, such as a Baker cyst, that occur in the popliteal space. It accurately determines the size of the aneurysm and the presence or absence of intramural thrombus. Duplex scanning can detect a thrombosed aneurysm and is helpful in the evaluation of lower extremity ischemia in which thrombosis of an aneurysm is suspected. If a nonoperative approach is elected for a patient with a small aneurysm, ultrasonography is the most appropriate method of follow-up.

Arteriography is not a sensitive test for the diagnosis of popliteal aneurysms, but it is important as a preoperative imaging study to evaluate the status of the runoff vessels. The presence of laminated intraluminal thrombus makes arteriography a poor diagnostic test for popliteal aneurysms, a situation analogous to the diagnosis of aortic aneurysms. Distal embolization from the aneurysm frequently affects the patency of the runoff vessels, which affects graft patency after surgical reconstruction. It is essential to know the anatomy and status of the runoff vessels before proceeding with reconstruction of a popliteal aneurysm.

Treatment and Results

Management Decisions

The treatment of popliteal artery aneurysms is operative repair for all patients with symptomatic aneurysms and asymptomatic aneurysms that are greater than 2 cm in diameter or contain intramural thrombi. The incidence of limb loss is extremely high if the patient has ischemic symptoms.[2, 12, 14, 17, 19] Reilly[12] reported a 35% primary amputation rate for 66 patients presenting with acute aneurysm thrombosis, with another 15% requiring amputation after early graft failure. Their operative mortality rate was 5.4%. Other surgeons have had similar experiences, and have reported major amputation rates of 16% to 43% for patients presenting with severe ischemia from acute aneurysm thrombosis.[2, 13, 14, 16–18] Most amputations are at a level above the knee. An excellent limb-salvage rate is obtained with elective reconstruction.

In a series of 80 symptomatic and asymptomatic patients undergoing elective reconstruction, Varga and colleagues[16] reported no operative mortality or limb loss and a 99% early graft patency rate. The University of Michigan reported similar early results, with no graft thrombosis or amputations in 17 asymptomatic patients undergoing elective reconstruction.[18] The Mayo Clinic compared limb salvage for patients with popliteal aneurysms who presented with acute ischemic symptoms, chronic ischemia, or no symptoms. At 1 year, the limb-salvage rates were 73%, 98%, and 100%, respectively.[10] In a series from the Cleveland Clinic, patients with asymptomatic aneurysms undergoing elective repair had a 10-year limb-salvage rate of 93%, compared with 79% for patients with symptomatic aneurysms undergoing elective repair.[1]

Long-term graft patency is related to the presence or absence of preoperative ischemic symptoms. The reported 5-year graft patency rates for asymptomatic patients undergoing elective reconstruction is between 82% and 97%, compared with 39% to 70% for symptomatic patients.[1, 13, 14, 17] The status of the runoff vessels also has a significant affect on long-term graft patency and limb salvage. In our series of 45 aneurysms treated with bypass grafting, 5-year graft patency and limb-salvage rates were 71% and 90%, respectively (Fig. 30–1). Factors favoring graft patency and limb salvage included the presence of two-or three-vessel runoff, compared with patients with single- or no-vessel runoff ($P < 0.025$ for graft patency, $P < 0.003$ for limb salvage;

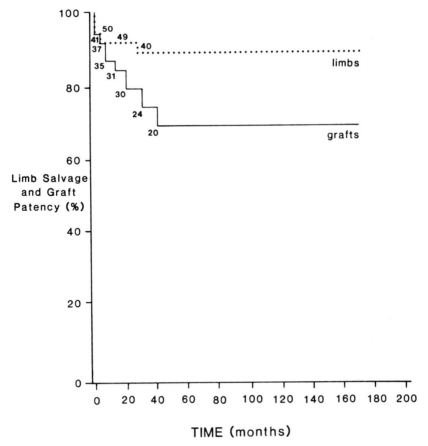

Figure 30–1. Cumulative time-to-event graft patency and limb salvage in 33 patients with popliteal artery aneurysms. Fifty-four limbs and 45 bypass grafts at risk were monitored for mean of 62 months (range, 1 to 172 months). The 5-year cumulative graft patency rate was 71%, and the limb salvage rate was 90%. The 30-day cumulative graft patency rate was 95%, and the limb salvage rate was 94%. (From Carpenter JP, Barker CF, Roberts B, et al. Popliteal artery aneurysms: current management and outcome. J Vasc Surg 1994;19:65.)

Fig. 30–2) and presence of a patent aneurysm ($P < 0.005$ for graft patency and limb salvage; Fig. 30–3) at the time of repair.[2] Other surgeons have reported similar results.[1, 14] The Cleveland Clinic series showed that patients with one or two palpable pedal pulses after reconstruction had a 10-year graft patency rate of 64%, compared with 32% for those with only a palpable popliteal pulse.[1] Shortell and colleagues[14] found that distal runoff did not affect early graft patency, but after 3 years, patients with good runoff had an 89% graft patency rate, compared with 40% for those with poor runoff. The choice of conduit for reconstruction also has a dramatic effect on long-term patency. The 5-year patency rate for saphenous vein grafts is 77% to 94%, but that for prosthetic grafts is 29% to 42%.[1, 12, 13]

The management of patients presenting with acute limb-threatening ischemia due to acute thrombosis of a popliteal artery aneurysm has changed. In this setting, we have found preoperative thrombolytic therapy to be beneficial as an alternative to emergent thrombectomy and aneurysm repair.[2] Thirty-three patients with 54 popliteal artery aneurysms were studied at the Hospital of the University of Pennsylvania, with a mean follow-up of 62 months. Seven patients diagnosed with thrombosis of the aneurysm and all runoff vessels were treated with preoperative thrombolytic therapy. These patients were

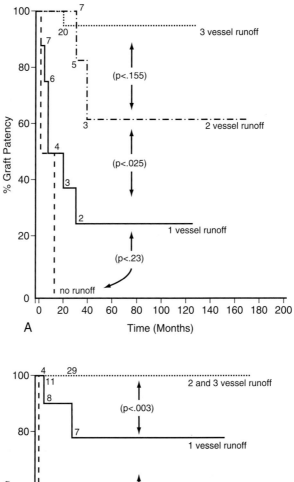

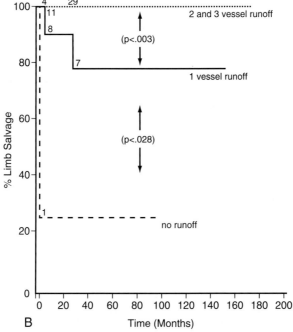

Figure 30–2. Time-to-event analysis of the effect of runoff on graft patency and limb salvage in patients with popliteal artery aneurysms. *A,* Graft patency was significantly better for patients with two ($P < .155$) or three ($P < .025$) patent runoff vessels than for those with single-vessel or no runoff. There was no significant difference between the graft patency of patients with single-vessel runoff and those with no runoff ($P < .23$). *B,* Limb salvage was significantly better for patients with two- or three-vessel runoff than for patients with single-vessel or no runoff ($P < .003$). No limbs were lost in patients with two or three patent runoff vessels. Significantly better limb salvage rates were found for patients with single-vessel runoff than for patients with no patent runoff vessels ($P < .028$). (From Carpenter JP, Barker CF, Roberts B, et al. Popliteal artery aneurysms: current management and outcome. J Vasc Surg 1994;19:65.)

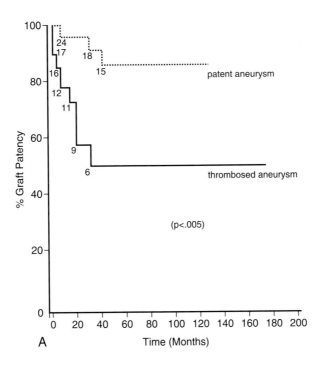

A

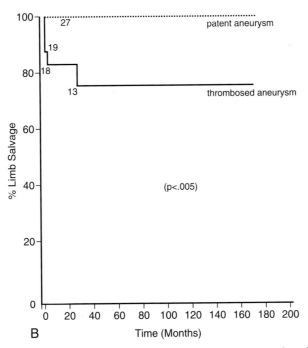

B

Figure 30–3. Time-to-event analysis of the effect of aneurysm patency or thrombosis, as determined by angiography and ultrasonography, on graft patency and limb salvage. *A,* Graft patency was significantly better in patients undergoing repair of patent popliteal artery aneurysms than in those undergoing repair of thrombosed aneurysms ($P < .005$). *B,* The limb salvage rate was significantly better for patients with patent aneurysms ($P < .005$). No amputations occurred in patients with patent aneurysms. (From Carpenter JP, Barker CF, Roberts B, et al. Popliteal artery aneurysms: current management and outcome. J Vasc Surg 1994;19:65.)

compared with 14 patients with thrombosed aneurysms treated with emergency surgery and no thrombolytic therapy. Complete clearing of thrombus from the distal circulation was achieved in six patients and in two of three runoff vessels in the remaining patient. The patients receiving preoperative thrombolytic therapy had better graft patency ($P < 0.005$) and limb salvage ($P < 0.01$) than comparable patients treated with emergency operations (Fig. 30–4). Six patients eventually required amputations; none had received thrombolytic therapy. We believe that by restoring patency to the runoff vessels, long-term graft patency and limb salvage are improved.

The management of patients with asymptomatic popliteal aneurysms is somewhat controversial. Several series have addressed the natural history of asymptomatic popliteal aneurysms. In 1953, the Mayo Clinic reported a 76% complication rate during 5 years for 21 asymptomatic patients with popliteal aneurysms.[5] Later series have demonstrated that 18% to 100% of asymptomatic patients with popliteal aneurysms eventually develop ischemic symptoms and require surgery, with as many as 13% of cases resulting in amputation (Table 30–3).

As the length of the follow-up period increases, so does the incidence of complications. Roggo and colleagues[13] followed 45 asymptomatic patients for up to 16 years; all patients eventually developed symptoms, 50% within 2 years and 75% within 5 years. Dawson and coworkers[3] found that 57% of asymptomatic patients with popliteal aneurysms ultimately required surgery, 83% within 2 years. Lowell and associates[10] identified size larger than 2 cm, poor distal runoff, and thrombus within the aneurysm as risk factors for the development of ischemic complications in patients with asymptomatic popliteal aneurysms. These studies demonstrate that the risk of complications, including limb loss, from asymptomatic popliteal aneurysms is high and increases as the length of follow-up increases. In view of the excellent results with elective reconstruction of popliteal aneurysms and the high rate of complications for asymptomatic aneurysms, it is difficult to justify routine nonoperative management. Most surgeons recommend elective repair of asymptomatic popliteal artery aneurysms larger than 2 cm in diameter in good-risk patients.[6, 10] Others suggest repair of popliteal artery aneurysms of any size with mural thrombus detected by ultrasonography.

Surgical Management

Popliteal artery aneurysms are usually repaired by bypassing the aneurysmal segment of the popliteal artery and ligating the aneurysm proximally and distally to prevent further thromboembolic events. Aneurysms that compress veins or nerves must be opened rather than excluded to decompress the aneurysm and relieve the extrinsic compression on adjacent structures. Occasionally, it is necessary to resect part of the aneurysm to provide adequate relief from the extrinsic compression, but it is unusual to have to resect the entire aneurysm. Resection of the aneurysm carries the risk of injury to the veins and nerves in the popliteal fossa and must be undertaken with care.

The technique of endoaneurysmorrhaphy can be used. The aneurysm is opened, and the graft is placed inside the aneurysm in a fashion similar to that used to repair aortic aneurysms. This type of reconstruction is particularly useful when the posterior approach to the popliteal artery is used.

Popliteal aneurysms can be approached from a medial or posterior approach. The medial approach to the popliteal artery with the patient in the supine position is appropriate for extensive popliteal artery aneurysms and

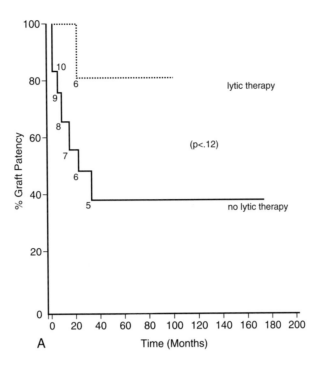

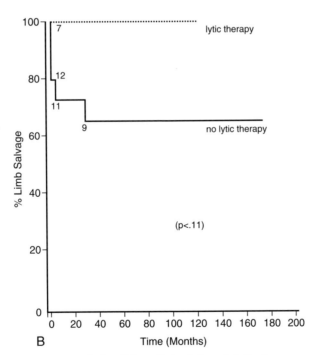

Figure 30–4. Time-to-event analysis of the effect of thrombolytic therapy on patients with thrombosed popliteal artery aneurysms. Although trends toward improved graft patency *(A)* and limb salvage rates *(B)* were detected with thrombolytic therapy, these values did not achieve statistical significance ($P < .12$ and $P < .11$, respectively). When a subgroup of patients diagnosed with thrombosed aneurysms and no patent runoff vessels was analyzed for the effect of thrombolytic therapy, the graft patency and limb salvage rates were significantly better for patients treated with thrombolytic therapy ($P < .005$ and $P < .01$, respectively). (From Carpenter JP, Barker CF, Roberts B, et al. Popliteal artery aneurysms: current management and outcome. J Vasc Surg 1994;19:65.)

Table 30–3.
Natural History of Asymptomatic Popliteal Artery Aneurysms Not Treated With Surgery at the Time of Diagnosis

Author	Patients (n)	Development of Ischemic Complications (%)	Resulting in Amputation (%)
Anton et al.[1]	15	27	13
Dawson et al.[3]	21	57	
Lowell et al.[10]	67	18	4
Roggo et al.[13]	45	100	
Varga et al.[16]	58	31	2
Vermilion et al.[17]	26	31	8
Whitehouse et al.[18]	17	18	12
Wychulis et al.[19]	87	31	3

is preferred by most surgeons. It is easier to harvest saphenous vein when this approach is used, and exposure is wider, providing easy access distally to the trifurcation and proximally to the superficial femoral artery. If an unexpected intraoperative finding necessitates a distal bypass procedure, it can be performed without repositioning the patient. The medial head of the gastrocnemius muscle often must be divided to facilitate exposure for large aneurysms.

The posterior approach to the popliteal artery with the patient in the prone position is an option for aneurysms limited to the popliteal fossa. This approach has limitations. Proximal exposure of the superficial femoral artery and distal exposure of the runoff vessels are limited, restricting the use of this approach to small aneurysms without proximal or distal extension. Harvesting saphenous vein is difficult with the patient in the prone position, and a separate incision is required. The advantages of this approach include easy access to the aneurysm, less risk of injury to the associated nerves and veins, and a shorter recovery period for most patients.

Because the bypass is often to the infrageniculate outflow vessels, autogenous vein reconstruction is preferred over prosthetic grafts. The long-term results with autogenous vein grafts are superior to those with prosthetic grafts. Because popliteal aneurysms often extend to the superficial femoral artery, this vessel is used as the source of inflow for the bypass in order to originate the graft proximal to the diseased segment of the artery. The status of the runoff is an important determinant of long-term graft patency. Preoperative arteriography in mandatory to visualize the runoff vessels and help select the most appropriate bypass outflow vessel.

Endoluminal stent grafting of popliteal artery aneurysms has been reported.[8, 11] Stents can be placed through the transfemoral route or retrograde by an infrageniculate approach. These procedures can be done under local anesthesia and avoid the large incisions required for traditional open reconstructions. The long-term patency of prosthetic stents grafts is unknown, but based on the known patency rates of prosthetic grafts placed using open techniques, patency of endoluminal stent grafts may be inferior to that of vein grafts. These techniques should be limited to high-risk patients who cannot tolerate open procedures.

Conclusions

Popliteal artery aneurysms are managed best by elective repair of before symptoms develop. Patent aneurysms with good distal runoff have the best long-term results. Good-risk patients with an acceptable life expectancy should undergo elective repair of all symptomatic popliteal aneurysms, asymptomatic aneurysms larger then 2 cm in diameter, or asymptomatic aneurysms with evidence of intraluminal thrombus detected by duplex ultrasonography at the time of diagnosis. In the difficult situation of the thrombosed popliteal artery aneurysm associated with acute leg ischemia, thrombolytic therapy safely and effectively provides patients with a more favorable alternative than emergency surgery. The improved runoff status provided by preoperative thrombolytic therapy produces more durable operative results, with greater limb salvage and longer graft patency, than emergent surgery.

References

1. Anton GE, Hertzer NR, Beven EG, et al. Surgical management of popliteal aneurysms: trends in presentation, treatment, and results from 1952 to 1984. J Vasc Surg 1986;3:125.
2. Carpenter JP, Barker CF, Roberts B, et al. Popliteal artery aneurysms: current management and outcome. J Vasc Surg 1994;19:65.
3. Dawson I, van Bockel JH, Brand R, et al. Popliteal artery aneurysms: long-term follow-up of aneurysmal disease and results of surgical treatment. J Vasc Surg 1991;13:398.
4. Evans WE, Conley JE, Bernhard V. Popliteal aneurysms. Surgery 1971;70:762.
5. Gifford RW Jr, Hines EA Jr, Janes JM. An analysis and follow-up study of one hundred popliteal aneurysms. Surgery 1953;33:284.
6. Halliday AW, Wolfe JH, Taylor PR, et al: The management of popliteal aneurysms: the importance of early surgical repair. Ann R Coll Surg Engl 1991;73:253.
7. Hollier LH, Stanson AW, Gloviczki P, et al. Arteriomegaly: classification and morbid implications of diffuse aneurysmal disease. Surgery 1983;93:700.
8. Joyce WP, McGrath F, Leahy AL, et al. A safe combined surgical/radiological approach to endoluminal graft stenting of a popliteal aneurysm. Eur J Vasc Endovasc Surg 1995;10:489.
9. Lawrence PF, Lorenzo-Rivero S, Lyon JL. The incidence of iliac, femoral, and popliteal artery aneurysms in hospitalized patients. J Vasc Surg 1995;22:409.
10. Lowell RC, Gloviczki P, Hallett JW, et al. Popliteal artery aneurysms: the risks of nonoperative management. Ann Vasc Surg 1994;8:14.
11. Marin ML, Veith FJ, Panetta TF, et al. Transfemoral endoluminal stented graft repair of a popliteal artery aneurysm. J Vasc Surg 1994;19:754.
12. Reilly MK, Abbott WM, Darling RC. Aggressive surgical management of popliteal aneurysms. Am J Surg 1983;145:498.
13. Roggo A, Brunner U, Ottinger LW, et al. The continuing challenge of aneurysms of the popliteal artery. Surg Gynecol Obstet 1993;177:565.
14. Shortell CK, DeWeese JA, Ouriel K, et al. Popliteal artery aneurysms: a 25-year surgical experience. J Vasc Surg 1991;14:771.
15. Szilagyi DE, Schwartz RL, Reddy DJ. Popliteal arterial aneurysms: their natural history and management. Arch Surg 1981;116:724.
16. Varga ZA, Locke-Edmunds JC, Baird RN. A multicenter study of popliteal aneurysms. J Vasc Surg 1994;20:171.
17. Vermilion BD, Kimmins SA, Pace WG, et al. A review of one hundred forty-seven popliteal aneurysms with long-term follow-up. Surgery 1981;90:1009.
18. Whitehouse WM Jr, Wakefield TW, Graham LM, et al. Limb-threatening potential of arteriosclerotic popliteal artery aneurysms. Surgery 1983;93:694.
19. Wychulis AR, Spittell JA Jr, Wallace RB. Popliteal aneurysms. Surgery 1970;68:942.

Index

ISBN 0-7216-7675-8

90038

9 780721 676753